The Rise and Fall of HMOs

The Rise and Fall of HMOs

An American Health Care Revolution

Jan Gregoire Coombs

THE UNIVERSITY OF WISCONSIN PRESS

The University of Wisconsin Press
1930 Monroe Street
Madison, Wisconsin 53711

www.wisc.edu/wisconsinpress/

3 Henrietta Street
London WC2E 8LU, England

Library of Congress Cataloging-in-Publication Data
Coombs, Jan.
The rise and fall of HMOs: an American health care revolution / Jan Gregoire Coombs
p. cm.
Includes bibliographical references and index.
ISBN 0-299-20240-2 (hardcover: alk. paper)—
1. Health maintenance organizations—United States—History. 2. Health maintenance
organizations—Wisconsin—History. 3. Health care reform—United States—History.
[DNLM: 1. Marshfield Clinic. 2. Health Maintenance Organizations—history—United States.
3. Health Maintenance Organizations—history—Wisconsin. 4. Health Care Reform—
history—United States. 5. Health Care Reform—history—Wisconsin. 6. Organizational
Case Studies—United States. 7. Organizational Case Studies—Wisconsin.
W 132 AA1 C775r 2004] I. Title.
RA413.5U5C677 2004
362.1′042584—dc22
2004012819

for Guerdon with all my love

Would the best off accept particular social or economic arrangements if they believed, at any moment, they might find themselves in the place of the worst off?

John Rawls, 1971

Contents

Preface

When I started to work on this book in the early 1990s, relatively few people were familiar with health maintenance organizations or their acronym, HMO. A decade later nearly everyone seems to blame HMOs, or what we now call "managed care," for all that is wrong with the U.S. health care system. As the twenty-first century begins, Americans wonder why the system that they used to trust has failed and what they can do to revive it. My answers to those questions could fill a book, indeed, this book. I have no crystal ball to predict the next phase of this nation's health care revolution, but I can explain how the HMO movement created our current problems and suggest some cures.

HMOs have antecedents in nineteenth-century America but did not gain legitimacy and develop into a movement until the federal government adopted them in the early 1970s. HMOs were quite different from traditional insurance companies when the movement began. Insurers like Blue Cross and Blue Shield usually paid private practitioners and community hospitals the full cost of any medical services that they provided to policyholders, but commercial indemnity insurers simply reimbursed policyholders for a predetermined portion of their medical expenses. Traditional insurers made no effort to influence medical decisions or evaluate their policyholders' medical needs or care. Moreover, insurers based their fee-for-service payments on liberal standards determined by the medical profession and the hospital industry. HMOs, on the other hand, assumed full responsibility for financing and providing all the preventive, diagnostic, and treatment care that their subscribers needed in exchange for a predetermined monthly premium. Some of these prepaid health care plans employed doctors and owned hospitals, but others contracted with independent providers to serve subscribers. In either case, HMO administrators tried to control, or at least influence, medical decision making in order to ensure high-quality, cost-efficient care for subscribers that did not exceed the revenue from premiums.

Relatively few people had an opportunity to participate in HMOs until the early 1980s, when an economic recession forced employers, who pay for most of the private health care in the United States, to reduce the cost of their workers' health care and other benefits. Many companies continued to offer health care benefits despite the recession but switched to HMOs and other forms of prepaid care that were thought to be more cost efficient than traditional fee-for-service care. Economic pressures and entrepreneurial ingenuity gradually extended the HMO rubric to include a wide variety of organizations that bore little resemblance to earlier prepaid plans. By the end of the twentieth century many HMOs and insurance companies were indistinguishable. Both were contracting with loosely organized networks of providers, and their primary administrative focus was the management of costs rather than patient care.

Fallout from the Health Care Revolution

For all their problems HMOs and the newer managed care organizations have had many positive influences on U.S. medical care. These prepaid health plans have shifted away from traditional reimbursement systems, which encouraged wasteful spending. The newer plans encourage doctors to become more conscious of costs. They have encouraged the development of evidence-based, scientifically determined medical treatment guidelines, which far too many doctors continue to disregard because of misplaced views about professional autonomy. These plans encourage the formation of new group practices well suited to coordinating patient care. And some of the better health plans have demonstrated the distinct advantages of primary care, preventive health services, and conservative treatment.

On the negative side the HMO movement introduced intense economic competition into the U.S. health care system, creating a powerful industry of for-profit managed care organizations, hospitals, and other providers. The movement spawned a new breed of health care administrator, who produces lucrative returns for investors by reducing services to subscribers and refusing to enroll applicants with significant health problems.

By 2002, only 1 in every 4 Americans belonged to some kind of HMO, but nearly every private and public insurance program was using managed care strategies. HMOs never fulfilled the aspirations of their early advocates, who expected them to slow spiraling health care costs, increase access to health care, and improve the nation's health. Instead, the portion of the U.S. gross domestic product (GDP) that is devoted to health care more than doubled, from 7.1 percent in 1970 to 15.3 percent in 2003.

Progress made since 1970 in the prevention, diagnosis, and treatment of disease is irrelevant for the millions of Americans who lost their insurance coverage and access to affordable care during the HMO revolution. The United States regularly spends more money on health care per person and as a percentage of its GDP than any other Western industrialized nation. According to the World Health Organization, however, Americans have the lowest life expectancy and highest infant mortality rates, as well as the highest proportion of uninsured citizens. More than forty-five million low-income U.S. workers and chronically ill individuals are unable to purchase health insurance. These individuals are much more vulnerable than the uninsured of the 1980s and 1990s because competition among health care providers has seriously eroded their access to charity care and other traditional safety nets. Many reliable sources, including the Robert Wood Johnson Foundation and the Health Insurance Association of America, predict that rising health care costs will leave at least 1 in 5, and perhaps as many as 1 in 4, Americans uninsured by 2009.

The health care world has changed for doctors as well as for insurance providers and patients. The changes would not surprise the physicians who fought HMO development because they feared that lay administrators would take control of medical decisions. Doctors entering the workforce in 2004 were more likely to be corporate employees than private practitioners. Compared to their predecessors, many have considerably less income and decision-making autonomy. Moreover, insurers in the public and private sectors now require physicians to demonstrate the monetary and therapeutic value of their work. Because of tight budgets doctors have had to become aggressive advocates for their patients in order to retain the trust that is easily lost in the competitive marketplace.

This book presents the U.S. health care revolution from two perspectives. From a national perspective it shows how the HMO movement transformed medical care from a cottage industry of private practitioners and benevolent community hospitals into a for-profit corporate enterprise whose officers care more about rewarding investors than helping the sick. At another level this book focuses on a unique physician-operated health care organization that joined the HMO movement, fought many battles during the revolution, and compromised some of its principles but won major victories for its patients. Doctors at the Marshfield Clinic in Wisconsin stand in sharp contrast to many of their peers because the Marshfield doctors embraced prepaid health care and control their own destiny.

Marshfield's Relevance as a Case Study

The Marshfield Clinic is a highly regarded multispecialty clinic in central Wisconsin. It organized a prepaid health plan in cooperation with Saint Joseph's Hospital in Marshfield and Blue Cross Associated Hospital Services of Wisconsin two years before enactment of the Health Maintenance Organization Act of 1973. The plan, known as the Greater Marshfield Community Health Plan (GMCHP), was a groundbreaking experiment that provides many striking contrasts with other health plans. It did much of what the advocates of prepaid plans in the 1970s hoped HMOs would accomplish. In addition, it had a remarkably successful run, even when compared with other new or well-established health plans in large metropolitan centers.

The clinic doctors who organized GMCHP envisioned a rural health care utopia that would encompass everyone who lived in their service area. Other HMOs marketed themselves almost exclusively to employers and served workers and their families, who tended to be relatively healthy. However, GMCHP sought to enroll entire communities, including poor, sick, and elderly families and individuals. After receiving long-awaited federal funding for a family health center program in the early 1970s, the clinic refused to start its program until federal authorities allowed low-income families to participate in GMCHP on an equal basis with other subscribers. Because of that and other innovations, Marshfield's Family Health Center became a model and resource for community health centers throughout the nation.

The clinic also played a leadership role in encouraging other HMOs to become involved with other federal programs in the 1970s and early 1980s, when most health plans were ignoring federal pleas to enroll Medicaid and Medicare beneficiaries. After promoting passage of enabling legislation by the Wisconsin legislature, GMCHP became the first HMO in the state to provide prepaid care to Medicaid patients. Marshfield's health plan was also one of the first in the nation to participate in a federal project that evaluated HMO care for Medicare beneficiaries, and it served more of them than all other HMO participants in that project. In the 1990s federal administrators and national accreditation teams called Marshfield Clinic a model for rural health care delivery. In addition, its health plan frequently topped state and national report cards for membership satisfaction.

Despite its successes, the clinic offers valuable and unique opportunities to illustrate the tremendous variety of problems that physicians experienced as they adjusted to prepaid care. The Marshfield Clinic is, in effect, a single battlefield, a microcosm of the larger revolution: Its objectives, strategies, successes, and failures were played out repeatedly on a larger scale nationwide. This book had a false start in 1988 when Dr. Russell F. Lewis, one of GMCHP's founders and its medical director for seventeen years, asked me to write a history of the Marshfield health plan. Lewis was familiar with several of my published papers on medical care and social conditions on the central Wisconsin frontier in the 1880s. As an inducement for me to accept his proposal, he offered his entire collection of correspondence and other papers related to the health plan. After several years of searching through census microfilm and dusty archives for scraps of information about early frontier life, the possibility of using intact files and interviewing people who had actually participated in historical events was irresistible. I agreed to tackle the project on the condition that I would be free to report whatever I found and could use Marshfield's experience as a case study within the context of national events.

Administrators of the Marshfield Clinic had readily allowed Lewis to retain his health plan files when he retired, but they were reluctant to allow anyone, including me, the wife of another clinic physician, to see or publish information from those files. I therefore turned to other projects until 1992, when my recently retired husband and I moved to Madison, where Lewis had moved a few years earlier. When we happened to meet one day, Lewis said that he was still eager for me to work on GMCHP's history and suggested that I start, with or without the clinic's approval. When he finally informed the clinic of what I was doing, Blue Cross of Wisconsin was rummaging through the clinic's corporate files for damaging evidence for an antitrust lawsuit. Any harm that I might cause by revealing corporate secrets seemed inconsequential in comparison. Moreover, a new set of clinic administrators welcomed my interest, gave me full access to the files, and encouraged me to interview anyone in the organization.

I spent the next six years cataloging Lewis's papers; reading everything

I could find about health care delivery, financing, administration, and leg-islation since the 1930s; and interviewing major players in Marshfield's health plan and the national HMO movement. As I began writing, I fre-quently asked individuals whom I had interviewed, and others who had worked or were still working for the clinic, to confirm the factual content of my work. No one ever asked me to change my subjective interpreta-tions. Clinic physicians and staff respected my integrity as a medical his-torian and my need to report and interpret the facts as I saw them. After verifying the factual content of one chapter, a senior administrator told me, "There is some very embarrassing information here, but everything is true and part of our history."

Hollywood producers will never make this book into a movie because it is totally devoid of sex. However, it has all the other markings of high drama: ambition, greed, altruism, political and legal machinations, frus-trations, setbacks, and strong, sometimes ruthless, personalities.

Acknowledgments

This book consumed much of my life for more than ten years and was, in retrospect, a fascinating experience. Michael Gordon introduced me to the joys of historical research and writing in 1983 when the Wisconsin Historical Society invited me to participate in its first Community Historians in Residence Program. Ronald Numbers, of the Medical History and Bioethics Department at the University of Wisconsin–Madison, helped me start my first medical history project while I was in the society's program. The American Association of State and Local History awarded me a grant to pursue that project the following year, and I have been hooked on medical history ever since. I continue to appreciate Ron's sage advice and advocacy on my behalf.

Many people contributed to the creation of this book. Dr. Russell F. Lewis planted the seed and nourished it with his vast collection of papers and endless hours of interviews. Gregory Nycz shared with me his encyclopedic knowledge of the HMO movement and his passionate concern for disadvantaged rural populations.

Many others who had a role in this story agreed to interviews, supplied me with materials, and read (and sometimes reread) drafts of various chapters. Among the Marshfield Clinic physicians who helped me were Gerald E. Porter, Dean A. Emanuel, Nelson A. Moffat, William Mauer, G. Stanley Custer, Richard Leer, Frederic Westbrook, Sue Turney, Richard Sautter, Humberto Vidaillet, and Robert A. Carlson. Staff members who gave freely of their time and knowledge included Reed Hall, Ronald Pfannerstill, Robert DeVita, Donald Nystrom, James Coleman, Scott Polenz, Robert Mimier, William Mineau, David Gruel, Charles Paine, Rhonda Kopelski, Pam Johnson, Kathy Parbel, Alan Zimmerman, Alana Ziaya, Barbara Bartkowiak, Irene Johnson, Dave Bushee, and John Smiley.

I am also grateful to Leo Suycott, Joseph Voyer, and David Neugent, former officers of the Blue Cross Plan in Milwaukee, who agreed to sit for taped interviews and provided many insights into their involvement with the Greater Marshfield Community Health Plan.

Several other individuals in Marshfield also submitted to interviews. They included Dave Jaye of Saint Joseph's Hospital, Dr. Robert Coopmans, Patrick Felker, Carl Meisner, and Sarah Hansen. Melvin Laird, the former member of Congress and secretary of defense, found time to chat with me while I was in Washington, D.C., and I received additional assistance from Richard Bohrer of the U.S. Public Health Service, and Judy Cahil and Erin Carlson at what was then the Group Health Association of America.

Individuals from the broader Wisconsin community who gave me information included Earl Thayer, formerly of the State Medical Society of Wisconsin; Tim Size of the Rural Wisconsin Hospital Cooperative; and David Kindig and Ralph Andreano of the University of Wisconsin–Madison.

I am also indebted to Dorothy Whitcomb and Michaela Sullivan-Fowler in the Medical History Department of the Middleton Health Sciences Library. Other librarians, far too numerous to mention here, patiently assisted me year after year at the Wisconsin Historical Society Library, Memorial Library, Law Library, Cooperatives Library, Pharmacy Library, and Social Work Library on the University of Wisconsin–Madison campus, and at Wisconsin's Reference and Loan Library, Law Library, and Legislative Reference Bureau.

Comments from scholars who read my manuscript before its acceptance by the University of Wisconsin Press contributed much to its organization. However, I am most grateful to Rosemary Stevens of the University of Pennsylvania for her constructive criticism and suggestions, which forced me to say not only what I knew but also to express my views about certain issues described in this book. My daughter Tracy, who has never forgiven me for making her the middle child in our family, took infinite pleasure in marking up my many drafts to make my words say what I meant rather than what I had written. Although many individuals helped mold this work into its present form, I accept full responsibility for any errors, omissions, or other failings that the reader may find.

During the decade that it took to write and research this book, my family and friends seemed encouraging and supportive but probably thought me mildly deranged for working so long and hard without assurance of publication. My husband, Guerdon, suspected the worst and therefore treated me with far more patience, kindness, and understanding than I deserved.

The Rise and Fall of HMOs

Introduction

American Health Care Insurance before 1970

> The greatest need is not to find more money for the purchase of medical care, but to find newer and better ways of budgeting the costs and spending the money wisely and effectively.
>
> Isidore S. Falk, 1936

The term *health maintenance organization* was coined in 1970, but historians trace the concept of prepaid health care to the 1800s, when railroads, lumber, mining, and textile firms hired "company doctors" to treat their injured employees. Many groups of workers, immigrant societies, and fraternal organizations also contracted with physicians to care for members and their families for as little as $1 per year.[1] At the start of the twentieth century, when most Americans still lived on farms or in small rural communities, contemporary observers estimated that physicians holding contracts with manufacturers, municipal agencies, or fraternal organizations served one-quarter to one-third of the residents of some cities.[2] Medical societies considered these forms of "contract practice" to be demeaning because such jobs were usually awarded to the lowest bidders without regard for their professional qualifications.[3]

Two prototypes of modern-day prepaid care appeared in the early 1920s. In Elk City, Oklahoma, Dr. Michael Shadid organized the Farmers Union–Cooperative Health Association, which became a popular model for consumer-run health care cooperatives. Drs. Donald Ross and H. Clifford Loos, owners of the Ross-Loos Clinic, developed a prepaid health

3

plan for the employees of the Los Angeles Bureau of Water and Power, and it later served as a model for physician-operated plans.[4] All three doctors were outspoken advocates of prepaid care, and their peers criticized their innovations as forms of contract practice and regarded them as professional outcasts.[5]

Relatively few Americans bought health insurance in the early 1900s because medical services were inexpensive, and patients often found home remedies just as effective. Several companies offered indemnity policies that reimbursed policyholders for some portion of their medical care, but most people paid their doctor and hospital bills with cash.[6] Families with little income tried to compensate their caregivers with goods or services or relied on charity. Doctors and hospitals routinely covered their losses from charity care by charging affluent patients more.

Advances in scientific medicine in the 1920s raised consumers' expectations and demands for health care services, but new technologies also increased medical costs by requiring greater investment in professional education and equipment. Although nearly 90 percent of Americans still financed their own care in the late 1920s, medical costs quickly exhausted family resources when members became seriously ill.[7]

Early Efforts to Reform Health Care Financing

The Committee on the Cost of Medical Care, composed of about sixty nationally prominent health professionals and laypersons, organized in 1927 to address the needs of Americans who could not afford the new, improved standard of medical care. The committee issued its final report five years later. "As a result of our failure to utilize fully the results of scientific research," the committee concluded, "the people are not getting the service they need—first because in many cases its cost is beyond their reach, and second because in many parts of the country it is not available."[8] A majority report recommended that doctors and other health care professionals form groups so that they could provide a comprehensive array of preventive and therapeutic services. The committee thought that funding for these services should come from periodic insurance payments and taxes, which would distribute the financial burden of illness evenly throughout the population.[9]

A majority of committee members supported the concept of health insurance because the "frequency of sickness and cost of medical care are predictable for groups of people but not for individuals."[10] They favored group medical practices over independent practitioners because the committee's investigators found that doctors in medical groups shared expensive facilities and equipment and were better able to coordinate patient care.[11] In order to meet health care needs in rural areas, where most Americans still lived, committee members envisioned networks of widely scattered clinics that would be staffed by small groups of doctors and affiliated with fully equipped centers in nearby cities.[12] Many of the committee's ideas about insurance, government subsidies, and group medical practices are still relevant and widely accepted in the twenty-first century. Moreover, the committee's ideas for improving rural health services are still very practical.

Reaction to the committee's recommendations was swift and strong. Leaders of the American Medical Association (AMA) and several physicians on the committee vehemently disagreed with the conclusions.[13] They condemned any form of corporate medical practice that would be financed through private or public intermediary agencies. Such measures, they said, would limit patients' choice, increase the cost and lower the standards of medical care, encourage illness, degrade the medical profession, and lead to a "compulsory system of care." Organized medicine continued to use these very arguments to oppose nearly every health care reform proposed during the next six decades.[14]

Nonetheless, the recommendations of the committee had far-reaching consequences for U.S. health care in both the private and public sectors. Almost immediately, the committee's final report convinced federal policy makers that Americans who had no access to reliable medical care were as deprived as those who lacked adequate food or shelter. Consequently, President Franklin D. Roosevelt's Federal Emergency Relief Administration (FERA) formally recognized medical care as a basic human right in 1933, declaring that "conservation and maintenance of the public health is a primary function of our Government."[15] FERA then used that mandate to fund medical services to indigent patients through existing state and local agencies.[16] That modest depression-era program planted a seed that eventually blossomed into a great profusion of publicly funded health care programs.

The seed was slow to take root, however. When Roosevelt decided to include health and disability insurance in his pending Social Security legislation, he asked Isidore Falk and Edgar Sydenstricker to help him draft those sections. Falk was a prominent member of the Committee on the Cost of Medical Care, and Sydenstricker was Falk's coworker at the Milbank Memorial Fund, a national foundation that supported nonpartisan analysis, study, and research on significant issues in health policy (and continues to do so today). The AMA, together with its state and local affiliates, promptly attacked their proposals for compulsory health insurance. Others called the legislation, which was based on the committee's recommendations, socialistic. Fearing that the insurance package would jeopardize passage of his entire Social Security program, Roosevelt had it removed from the final bill. Instead of widely available health and social welfare benefits, the Social Security Act of 1935 authorized a patchwork of ten programs, including federal old age insurance and grants to states for unemployment compensation, aid to dependent children, and maternal and child welfare.[17] Such compromises, made in fear of organized medicine's political opposition, became a thoroughly ingrained characteristic of federal health care legislation.

The Rise of Private Health Insurance

The government's failure to adopt the committee's recommendations or enact meaningful health care legislation in the 1930s, coupled with industrial mobilization during World War II, pushed the nation into the private work-related health insurance system that prevails today. It began in 1942, when the War Labor Board provided incentives that enabled companies to offer fringe benefits—but not higher wages—in order to attract and retain employees for the war effort. When the war ended, 1 in 4 Americans was covered by an on-the-job policy that helped to pay his hospital bills. The Taft-Hartley Act further expanded coverage for workers and their dependents, as did a Supreme Court ruling against Inland Steel in the late 1940s that gave labor unions the right to negotiate benefit plans as a condition of employment.[18]

Many Western industrialized countries nationalized their health services in the 1950s so that all citizens would have access to care. But in the United States in 1953, Congress and the Internal Revenue Service institutionalized the link between private health insurance and work by making company contributions to employee benefit plans tax deductible. In effect, health insurance and other on-the-job fringe benefits became a massive and well-entrenched government subsidy for the employed.[19]

Workers' demands for better health care coverage stimulated development of the nonprofit Blue Cross hospital and Blue Shield surgical care plans in the 1930s. The nonprofit Blues used a community rating system recommended by the Committee on the Cost of Medical Care to spread risks over large groups of people, and they reimbursed providers directly for their services. In contrast, commercial indemnity carriers based their rates on age, sex, health status, and other actuarial variables, and they reimbursed policyholders for some portion of their medical expenses. When commercial carriers sought to gain a greater share of the growing health care market in the 1940s, their pricing formulas enabled them to attract young, healthy subscribers with low-cost policies. Left with progressively older, less healthy, and more expensive risk pools, the Blues had to the raise the premiums for their remaining policyholders. Most Blues abandoned community rating in the 1950s, when they began to sell risk-adjusted policies priced beyond the means of many sick and elderly patients. Within another decade policies offered by the nonprofit Blues and commercial carriers were indistinguishable.[20]

The growing availability of private health care insurance for workers and their families during the late 1950s and early 1960s spawned what some have called the "golden age of American medicine."[21] Consumers' expectations and demand for medical services reached an all-time high. Blue Cross and Blue Shield plans, which set reimbursement standards for the industry, were controlled by hospital boards and physicians, who compensated themselves generously. Amid a seeming abundance of health care resources, hospitals enlarged their facilities and bought expensive equipment, while doctors ordered tests and treatments without concern for costs. High reimbursement levels enabled physicians and hospitals to provide charity care to patients unable to pay for services.[22] Some observers viewed such arrangements as informal social welfare. Others thought that the system demeaned economically disadvantaged patients and furnished less-than-optimal care.

Coincidental with the rise of private health insurance companies, local consumer cooperatives in various parts of the county organized their own health plans during the 1930s, 1940s, and 1950s. These health care cooperatives were considered another type of business that consumers could operate to their advantage, just like feed stores, fuel outlets, and power companies. The earliest health plans were located in farming communities, but the idea later spread to labor unions and groups of urban workers. The managing boards of consumer cooperatives hired doctors to serve their members, who paid a monthly fee that covered all the medical care that they and their families would require.

The cooperative movement had its heyday in the first half of the twentieth century, and health care became its fastest-growing sector after a federal court found the AMA guilty of obstructing consumer-sponsored health plans and ruled that "health is too important to be wholly entrusted to the doctors." Between 1941 and 1946 the number of health cooperatives more than doubled, to sixty-eight programs with 140,000 members.[23] Most of the rural programs did not last long, but a few urban organizations became large and influential. These included the Group Health Cooperative of Puget Sound in Seattle; the Health Insurance Plan of Greater New York; the Labor Health Institute in St. Louis; the Group Health Association in Washington, D.C., and the Group Health Cooperative in St. Paul.

The Cooperative Health Federation of America was organized in 1946 to establish standards for prepaid organizations and to promote cooperative health care. In 1951 the federation began to sponsor the annual Group Health Institute, which presented information about health promotion and management of health cooperatives for member organizations. After joining with other like-minded organizations and undergoing a few name changes, the federation emerged as the Group Health Association of America (GHAA) in 1959 and moved its national office to Washington, D.C., in 1965. By then the association represented twenty-one prepaid health care plans and seventy-five supporting organizations but not Kaiser Permanente Health Plan, the largest prepaid organization in the nation.[24]

Kaiser Permanente began when the steel maker Henry J. Kaiser arranged for a few doctors to provide prepaid care to his workers and their dependents at the Grand Coulee Dam construction site in the late 1930s. Later, during World War II, Kaiser hired doctors to care for steelworkers at his shipyards.[25] By the late 1960s the Kaiser Foundation Health Plan, Kaiser Foundation Hospitals, and Permanente Medical Groups had six regional divisions operating in northern and southern California, Oregon, Hawaii, Ohio, and Colorado. Kaiser Permanente finally joined GHAA in 1969 but only after the national association dropped its requirement that member organizations be consumer controlled. Because the Kaiser Health Plan's six divisions served more than half of prepaid subscribers in the nation, it quickly became a major force in the association.[26] But I'm jumping ahead of my story.

The Rise of Public Health Insurance

In addition to fighting health cooperatives and prepaid care throughout the 1940s, 1950s, and early 1960s, the AMA invariably sidetracked or diluted federal efforts to fund health care for people who were old, poor, or lacked work-related benefits.[27] Access to federally subsidized medical care finally became a reality for millions of elderly and low-income Americans when President Lyndon B. Johnson signed the amendments to the Social Security Act in 1965 that created Medicare and Medicaid.[28] However, the concessions that Johnson made to the AMA and American Hospital Association in order to gain support for his legislation proved very costly.

Federal and state costs for Medicare and Medicaid rose about 20 percent each year between 1966 and 1970. The enormous demand for medical services by previously deprived populations was only partly responsible for that spending increase. Johnson's concessions had entrusted the financial administration of Medicare to insurance intermediaries (usually Blue Cross Hospital Plans and Blue Shield Surgical Care Plans) and the administration of Medicaid to the states.[29] The insurance intermediaries were generous with the public purse in reimbursing hospitals, which enabled them to further expand their facilities, and in reimbursing physicians, who prospered as never before. With financial barriers to elderly and indigent care removed, and insurance companies in charge of the till, the federal government quickly became the nation's largest purchaser of health care services.[30] High reimbursement levels for physician and hospital services quickly spread into the private sector as well.

By the late 1960s policy makers faced what many called a national health care crisis; it involved skyrocketing costs, severe shortages of health care personnel, and unevenly distributed medical resources. Although more Americans than ever had access to public or private health insurance, millions of others still lacked adequate care because they lived in medically underserved inner cities or rural areas. As in the 1930s, many reformers sought to change the way in which medical care was financed and delivered.

Calls for Prepaid Health Care

This time, the GHAA was in the forefront of reform activity. Prepaid health care covered only 4 percent of the nation's population in the late

1960s, but it had many ardent advocates, including Wilbur Cohen, a key player in virtually every major piece of federal social legislation since the Social Security Act of 1935 and Johnson's last secretary of health, education, and welfare (HEW).[31] During congressional debate about Medicare and Medicaid, Cohen tried without success to link those two programs with reforms featuring prepaid care.[32] Many lawmakers and HEW staffers shared Cohen's views but feared his proposals would jeopardize enactment of Medicare and Medicaid. They took up his call for federal support of prepaid health care only when the enormous costs of Medicare and Medicaid became apparent in 1967. Despite a groundswell of support, it took Congress six years to fund the development of prepaid plans and another decade before such plans began to have a significant influence on U.S. health care.

The chapters that follow trace the HMO movement in chronological order from the 1970s to the end of the century, pausing occasionally to examine major events and health care issues from a national perspective or from the perspective of the Marshfield Clinic. In chapter 1, I describe the enormous problem that Marshfield encountered while starting its health plan, difficulties that were emblematic of the failure of many new health plans in the early 1970s, before and after federal legislation to encourage their development.

As the Greater Marshfield Community Health Plan began, the battle to gain passage of HMO legislation raged in Washington. Chapter 2 traces the three-year gestation of the 1973 Health Maintenance Organization Act and subsequent attempts to make it workable. Because President Richard Nixon did not support HMO development after reelection, his administration did not spend much of the money that Congress appropriated.

Chapter 3 returns to central Wisconsin to look at conditions of rural poverty and efforts to furnish care to low-income residents. Marshfield's Family Health Center worked closely with its federal sponsor, the U.S. Public Health Service, to develop a prepaid model for urban and rural health centers that provided more comprehensive benefits to underprivileged patients. This chapter also considers the advantages and problems associated with the consumer advisory and governing boards required by many federally funded programs, including the one for HMO development.

Early prepaid prototypes such as health care cooperatives and Kaiser Permanente Health Plans relied on staff physicians to serve their subscribers. As HMOs mutated, however, they increasingly contracted with independent providers for their services. Chapter 4 illustrates the difficulties that HMOs encountered when dealing with independent practitioners. It also explains why the HMO movement made few inroads into rural areas and failed to become a dominant force in U.S. health care.

Advocates hoped that federal HMO legislation would reduce public health care expenditures by encouraging prepaid enrollment of Medicaid and Medicare beneficiaries. Chapter 5 tracks Marshfield's ill-fated experiences through the late 1970s and early 1980s to show why HMOs were and still are reluctant to enter contracts with Medicaid and Medicare.

A lack of technical assistance and shortage of experienced administrators contributed to the high failure rate of new HMOs before and after enactment of the HMO Act. Better-equipped managers became available only after Congress appropriated funds for training in the late 1970s. Chapter 6 identifies several administrative requirements for a successful HMO and shows why data processing is particularly critical for controlling costs and ensuring quality of patient care in prepaid systems.

Chapter 7 evaluates HMOs in 1980 by using the definitions of quality and measurements of performance available at that time. Many studies concluded that prepaid health care was equal to or better than that found in traditional systems. New evidence also suggested that HMO patients who received fewer tests and more conservative treatment, including less time in hospitals, recovered faster than their fee-for-service counterparts.

Just as the federal government was withdrawing its support from HMO development in the early 1980s, an economic recession created a highly competitive, commercialized climate throughout the health care industry. Chapter 8 demonstrates how competition among central Wisconsin insurers destroyed GMCHP's ability to provide affordable care to its poorest and sickest subscribers. A review of Marshfield's problems with some affiliated providers during this financially difficult period reveals why all physicians, not just those on medical licensing and examining boards, need to protect the public from poorly trained and unethical doctors.

Competition for central Wisconsin's prepaid market and changing corporate goals among GMCHP's partners ultimately led to the dissolution of that health plan. Chapter 9 describes the conflict between the

Marshfield Clinic and Blue Cross, as well as the struggles among the clinic's leaders, that led to the demise of GMCHP. Creation of another health plan solely owned and operated by the clinic quickly followed.

Chapter 10 follows a five-year antitrust lawsuit filed by Blue Cross and its HMO against the Marshfield Clinic for refusing to enter into a new financial arrangement on Blue's terms. This case had far-reaching implications for antitrust enforcement in the health care field but failed to settle many outstanding issues.

Debate about managed competition and provider accountability during the early 1990s had enormous influence on the health care industry. Chapter 11 explains why continuing federal and state efforts to encourage HMO enrollment among Medicare and Medicaid beneficiaries and other disadvantaged populations were largely unsuccessful. Chapter 12 describes how employer demand for less expensive health benefits caused the unprecedented competition by and growth of for-profit health care in the private sector.

Concern among major health care purchasers—employers and government agencies—and patients created the demand for provider accountability. Chapter 13 examines how the HMO industry, employers, legislators, government, and physicians developed new ways of measuring and improving the value of health care services, and it considers the effects that these revolutionary changes had on the practice of medicine

Despite improvements in the delivery and quality of medical services by the late 1990s, the U.S. health care system was in crisis by 2000. Chapter 14 summarizes what critics and reformers had to say about the system's problems, their causes, and potential cures. The concluding chapter reviews some lessons that I've learned from my study of the HMO movement and some conclusions that I've drawn from the Marshfield Clinic's experiences.

Chapter 1

Dreams of a Medical Utopia

Of all the things I've done, I expect to be remembered only for the Hospitals and Health Plan. They're the things that are filling the peoples' greatest need—the need for good health care at a cost that the average family can afford.

Henry J. Kaiser, 1971

Reformers of almost every political persuasion agreed that passage of Medicare and Medicaid in 1965 had created an immense national health care crisis by the late 1960s. Most assumed that slowing spiraling health care costs, relieving physician shortages, and redistributing medical resources would require drastic measures. Literally, hundreds of groups representing a broad spectrum of interests conferred and offered recommendations. Recalling proposals made by the Committee on the Cost of Medical Care nearly four decades earlier, some groups called upon doctors and hospitals to form prepaid health care plans. Other groups repeated demands made many times since the 1930s for the federal government to nationalize health care services. Still others argued for a combination of both solutions.

While Congress debated how best to deal with the growing crisis, some insurers, physicians, and hospitals took matters into their own hands. By the time the Health Maintenance Organization Act of 1973 was implemented in 1974, they had started more than 120 new prepaid health plans. The private sponsors of these nascent plans faced enormous difficulties because relatively few technical or financial resources were available. Central Wisconsin's Greater Marshfield Community Health

Plan (GMCHP), which opened its doors in 1971, experienced nearly all the problems typical of that period. Having a well-established group practice involved in that plan clearly facilitated the organizational process. But Greater Marshfield also encountered some unusual difficulties because the doctors at the Marshfield Clinic had what many observers believed were unreasonable expectations for their health plan.

A Call to Action

U.S. Rep. Melvin R. Laird, the ranking Republican on the Subcommittee on Health of the House Appropriations Committee, visited central Wisconsin in January 1968 to address a medical society meeting in his district. Laird brought his audience some disquieting news. "The federal government," he warned, "is going to nationalize medical care within the next few years unless the profession itself takes responsibility for controlling runaway medical costs." If the doctors in his audience wanted to try a new approach to delivering health care, he said he would arrange for some planning assistance from Washington.[1]

Laird had addressed the group at the invitation of Dr. Russell F. Lewis, a boyhood friend of Laird's and president of the Marshfield Clinic. On the way home to Marshfield after that meeting, Laird urged Lewis to involve the clinic in an experimental prepaid health care program patterned after the Kaiser Permanente Medical Care Plans on the West Coast. Laird explained that the results of such an experiment would have great value because the Marshfield Clinic had a patient population vastly different from that of existing prepaid plans. Kaiser Permanente, Group Health Cooperative of Puget Sound, and the Health Insurance Plan of Greater New York, for example, served urban workers and their dependents, whereas the clinic's clientele included many poor farm families and Medicare and Medicaid beneficiaries.[2] (The Marshfield Clinic had been operating a small prepaid program with the Felker Manufacturing Company of Marshfield and Time Insurance Company of Milwaukee since 1964, but the arrangement was primarily a bookkeeping convenience. Time Insurance collected premiums and paid all employee medical bills, and the Felker Company paid Time for cost overruns at the end of each year.)[3]

Lewis accepted Laird's challenge because he was eager to help his friend prevent passage of the national health insurance legislation under consideration by Congress at the time. Dr. Ben Lawton, a surgeon who was vice president of the clinic, was equally enthusiastic about Laird's proposal for entirely different reasons. As a self-described "card carrying liberal Democrat," Lawton thought that the Marshfield experiment would provide valuable information about prepaid rural health care when Sen. Edward M. Kennedy succeeded at nationalizing American medicine. Although their motives were dissimilar, both Lawton and Lewis envisioned a health plan that would provide low-cost comprehensive care to all thirty-five thousand people living in and around Marshfield.

The Marshfield Clinic was one of several multispecialty clinics that had sprung up during the first half of the twentieth century in Midwestern rural trade centers. These clinics offered an array of specialized medical services usually available only in large cities. Most were patterned after the Mayo Clinic, established by Dr. William W. Mayo and his two sons in Rochester, Minnesota, in 1887.[4] Wisconsin had a few other group practices that were organized as limited partnerships by 1916, but the six physicians who founded the Marshfield Clinic that year were the first to receive a business corporation charter from the state.

The American Medical Association (AMA) and its local chapters condemned corporate medicine as inappropriate and "unethical" because it "distracted from the practice of medicine."[5] The State Medical Society of Wisconsin finally convinced state legislators to outlaw corporate medical practice in 1920, but Wisconsin's attorney general gave an exception to the clinic because it already held a charter. State lawmakers reversed their opposition to corporate medicine after World War II when returning physician-veterans touted the benefits of specialization and shared practices. Group practice finally gained national legitimacy after the U.S. Department of Health, Education and Welfare (HEW) sponsored a national conference in 1967 extolling the advantages of such delivery systems. Three years later the AMA joined the American Association of Medical Clinics and the Medical Group Management Association in publishing guidelines for the efficient management of group practice clinics.[6]

During the Marshfield Clinic's first fifty years, its staff quadrupled to sixty-three specialists, while the city of Marshfield's population doubled to fifteen thousand. By 1966 the clinic was one of the nation's three largest multispecialty clinics located in a rural community; the others were the Scott and White Clinic in Temple, Texas, and the Geisinger Clinic in

Danville, Pennsylvania. Marshfield Clinic physicians and a few solo practitioners in the community admitted patients to Saint Joseph's Hospital,
founded in 1890 by a small group of Bavarian nuns from the Sisters of the
Sorrowful Mother. By the late 1960s their four hundred–bed hospital averaged twelve thousand admissions a year. The hospital and clinic made
health care Marshfield's largest industry.[7]

The Marshfield Clinic is unconventional in many ways. Its governance
is democratic; each doctor on the staff has one vote on the corporate board
of directors, which owns and operates the clinic. The doctors elect most of
their officers each year, and the office of president has a limited term.[8] In
1954 they took the highly unusual step of giving themselves equal compensation, even though surgeons and other procedure-oriented specialists usually commanded much higher salaries than pediatricians and internists.[9] The physician staff based its decision on a conviction that the
services of the various doctors were of equal value to their patients and the
organization, regardless of the income that they generated for the clinic.[10]
Many Wisconsin physicians believed that the clinic doctors were socialists
because of their uniform salary plan.

Shortly after Laird's visit in 1968 Lewis contacted the State Medical
Society of Wisconsin to determine whether its Blue Cross and Blue Shield
plan, the Wisconsin Physicians Service, would be willing to participate in
a prepaid project. The society's staff was enthusiastic, but its physician
leaders rejected Lewis's offer because they had an aversion to any kind of
prepaid care. Lewis then offered a similar proposal to two central Wisconsin insurance executives, Robert F. Froehlke, vice president of Sentry
Insurance in Stevens Point, and T. A. Duckworth, president of Employers
Insurance of Wausau. Both men agreed to consider such an experiment.[11]

Lee Sherman Dreyfus, president of Wisconsin State University at
Stevens Point and a future governor, had been promoting regional cooperation in central Wisconsin for some time. His "ruraplex" concept identified
Stevens Point as the regional center for higher education, Wausau and Wisconsin Rapids as manufacturing centers, and Marshfield as the center for
medical care. Central Wisconsin doctors disliked the ruraplex idea because
it reinforced the clinic's growing influence.[12] When Lewis polled them
about participating in an area-wide prepaid health care experiment, many
saw his plan as another attempt to promote the clinic's regional preemi-
nence. They therefore refused to approve of, or participate in, such a plan
unless subscribers were free to see physicians of their choice.[13]

When the Wisconsin Physicians Service learned that Sentry and Employers were cooperating with the clinic, its governing board instructed its staff to participate in planning discussions so that the service could monitor the clinic's activities.[14] During the next few months representatives from the clinic, Sentry, Employers, and Wisconsin Physicians Service met several times to discuss such issues as reimbursement methods, physician participation, patient choice, sharing of risks, and arrangements for enrolling people too poor or sick to afford premiums. They never reached consensus on a single issue because, Lewis said, "what we [the clinic doctors] were talking about had more to do with social conscience than with good business sense."[15]

The clinic and the three insurers finally asked Laird to arrange a meeting with federal health care agency staffers in Washington so that they could get some expert advice about prepaid care. Laird obliged and set up with three meetings: a morning session with representatives from the Comprehensive Health Planning Agency, the Regional Medical Program, the Office of Economic Opportunity (OEO), the Mental Health Services Administration, and several other groups; a luncheon with Sen. Gaylord Nelson, D-Wis., and HEW secretary Wilbur Cohen and several of his senior aides; and an afternoon conference with high-level administrators in the Social Security, Medicare, and Medicaid programs. Just before Lewis left for Washington, a deputy director at the National Institutes of Health advised him that the HEW aides were "extremely knowledgeable in their fields and . . . would have firsthand knowledge of most [prepaid] projects in the United States."[16]

The scope of central Wisconsin's proposal surprised federal administrators, and the Wisconsin delegates quickly learned that the administrators were not equipped to give advice about prepaid care or provide financial support. If and when funding became available for the Wisconsin venture, it would have to come from a variety of sources.[17] Three months after the meeting at HEW a liaison assigned to Lewis instructed him to prepare a proposal defining exactly what he and his committee intended to do so that the HEW staff could decide whether his project was "interesting and fundable."[18] Although Cohen visited Marshfield with Laird several months later to tour the clinic and Saint Joseph's Hospital, HEW never responded to Lewis's proposal.

The only tangible results to emerge from those Washington meetings were small grants for two surveys. An OEO grant funded a door-to-door survey to evaluate the medical care and financial status of people living within the Marshfield Clinic's immediate service area. Dr. Gerald E. Porter, a pediatrician, had proposed such a survey because he thought that the clinic's emphasis on specialty care failed to meet the medical needs and pocketbooks of local families.[19] The survey, published in December 1969, found that local residents were considerably poorer, less healthy, and more disabled than their counterparts in urbanized regions of the state. Family size in central Wisconsin was larger than the state average, but income levels were well below. More than half of all households had annual incomes of $5,000 to $8,000—too high for Medicaid entitlement but too low for families to afford private insurance coverage. All the industries around Marshfield had low wage scales. Dairy farms throughout the area were generally small and often barely profitable. Forty percent of farmers and their spouses held nonfarming jobs. The report confirmed Porter's suspicion that many people living within fifteen miles of the clinic lacked routine medical care.[20]

HEW funded a second study to evaluate health care needs, services, and resources in five central Wisconsin counties. The consultants hired for this study noted in their report that the "Marshfield Clinic, with its high concentration of specialty services, is unique for an essentially rural region and without a counterpart elsewhere in the United States." Almost in passing, they suggested that the clinic involve area doctors in forming a "foundation" to provide prepaid care to area residents.[21] As a model, they recommended the San Joaquin Foundation for Medical Care, organized in 1954 by the San Joaquin County Medical Society of Stockton, California. Approximately twenty such foundations were operating or in some stage of planning by 1960. Organized medicine approved of prepaid plans operated by medical foundations because their physicians worked independently and received fee-for-service reimbursements, and their subscribers were free to choose any doctor affiliated with the sponsoring medical society.[22] By the time the HEW-funded report was released in August 1970, the clinic's leaders had embarked on an entirely different sort of arrangement.

By October 1968, nine months after Laird issued his challenge to the doctors in his district, discussions between the clinic and the insurance carriers were stalled. At a meeting with friends from Wisconsin Physicians Service, Sentry, and Employers, Laird warned, "The federal government will start to build or purchase hospitals and medical facilities within five to seven years if the private system does not develop proper cost control mechanisms." He urged the insurers to concentrate their efforts on using prepaid health care to reduce costs rather than trying to accommodate the poor. They were to let him know within a few weeks whether they intended to continue or abandon the prepaid project. He emphasized that any venture would have to be voluntary and enthusiastically supported by the organizations involved, especially the medical profession.[23]

Laird subsequently told Lewis that he "didn't want to push people into anything." If central Wisconsin doctors and insurers were unwilling to experiment with cost-control measures, an HMO study could just as easily be done in Cleveland or Milwaukee.[24] Lewis concluded from their conversation that Laird had lost his enthusiasm for the clinic's project after hearing complaints from several independent practitioners in his congressional district.[25]

Nothing more happened until December 1968, when Dr. Paul M. Ellwood Jr. invited Lewis to a conference on prepaid care in Minneapolis. Ellwood was executive director of the American Rehabilitation Foundation and an ardent advocate of prepaid health care. After hearing Kaiser Permanente representatives describe their programs, Lewis wrote Ellwood to take issue with the way Kaiser controlled its costs. Among other things, Lewis believed that the practice of limiting subscribers' choice of physicians was improper.[26] Lewis later changed his views, but "at that time," he wrote, "most of us thought Kaiser's methods for saving money resulted in poor medicine."[27]

The prospects for starting any kind of prepaid health care plan in Marshfield looked dismal at the end of 1968. Several key players were no longer around. President-elect Richard Nixon had drafted Laird to be his secretary of defense. Froehlke, who had already left Sentry, would soon follow Laird to Washington as secretary of the army. And Duckworth was no longer at Employers. Negotiations with Wisconsin Physicians Service ground to a halt when it became apparent that the State Medical Society's insurance program wanted to influence negotiations rather than participate in the clinic's plan.[28] Years later Earl Thayer, who had represented both the state society and its insurance plan at those meetings, recalled that his bosses were afraid that imposition of cost controls by Sentry and Employers would unduly interfere with the practice of medicine. "Fundamentally," he said, the State Medical Society's leaders "wanted no part of prepaid care because they were convinced it would destroy the foundations of professional free enterprise and the 'godlike supremacy' of doctors."[29] Thayer also said that Sentry and Employers retreated from the project because they were concerned about enrolling people in poor health and losing their profitable group contracts if the clinic's plan proved attractive to employers.[30] As it turned out, Sentry and Employers' new executives were far less interested than their predecessors in working with the clinic and had begun to organize their own prepaid plans instead.[31]

In 1969 members of the Marshfield Clinic's board of directors picked the two most outspoken advocates of prepaid health care to lead them. They elected Ben Lawton president and named Lewis, who had served his maximum allowable number of terms as president, to the newly created post of medical director. The two doctors had vastly different personalities but complemented one another well. Lawton was altruistic, outspoken, and autocratic. Lewis was equally uncompromising in his social convictions but, unlike Lawton, cultivated friendships and used quiet persuasion to pursue his goals. Both men were incredibly hard workers and shared a common vision of the clinic's future.

Shortly after the clinic election, a U.S. Public Health Service (USPHS) delegation from Chicago appeared in Marshfield without notice. The USPHS people said that the purpose of their visit was to help clinic administrators compare fee-for-service reimbursements with capitation payments (uniform payments for whatever services were required) in a rural setting.[32] Nothing came of their visit, however, and the clinic's plans for prepaid care languished until year's end when more visitors suddenly appeared.

Marshfield Clinic Joins the Blues

Leo E. Suycott, president of the Milwaukee-based Blue Cross Associated Hospital Service, and David Neugent, his vice president of marketing, visited Lewis and Lawton in December 1969. They proposed to help the clinic start a prepaid group practice plan in partnership with Saint Joseph's Hospital. The plan would be similar to one that they were organizing with some doctors and a hospital in Milwaukee and others that they hoped to start in Madison and Green Bay.[33] Suycott said that he and Neugent would also represent Blue Cross's Milwaukee affiliate, Blue Shield Surgical Care, in negotiations.

The Milwaukee-based Blues had been competing with the Wisconsin

Physicians Service, the State Medical Society's Blue Cross and Blue Shield plan, in Madison since the 1940s. Lewis and Lawton were active in the State Medical Society but chose to ignore the feuding between the two camps. "By the time Milwaukee's Blue Cross came to the clinic," Lewis said, "our doctors were convinced that we had to do something. A lot of people in Marshfield felt they couldn't afford medical care, and we thought a reasonably priced prepaid plan would help them budget for care."[34]

Suycott was equally motivated by high medical costs. He and Neugent had increased their company's enrollment to nearly one million subscribers in the late 1960s, but rising costs were eroding the company's profits.[35] Suycott thought that Lewis and Lawton were initially suspicious of his company's intentions. He assured them that he, a newly licensed pilot, and Neugent, a very reluctant passenger, would not have flown up to Marshfield through dense fog in a rented plane if they did not intend to work out an arrangement with the clinic. Suycott's display of determination and risk taking would characterize much of his subsequent involvement with the Marshfield health plan.

Marshfield's location held great appeal for Suycott. He would soon have a plan in Milwaukee, and a prepaid arrangement with the highly respected Marshfield Clinic "in the cornfields of central Wisconsin" would give him a rural prototype as well. He anticipated that his company's close ties with the Sisters of the Sorrowful Mother, who were headquartered in Milwaukee and operated Saint Joseph's Hospital in Marshfield, would facilitate negotiations with the hospital's board. A Blue Cross–sponsored plan in Marshfield would also open new markets in central and northwestern Wisconsin, thereby expediting his company's plans to eventually cover the whole state.[36] Perhaps because of their own expansion strategies, Suycott and Neugent believed that Marshfield doctors wanted to enlarge their reputation and service area so that they could "be like the Mayo Clinic."[37]

The Marshfield Clinic's business was booming when negotiations with Blue Cross began in January 1970. The clinic's staff had grown to nearly ninety physicians who were either board-certified specialists or preparing for certification examinations. The thirty-five thousand residents in Marshfield's immediate market area accounted for only one-fifth of the clinic's revenue. Most patients came on their own initiative or by referral from an area that included the northern half of Wisconsin and Michigan's Upper Peninsula and sometimes points beyond.

Lewis and Lawton personally conducted most of the fifteen-month planning phase with Blue Cross. The clinic's doctor-directors unanimously approved a preliminary proposal at midyear and directed their two leaders to work out the details with the clinic's administrative staff and Blue Cross representatives.[38] Saint Joseph's Hospital, the health plan's third partner, played only a minor role in the planning discussions. Lewis believed that David Jaye, who was hired as hospital director in 1969, joined the partnership only at the urging of Blue Cross. "He didn't care about the plan," Lewis said. "He just didn't want the hospital to lose any money."[39] Nor did Jaye want to be managed or coerced by the clinic. Suycott said that he "tried to referee the situation," because the two institutions "took advantage of one another" and were "very antagonistic."[40]

Conflict between hospitals and their attending physicians is a long-standing tradition. American physicians like to use hospitals as an extension of their private practice, a workshop where they treat patients. Yet hospitals are independent corporations whose lay governing boards grant physicians the "privilege" of working in their institutions. Conflicts arise from a clash of interdependent needs. Doctors have to do some of their work in a hospital setting and want to control their work environment. Hospital boards want to protect their institutional power structure but depend upon doctors to provide clientele.[41] The inevitable hospital-physician conflict was perhaps more intense in Marshfield because clinic doctors provided Saint Joseph's Hospital with nearly all its patients. Despite his concerns about the clinic, Jaye deferred most decisions about the plan to the two other partners. The two exceptions were financial matters affecting the hospital and theological issues related to certain medical practices, such as abortions and sterilizations.[42]

Tough Planning Decisions

The partners had to make many difficult planning decisions. Defining the geographic enrollment area for what eventually became the Greater Marshfield Community Health Plan was a particularly sensitive issue. The clinic's leaders initially planned to limit enrollment to an area within a fifteen-mile radius of Marshfield so as not to invade the practice territories of other physicians upon whom they relied for referrals. That strategy proved impractical because many potential subscribers used doctors in nearby communities. Some worked in Marshfield but used doctors where they lived; others lived and worked in Marshfield but used doctors located elsewhere because they felt the waiting time for clinic appointments was too long. Lewis and Lawton decided to accommodate these potential subscribers by inviting independent physicians in neighboring towns to affiliate with GMCHP on a fee-for-service basis. The Marshfield Clinic also established a family medicine department and hired its first family practitioner in June 1971 so that local residents could receive prompt attention for minor ailments.

Many area physicians distrusted the clinic's motives and worried that affiliation with the health plan would have a negative effect on their practices. Conversely, some clinic doctors believed that the independent practitioners, who worked in comparative isolation and often did not realize how much their practices deviated from accepted norms, would adversely affect the quality of subscribers' care. When the clinic doctors finally agreed to accept affiliates, three highly regarded physicians in a small group practice twenty miles north of Marshfield were the first to sign up; other doctors soon followed their lead.

Blue Cross contributed considerable insurance expertise to the health plan's development process, and the clinic hired William Shearer from the Ross-Loos Clinic, which had been running a prepaid plan in Los Angeles for many years, for additional assistance. Lewis and Lawton ignored much of the advice from these sources, however, because it did not fit the kind of plan that they envisioned. For example, the doctors were determined to enroll as many residents as possible, even though Shearer warned that their health plan would not survive if they opened its doors to everyone.[43] And the doctors insisted that GMCHP distribute the cost of treating seriously ill patients throughout its enrolled population, even though by the 1960s most Blue Cross plans had abandoned community rating as competitively disadvantageous.

The clinic's leaders also wanted their health plan to incorporate several other features that were unsound from an insurance perspective. Against the advice of its actuaries, Blue Cross agreed to all the doctors' requests. For example, GMCHP subscribers who purchased their own insurance were allowed to pay the same premium as group subscribers, even though direct-pay policies cost more to administer and tended to attract unhealthy applicants. In fact, the additional costs associated with direct-pay policies were such that most prepaid health care plans enrolled only groups.[44]

Blue Cross also allowed childless couples to purchase two single policies rather a more expensive family policy. Insurers usually required all
married couples to pay family premiums because they assumed that
couples with no dependents were likely to be older and require more
medical services than those with children at home. Although some plans
varied the cost of family premiums according to the number of dependent
children, most plans charged a uniform family rate because children consumed relatively few services.[45]

Determining GMCHP's rate was one of the more contentious issues.
One actuarial expert called premium determination "both an art and a science," but rate setting in Marshfield was neither.[46] Blue Cross actuaries
tried to set the rate sufficiently high to cover anticipated costs. The clinic
doctors wanted to offer comprehensive services at affordable rates and
were adamantly opposed to using copayments for services as a way to discourage overuse. Saint Joseph's Hospital simply refused to give the health
plan a meaningful discount because the hospital feared it would lose
money. Lawton, who often pounded his fist on the table to make a point,
invariably declared that any rates proposed by Blue Cross were too high
and would discourage enrollment.

When the dust settled, monthly premiums for the first year of operation were set at $17 for all single enrollees and $49.80 for all families with
dependents. GMCHP's first-year premiums were comparable to those of
well-established plans that offered fewer benefits, refused to accept nongroup enrollees, and required copayment for some services.[47] However,
clinic administrators were horrified to learn that Lewis and Lawton had
agreed to a reimbursement rate that was half the anticipated cost of providing outpatient services to subscribers.[48]

Reflecting on their early negotiations, Suycott said, "Ben [Lawton]
had some pet theories that were usually bad moves. We wanted the premiums to be higher so they would cover expenses, but we went along because we liked Ben. We took a shot at it. Greater Marshfield was a money
loser during the early years, but we were willing to take a risk."[49] Suycott
was apparently willing to take that risk because he wanted a successful
rural health care plan, and working with a facility like Marshfield Clinic
greatly improved his chances.

The clinic's leaders simply wanted to provide low-cost prepaid care to
area residents, especially those who were seriously ill, elderly, or poor. In
the months before GMCHP became operational, Lewis and Lawton made

many trips to Washington to confer with officials at HEW, OEO, and the Social Security Administration. They learned that federal laws for Medicare were in conflict with GMCHP's generous hospitalization benefits, and subsidized health care for poor rural families was apparently not available.[50] "We had the feeling that people in Washington met with us because of Laird's influence," Lewis said. "They sometimes gave us advice but never any money. The OEO-financed survey helped us to meet some people in that office, but our contacts there didn't pay off until much later."[51] An aide to Gaylord Nelson told Lewis that the clinic's program looked good, but almost no money was available for pilot projects. Part of the problem, he said, was a rapid turnover of agency administrators and priorities.[52]

While the clinic's leaders were trying to enlist cooperation from federal agencies, Neugent of Blue Cross was in Madison, urging Wisconsin health officials to enroll Medicaid recipients in GMCHP. He noted that such an experiment offered an excellent opportunity to compare the cost of prepaid capitation with Medicaid's usual fee-for-service reimbursement system.[53] While state health administrators were somewhat receptive to the concept, state statutes prohibited prepayment for services for Medicaid recipients.

Lewis and Lawton also met with the executive committee of the State Medical Society's Commission on Medical Care Plans in order to "cut down on some of the rumors" that the medical society was hearing about the clinic's program.[54] Some commission members worried that GMCHP would erode enrollment in the society's insurance plan, but their chair said that "times were changing" and it was appropriate for the clinic to try something new. Some months later the society tried something new when its insurance plan launched a prepaid plan in Wild Rose, a very small community ninety minutes south of Marshfield. The Health Maintenance Program initially involved only two physicians but soon expanded to include other independent practitioners in neighboring communities and counties.[55]

With the tacit blessing of the medical society's Commission on Medical Care Plans, the clinic's leaders signed agreements with Saint Joseph's Hospital and Blue Cross that formalized each partner's obligations to GMCHP. These documents were similar to those used by other Blue Cross–sponsored prepaid plans. The Milwaukee Blues agreed to provide marketing, actuarial, and financial services and to reimburse charges for services at Saint Joseph's Hospital and out-of-area hospitals that provided emergency or referral care; the Blues also agreed to pay for extended care and home nursing services after hospitalization. Blue Shield agreed to reimburse the clinic for outpatient services and to administer claims from out-of-area physicians who provided emergency and referral care. And the clinic agreed to use its capitated reimbursements for all outpatient services, including fee-for-service reimbursements to GMCHP's affiliated physicians.[56]

The clinic assumed financial risk for outpatient costs exceeding its capitation. Saint Joseph's Hospital lost money only if inpatient expenses exceeded its predetermined daily rate. And Blue Cross and Blue Shield agreed to cover the losses for all services not specifically assigned to the clinic or hospital. The agreements also called for the partners to periodically appraise their plan's operation and issue an annual report.[57]

Just before the plan opened for enrollment, GMCHP participated in a flurry of marketing efforts aimed at informing potential subscribers about the benefits of prepaid health care, a concept unfamiliar to most consumers. The partners invited community leaders to briefings and enlisted some of them to serve on an advisory committee. GMCHP's planners hoped that the committee members would inform their constituencies about the plan and act as conduits for subscriber complaints.

Lawton told participants at a Milwaukee workshop on consumer-sponsored group health plans that "our recent negotiations with Blue Cross and our local hospital have been most cooperative. We have hammered on the table for a whole year now, and I think we have an honest-to-God comprehensive prepaid group practice plan that will be operational in the near future."[58] Lewis was less optimistic. He told an interviewer, "We're going into this all the way but, frankly, I don't believe that prepaid group practice is going to save the health care system or the patient a cent."[59]

GMCHP officially began operation on March 1, 1971. Compcare, the Blue Cross plan in Milwaukee, did not start until two months later. The *Capital Times* in Madison touted GMCHP as the first HMO in Wisconsin and the first rural HMO in the county.[60] Suycott and Neugent thought that the development process had moved relatively fast in Marshfield because clinic doctors were accustomed to working together as a group and willing to defer to Lewis and Lawton on most decisions. The solo practitioners who participated in the Milwaukee Compcare Plan, were not as well organized or deferential to their lead negotiators.[61]

In the early 1970s HMOs generally assumed one of three organizational forms: a staff model, a group practice model, or an independent practice association (also called an IPA or foundation for medical care). Staff model HMOs hire or contract with a group of doctors to care for their enrollees. The early Kaiser plans invariably contracted with Permanente Medical Group doctors who worked exclusively for Kaiser. Group practice physicians own and operate their own HMOs, usually with other partners, as in the case of Greater Marshfield. Group practice models often provide fee-for-service care to patients not enrolled in their HMOs. Staff and group practice doctors generally receive a salary or a capitation based on the number of enrollees they serve. Centralized record keeping and peer interaction help staff and group model HMOs control cost and quality. IPAs, like Compcare, contract with solo practioners whose reimbursements are based on the cost of services they provide. Care and costs are more difficult to monitor in those circumstances. Blue Cross calculated that GMCHP's fifteen-month development phase, including travel and time-consuming negotiations with federal and state administrators, cost the company slightly more than $282,000, or $1.29 million in 2004 dollars.[62] Clinic administrators made no effort to calculate their portion of GMCHP's development costs.[63]

Some Successes, Losses, and Lessons

On the occasion of GMCHP's first anniversary celebration in May 1972, when it was fifteen months old, a Wisconsin newspaper called it "the largest rural prepaid community health plan in the nation."[64] With 13,665 subscribers in portions of three counties, GMCHP was also one of the largest newly organized plans anywhere in the nation.[65] HEW secretary Elliott Richardson had visited Marshfield earlier in the year, just after his department began to promote HMOs. He called GMCHP "a constructive program the rest of the United States will do well to emulate."[66] A local butcher and health plan subscriber told a news reporter that GMCHP was "the finest insurance ever invented, and the only thing I ever had that was worth a damn."[67]

Despite all the adulation, GMCHP lost more than $482,000 during its first sixteen months of operation. Its unorthodox policies, enrollment of too many subscribers with serious health problems, and overuse of outpatient services all were to blame. Nearly half of GMCHP's initial losses resulted from more use than anticipated by the clinic's employees and their families. Health care personnel routinely consume more care than other segments of the population because it is readily accessible. The clinic absorbed losses attributed to its personnel and their dependents because it had previously provided them with free care.[68]

GMCHP enrolled many direct-pay subscribers who required expensive medical care but failed to attract enough healthy employees in group contracts to offset the costs of its high-risk pool. Elsewhere, new HMOs were having trouble marketing to employee groups, but they rarely accepted direct-pay subscribers and, if they did, refused applicants with serious health problems. Group enrollment grew slowly in Marshfield because some employers held multiyear contracts with insurers and others simply wanted to see how the plan developed before making a change. The city's largest manufacturer was unable to participate because its national office purchased all employee benefits.

GMCHP lost $9,000 a month by allowing childless couples to purchase two single policies and suffered even greater losses from its open enrollment policy, which allowed individuals to join the plan throughout the year. As GMCHP's medical director, Lewis readily accepted sick patients into the plan and encouraged his obstetrical patients, including one woman who was eight months' pregnant, to enroll when they lacked insurance coverage. Don Nystrom, the health plan manager, said that "it was years before we put a nine-month waiting period into the plan for obstetrical care."[69] Lewis acknowledged that finances were not his strong suit, but "part of the reason for starting the plan was to care for people who were sick. It was quibbling to ask them to wait for an open enrollment period when they were already sick." He later recalled with considerable regret that "one person actually died while waiting to enroll."[70]

Other losses arose because local agents of competing insurance carriers encouraged sick clients to enroll in GMCHP but warned healthy customers to avoid the clinic's plan because HMOs "attract sick people and large families who abuse those plans."[71] After doing "some research" on the rumors that insurance agents were circulating, Joseph Voyer, a Blue Cross vice president in charge of fiscal affairs, told Lawton that he had found "two or three people who had sold their homes and moved into the area to get their potentially huge medical bills covered." In response, Lawton said that "volume would eventually solve the problem without having to stand on some patient's air hose."[72]

The clinic suffered heavy losses because GMCHP subscribers used far more outpatient services than predicted.[73] They visited doctors no more than people enrolled in well-established HMOs, but they had 30 percent more visits than the clinic's fee-for-service patients, whose use of the clinic had been used to calculate the premiums.[74] Although the subscribers' visitation rates were exceedingly high by Marshfield standards, the clinic's leaders refused to regulate utilization for two reasons. First, GMCHP was an experiment designed to determine the cost of high-quality prepaid care to a rural community, and limiting services that patients believed they needed might have had a negative effect on quality. Second, the clinic expected its physicians to treat all patients equally, regardless of cost, and expected its business office to help patients pay their bills.[75] Identifying the charts of GMCHP subscribers and suggesting that they be treated in a manner different from that extended to other patients would have been contrary to the clinic's policy.

Most HMOs are able to reduce hospital care, but GMCHP subscribers increased their hospital use, logging 60 percent more hospital usage than fee-for-service patients during the first year; Saint Joseph's Hospital lost $73,000.[76] Even so, GMCHP's hospitalization rates were just slightly higher than those reported by well-established plans.[77]

An independent study of prepaid hospital utilization attributed Marshfield's highly unusual increase to the salaried clinic doctors, declaring that they had no incentives to reduce admissions or length of hospital stays.[78] One would expect to find higher-than-average hospitalization rates in Marshfield because the clinic and hospital are tertiary referral centers, which attract seriously ill patients from a very large area.[79] In fact, Saint Joseph's utilization was less than half the state average in 1972.[80] Elsewhere, out-of-town patients were often hospitalized for their convenience while undergoing a battery of diagnostic tests or remained hospitalized longer than usual so that the medical staff could monitor their recovery. Many physicians also continued to hospitalize patients for tests and simple treatments. Long before GMCHP began operation, the clinic's doctors had reduced their reliance on inpatient care because their highly refined scheduling and delivery systems enabled them to test, diagnose, and treat most patients during a one-day visit.

Although GMCHP had relatively good utilization rates compared with other HMOs, Blue Cross asked the doctors during the second round of rate negotiations to further reduce their outpatient and hospital use.

Dr. David Ottensmeyer, who replaced Lawton as clinic president in January 1972, appreciated the need for such measures. "If we go on practicing medicine under this program just as we do under all other systems of re-muneration," he said, "we have done nothing but change the payment sys-tem. It is incumbent upon the physician to practice medicine in a way that will cost less. This offers us the only realistic method of making [a] profit from such a plan." Lewis said that he would encourage doctors to use nursing homes and home nursing services instead of hospital care when-ever appropriate, and Ottensmeyer appointed a utilization committee to explore other options for increasing efficiency.[81]

Lewis and Lawton continued to demand many actuarially unsound policies. In order to keep premiums as low as possible, however, they with-drew their insistence on marketing single policies to childless couples and agreed to limit open enrollment periods for individuals to two 30-day pe-riods each year. But when Blue Cross tried to impose a six-month waiting period on the coverage of preexisting conditions, Lewis said the insurance company received "violent opposition from some of us who felt that we were selling a community health plan, not an insurance program."[82] The doctors ultimately agreed to a six-month waiting period for preexisting conditions but only when subscribers left the plan and then reapplied when they got sick.

The clinic accepted a capitation for GMCHP's second year that was only slightly more than the cost of serving group contract subscribers, those who on average used the fewest services. The clinic could afford to discount its services because prepayment saved approximately 10 to 15 percent of its billing, collection, and bad debt costs, and the health plan accounted for only 10 percent of its revenue.[83] Because the doctors were content to break even, GMCHP's rates for its second year of operation compared favorably with those for HMOs in other regions of the country and with standard insurance policies in the Marshfield area that offered fewer benefits and required out-of-pocket expenditures.[84]

Troubles with the Blues

Before starting their health plan, the clinic's leaders had been warned to expect trouble if they partnered with Blue Cross. William Shearer, whose Ross-Loos Clinic plan operated in conjunction with Los Angeles Blue Cross, told Marshfield doctors that "insurance companies do not know or care about how we are notified about enrollment." If Blue Cross failed to provide immediate notification when people were enrolled or removed from the plan, Shearer said, the Marshfield Clinic would antagonize patients and "go broke" because of bookkeeping problems.[85] Dr. Paul Ellwood, the Minnesota prepaid care advocate, told Lewis that reports from other plans caused him to be gravely concerned about the clinic's becoming involved with Blue Cross.[86]

A clinic report issued eight months before the health plan started contained the most serious warning of all. Its author said that his department routinely had more problems collecting payment from Milwaukee Blue Cross and Surgical Care than from any other insurance carrier. Among his list of twenty-two complaints, he noted that the Blues had exceptionally long processing times and often made errors in denying claims and payments. Furthermore, their enrollment reports and advice to subscribers regarding coverage were unreliable. "Our public relations are ruined many times because of Blue Cross-Surgical Care errors," he said. "Since the first of the year, [one staff member] has spent approximately 90 percent of her time rectifying Surgical Care errors and explaining their slow payment procedures to patients."[87] The clinic's leaders had ignored all these warnings because they wanted to start a health plan and Blue Cross was the only insurer willing to work with them.

No one was surprised, then, when the clinic's accounting staff found numerous inaccuracies in Blue Cross capitation reports and billing procedures within a month after GMCHP started operation.[88] These bookkeeping problems compounded as time went on. In a letter to Neugent at Blue Cross, the clinic's health plan manager, Don Nystrom, said, "From the standpoint of most enrollees in the program, everything is what was promised. From the standpoint of those of us responsible for the day-to-day administration of the program, it is a complete and utter fiasco. Not only are the enrollment records unbelievably fouled up, the capitation report is a shambles."[89] Lewis wrote Neugent a conciliatory letter some days later, saying, "You have always been cooperative and if there are problems they must stem from our administrators, who apparently have problems with your administration. I'm not very excited about it personally."[90] Recalling these events later, Neugent said, "We had problems with the day-to-day administration. Russ [Lewis] understood, and Ben [Lawton] would get up and wave his arms. In the early years we worked things out, but there was a change in personalities later on—not a good combination."[91]

A few days later Lewis again demonstrated his preference for taking a broader view from above the administrative fray. Nystrom reported that

Blue Cross had breached its contract with the clinic by admitting four critically ill patients to the plan after an open enrollment period had closed. One was a woman in kidney failure who required hemodialysis. The second was a local businessman whose employer enrolled him in the plan belatedly and only after he required hospitalization overseas. The third was a recent college graduate who no longer qualified for coverage under her mother's policy but was allowed to purchase retroactive individual coverage when she was seriously injured in an automobile accident. And the fourth was a local politician. "I am not unsympathetic to families with unexpected high medical expenses," Nystrom said, "but there is not an insurance agent in town who would sell us fire insurance after the place is on fire."[92] "While you are technically correct," Lewis replied, "you perhaps still do not grasp that some of us are interested in giving coverage to everyone."[93] Nystrom, who had written off hundreds of thousands of dollars in charity care while working in the clinic's billing department, had great admiration for the clinic's beneficence, but his previous employment with the Internal Revenue Service had trained him to take a technical view of contracts. In his mind the clinic and Lewis, who "would have flunked Insurance 101," were clearly being deceived by Blue Cross.[94]

Clinic and Blue Cross administrators met almost monthly in Marshfield or Milwaukee in attempts to resolve their enrollment and accounting discrepancies, but problems persisted. Joseph Voyer of Blue Cross advised the clinic in August 1972 that computer programmers had not yet completed the complex task of calculating GMCHP's new rates. Because adjustments to the August capitations had to be done by hand, the clinic could expect more errors.[95] Lewis overlooked the bookkeeping problems until he realized that they were causing trouble for some subscribers. At that point he announced in a memo to staff, "I think we should check out our relationship with Blue Cross in so far as our contract is concerned, and seriously consider going to Wisconsin Physician Service or Sentry to ask if they would be willing to sell the same contract to people in this area. I think we should tell Leo Suycott we are going to tell Senator Kennedy and the people in Washington that they were right, that Blue Cross is incapable of handling this sort of a program."[96]

Suycott appointed an intramural task force to improve his company's administration of GMCHP, but nothing changed. By the end of 1973 Lewis was again considering an arrangement with other insurers.[97] Despite occasional lapses, Lewis was generally optimistic about the health plan's progress and grateful for the help that he had received from Blue Cross. "Problems with their record keeping were never a major concern," he said in retrospect. "Those things bothered 'the office,' but I just let them wash over. I was amazed at how nice Blue Cross was to us. I thought they were very fair."[98]

The Status of GMCHP and Other New HMOs in 1973

As 1973 ended, GMCHP's enrollment exceeded sixteen thousand subscribers, even though Medicare and Medicaid beneficiaries, and families too poor to afford the premiums, were unable to join the plan. Its service area included portions of four counties, and about two dozen primary care doctors from outlying communities had affiliation agreements with the plan.[99] The partners had recovered from their first-year losses, and the plan had a slight excess in revenue.[100] GMCHP's premiums had increased but compared favorably with those of other HMOs in the state and nation despite GMCHP's remarkably liberal enrollment policies. The clinic's staff had more than doubled in seven years, to 125 salaried specialists. The rapidly growing clinic and health plan, unique in a rural setting, were the subject of several studies and dozens of professional and lay reports, including one from HEW that described the clinic as the "avant garde of country medicine."[101]

A study of GMCHP's operation from July 1972 to July 1973 was apparently the first to compare utilization by group and nongroup enrollees in a community-rated prepaid health plan. Its findings were significant, particularly because much of the HMO legislation being considered by Congress contained language that required federally funded HMOs to use community rating and enroll all applicants, regardless of their health status. Unfortunately, the study was not published until three years later, well after passage of the HMO Act. It reported that direct-pay enrollees used more outpatient services and were admitted to the hospital more often than group enrollees, but the inpatient care of direct-pay enrollees tended to be less expensive than that of group subscribers. The expense of caring for direct-pay enrollees, who accounted for almost one-fourth of GMCHP's membership, increased premiums by 7.3 percent—approximately $1 a month for each subscriber.

The study's author regarded the additional cost as "not prohibitive" for employers who purchased group contracts because the utilization rates of direct-pay enrollees approximated those of group subscribers soon after direct-pay enrollees joined the health plan. "If HMOs are ever to conclusively demonstrate their viability as an alternative health care delivery system," he concluded, "they must do so by serving a true cross-section of the population. This study demonstrated that, at least in the case of GMCHP, open enrollment and community rating have not hampered the financial viability of the plan."[102] A few companies that resented paying extra to subsidize direct-pay enrollees switched their workers' insurance policies, but community rating did not deter growth in group enrollment during the late 1970s because employee unions liked GMCHP's liberal benefits and fought to join or remain in the plan.

GMCHP was one of more than 120 new prepaid health care programs that developed in the United States during the early 1970s before passage of the HMO Act of 1973. More than half of these plans were operating or in advanced planning stages when Richardson, the new HEW secretary, established an HMO project office in June 1971 and began to distribute grants and federally guaranteed loans to would-be HMO sponsors.[103] The office had awarded $16.5 million in planning and development grants to seventy-nine organizations by the time Congress decided that Richardson's funding activities were unauthorized and halted the program in 1973. The results of this project were disappointing. Thirty-seven sponsors judged their projects unfeasible during planning stages, and only thirty-five grant recipients had operating programs by 1974.[104]

Many HEW grantees had to terminate their planning phase or programs because their sponsors and staff lacked sufficient commitment and/or managerial skills or they could not recruit enough physicians.[105] Health reformers had worried that state statutes and administrative regulations would deter HMO formation, but few HEW projects encountered legal restrictions, presumably because the organizers of HMOs avoided states inhospitable to prepaid care.[106]

A lack of HMO managerial expertise troubled nearly all new health plans in the early 1970s. Potential sponsors sought advice from well-established organizations like the Kaiser Permanente Medical Care Plans on the West Coast, the Health Insurance Plan (HIP) of Greater New York, Group Health Cooperative of Puget Sound, and Group Health Association in Washington, D.C. As a result these plans and many of their smaller counterparts were besieged by insurance companies and others eager to learn about prepaid operations. Blue Cross snapped up all the places for Kaiser's HMO management conference in 1969 and other conferences held in Portland, Oregon, and at HIP in New York in 1970. The following year, representatives from nearly one hundred medical education institutions, large clinics, and foundations attended a Kaiser Permanente symposium on HMO management.[107]

Health plan medical directors who attended a 1973 HEW-sponsored conference in Denver called for more training programs for medical directors and administrators. The only formal training available at the time was a thirteen-week "advanced management program" offered by Harvard University. Several medical directors, some in brand new programs, complained about a constant procession of visitors wandering in and out of their offices in search of advice. Kaiser tried to reduce visits to its facilities by imposing high charges on casual visitors. The Harvard Community Health Plan set aside one day a month during which prospective HMO sponsors were allowed to visit by prearrangement.[108] These tales sounded familiar to Lewis, who had been inundated with inquiries even before his plan was operational. Ironically, HEW sent Lewis a letter just as GMCHP began, asking how the clinic could help other HMOs get started.[109]

Opposition from organized medicine and from doctors intent on preserving their fee-for-service practices proved lethal to many new plans in the 1970s. Nevertheless, physicians constituted the largest group of prepaid health care sponsors in the years immediately preceding the HMO Act. Although one-fifth of the nation's physicians were in group practice by the late 1960s, many of those groups consisted of a few specialists who simply shared equipment and office management.[110] Physicians who practiced in large multispecialty groups or at university medical centers were often at odds with their more conservative peers in organized medicine. They were also among the first to organize prepaid plans in the early 1970s, frequently using the Ross-Loos plan as a model.

Many academic physicians viewed prepaid programs as expanded opportunities for student education and community service. Harvard, Yale, and Johns Hopkins started three of the earliest university plans. The Harvard Community Health Plan began operation as a nonprofit charitable corporation in 1970 after receiving nearly $2 million in loans and grants from the Ford Foundation, USPHS, Rockefeller Foundation, and Commonwealth Fund. The program contracted with university hospital teaching centers, house staff, and attending faculty for inpatient and outpatient care. Several insurance carriers, including Blue Cross, provided marketing and other insurance services.[111] The Community Health Care Center Plan in New Haven, Connecticut, was affiliated with Yale University

and the Yale–New Haven Medical Center. It too had an insurance arrangement with Blue Cross. The impetus to start the Yale plan in the late
1960s came from organized labor groups in the community and Isidore
Falk, who had continued to promote prepaid care since serving on the
Committee on the Cost of Medical Care in the 1930s.[112] The Columbia
Medical Plan was formed in 1969 in cooperation with Johns Hopkins
Medical School and Johns Hopkins Hospital in order to provide medical
care to residents of the newly developed city of Columbia, Maryland. The
major players in that plan were James Rouse, the city's developer; the non-
profit Columbia Hospital and Clinics Foundation; Johns Hopkins Medical
Partnership; and Connecticut General Life Insurance.[113]

In order to compete with, or prevent development of, lay-controlled
HMOs, some physicians banded together to form prepaid plans modeled
after the San Joaquin Foundation for Medical Care in California.[114] These
foundations were also called independent practice associations, or IPAs,
because they allowed doctors to retain their professional autonomy. Like
HMOs, IPAs collected monthly payments from their subscribers but reimbursed physicians on a fee-for-service basis rather than a monthly head
count. IPAs generally withheld 10 to 15 percent of each doctor's payments
until the end of the fiscal year to cover unexpected costs, and they made
further disbursements only if sufficient funds remained in the plan. In addition, some plans required participating physicians to return a proportion
of their payments if huge losses occurred. IPA physicians generally had
few guidelines governing the way they practiced medicine, but the threat
of year-end cost overruns theoretically encouraged them to make cost-
conscious decisions.[115]

Consumer-sponsored plans were the second most popular type of
HMO to be developed in the early 1970s. Consumer cooperatives and labor unions had been responsible for starting most of the prepaid programs
before 1960. Historically, organized medicine opposed plans operated by
consumers because the AMA was afraid that lay boards would dictate how
their staff physicians practiced medicine. However, some consumer-run
plans organized in the early 1970s included federally subsidized neighborhood health centers, which had agreements with medical schools and
other health care providers to serve low-income families and groups with
special needs.[116]

Few of the new HMOs were able to fully replicate the Kaiser model
because they lacked sufficient resources to build or purchase their own

hospitals. Moreover, many doctors were unwilling to work in "close-paneled" group practices, which limited patients to physicians in the group. Hospitals often cosponsored but rarely initiated HMO development during the early 1970s because they anticipated difficulties with physician recruitment.[117] And just as doctors feared consumer-run plans, so they feared that lay members on hospital boards would try to control their practices.

Insurance companies were heavily involved in the sponsorship of new HMOs. Their major contributions were capital funding for development and the costs of operation, as well as assistance with insurance functions. The nonprofit Blues were much more active in this regard than commercial insurance carriers. The national Blue Cross Association (BCA) launched an aggressive nationwide campaign to corner the prepaid health care market after its representatives attended Kaiser's first HMO management training sessions in 1969. The program of the annual BCA leadership meeting the following year was carefully choreographed to convince local Blue Cross presidents that industry, labor, government, consumers, medical educators, and some physicians sought development of prepaid group practices—and that Blue Cross needed to "hop on the wagon." Leo Suycott was one of the key speakers at that meeting.[118]

Other meetings to promote HMOs followed in quick succession. In 1972, for example, an HMO workshop at BCA's national marketing meeting formulated guidelines to help local affiliates develop their own HMO policy statements. BCA also published a comprehensive manual on the development and operation of prepaid group practices that was widely distributed to increase public awareness about its leadership role in prepaid care. And BCA leaders took every opportunity to stress that HMO initiatives were a matter of survival in a rapidly changing marketplace.[119] BCA president Walter McNerney told a congressional hearing in 1972 that his company was involved with more than forty HMOs in two dozen states.[120] In addition to the Harvard Community Health Plan in Boston, and GMCHP and Compcare in Wisconsin, McNerney said his local affiliates were helping twenty-three other groups.[121] Within a year Blue Cross was marketing three different plans in Rochester, New York—an HMO, an IPA, and a federally funded health center.[122]

Leo Suycott told a congressional hearing on HMO legislation that the insurance functions necessary to operate a single HMO cost $300,000 to $500,000 annually. Based on those figures, an HMO needed 15,000 subscribers to break even and 25,000 to 30,000 enrollees to realize a profit.[123]

If such estimates were applied to programs operated by other sponsors, few health plans were meeting their costs in 1974. Nearly half of all HMOs and most of the new ones had fewer than 5,000 enrollees.[124] In fact, most of the nation's prepaid health care plans—except for a few very large programs—experienced difficulties in the early seventies. Shortly before passage of the HMO Act in 1973, 60 percent of the plans responding to a survey had problems with marketing and financial support, while half were having trouble with physician recruitment and opposition from the medical profession. Prospects seemed somewhat more promising in Wisconsin, where four of five newly formed HMOs reported enrollments of 15,000 to 20,000 subscribers.[125]

The Marshfield Clinic was able to overcome many of the development problems that other health plan sponsors encountered in that period once it found a cooperative insurance carrier. The three carriers that refused to deal with the clinic all started their own health plans, suggesting that they were not averse to prepayment but to conditions that the clinic wanted to impose on its plan, such as marketing to individuals and accepting applicants with health problems. Milwaukee Blue Cross agreed to the clinic's unusual demands and spent considerable amounts of time, effort, and money on the Marshfield plan because it wanted a rural HMO and a share of central Wisconsin's market.

Many of GMCHP's difficulties were caused by the clinic's wanting to do all things for all people. Despite good connections in Washington, the clinic's leaders were unable to enroll Medicare and Medicaid beneficiaries, and other low-income families, in their program. GMCHP's lack of management experience with prepaid plans was typical of most new HMOs. But the clinic's refusal to heed Blue Cross's actuarial advice would have doomed the development process had the carrier been less cooperative. Most observers thought that Lewis and Lawton were unreasonable in their determination to provide comprehensive, prepaid care to area residents regardless of their age, financial status, or medical needs. However, the clinic actually achieved that goal for a short time in the early 1980s.

The HMO Act of 1973 incorporated many lessons learned from new plans that developed and failed, with or without help from HEW project grants in the years just before its passage. But instead of assisting potential health plan sponsors, the long-awaited federal legislation nearly derailed the HMO movement.

Chapter 2

The HMO Act and Its Aftermath

Health care should be given to those who need it, not just to those who are fortunate enough to live where doctors are, [are] aggressive enough to insist on and arrange care, and affluent enough to pay for transportation and treatment.

Senator Edward M. Kennedy, 1972

The White House and Congress responded to rapidly rising public and private health care costs by introducing more than two dozen bills between 1970 and 1973.[1] The legislative process pitted Democrats' proposals for nationalized health care against Republican solutions that promoted free enterprise and competition. It also pitted reformers against lobbyists for the health care industry. Fearing that prepaid care providers would scrimp on services to save money, some reformers demanded regulations that would permit the government to monitor quality of care. Some special interest groups sought provisions mandating that the benefit packages of federally funded HMOs include such services as those offered by their group plans. Most old and new prepaid health plans lobbied for conditions that would enable them to compete successfully in the marketplace. Organized medicine, on the other hand, mustered its considerable influence and resources to subvert once again any legislation that might alter its traditional fee-for-service system or promote meaningful health care reform.[2]

The Marshfield Clinic's leaders tried to influence the course of the legislative debate through their personal connections with key players in Congress and the Nixon administration. On the surface, at least, the Greater Marshfield Community Health Plan (GMCHP) closely resembled the Republicans' vision of HMOs as it appeared in the initial version of the legislation sought by the White House. GMCHP combined the efficiencies of group practice with prepayment to serve a broad cross-section of its community, and it was competing successfully with other insurers by offering more and better services for comparable costs. However, the altruistic attitudes of clinic leaders more closely aligned Greater Marshfield with the Democrats' attempts to make health care accessible to all people, regardless of their health or finances. As the debate droned on, Marshfield became one of only a few special interest groups lobbying for the sick and poor, who would soon be abandoned by the Health Maintenance Organization Act of 1973, a piece of legislation that has been called a monument to the best in democratic politics and the worst in health care planning.[3]

Pressures to Reform the Health Care System

Melvin Laird and other congressional leaders were deeply concerned about staggering health care costs in 1968, but Richard M. Nixon devoted almost no time to domestic issues during his presidential campaign that year. Once in the White House he continued for many months to ignore rising inflation in health care and other sectors of the nation's economy.[4] Only after Robert Finch, secretary of health, education and welfare (HEW), warned Congress in July 1969 that "the nation is faced with a breakdown in the delivery of health care unless immediate concerted action is taken by government and the private sector," did Nixon acknowledge that the situation was "much worse" than he realized.[5] Finch submitted proposals to Congress that he believed would "create efficiency and economy" and "strengthen our ability to control some of the abuses in the [Medicare and Medicaid] programs," but the House Ways and Means Committee summarily rejected them as patchwork solutions.[6]

In fact, many members of Congress and dozens of special interest groups were calling for a broad overhaul of the nation's entire health care system. The Special Committee on Aging wanted Congress to adopt legislation that would provide comprehensive public insurance like Medicare and Medicaid for all segments of the population. The 1969 National Governors' Conference overwhelmingly endorsed New York governor Nelson A. Rockefeller's plan for national health insurance.[7] And the Committee of 100 for National Health Insurance, a blue-ribbon panel convened by United Auto Workers' president Walter P. Reuther, was drafting its own health care legislation to cover all Americans.[8]

After repeatedly hearing recommendations such as these, Lewis H. Butler, an assistant secretary at HEW, wrote to the presidential assistant John Ehrlichman. "Ultimately some kind of national health insurance should be enacted," Butler advised, "but the immediate problem is training more doctors and subprofessional people, and getting away from hospital-dominated care into more efficient systems."[9] Nixon chose not to address these issues in his State of the Union message to Congress in January 1970. Instead, he promised a "far-reaching set of proposals for making America's health care available more fairly to more people" without specifying what those proposals would be.[10]

Just days after Nixon's address, Sen. Edward M. Kennedy introduced the Committee of 100's Health Security Bill with strong bipartisan sponsorship from both houses of Congress. In a confidential memo to Dr. Roger Egeberg, assistant secretary for health and scientific affairs, Dr. Vernon H. Wilson, the newly appointed chief of the Health Service and Mental Health Administration at HEW, said he thought Kennedy's plan "was a well-conceived, comprehensive approach to solving the nation's health delivery problems."[11] With so many Republicans supporting Democratic initiatives, White House aides felt compelled to develop a health care proposal that Nixon could call his own.

Nixon's HMO Strategy

Dr. Paul M. Ellwood Jr. came to the administration's rescue in February 1970, when an HEW staffer invited him to a meeting to present his ideas for reducing federal health care costs. According to Ellwood, the White House could rely on continued or increased federal intervention through regulation, investment, and planning, or it could promote a prepaid health care industry that would be largely self-regulatory and would make its own investment decisions regarding resources such as facilities and staffing.[12] Ellwood recommended that the federal government promote a prepaid health care system that, unlike traditional systems, would motivate doctors and hospitals to control costs and keep patients healthy.[13] HEW policy makers liked Ellwood's ideas and asked him to prepare a proposal for White House review. Ellwood enlisted Scott Fleming from Kaiser

Permanente in Oakland, California, to help draft a document. While casting about for a catchy name that would make prepaid health care plans more marketable, they decided "health maintenance organization" was worth keeping.[14]

Assistant secretary Butler told White House aides that Ellwood's ideas embraced dearly held Republican values, such as free markets and competition to reduce government costs. Moreover, a health maintenance program would complement the president's income maintenance policy and legislation that he was seeking to provide a guaranteed income to working poor families with children. HMOs would be inexpensive to implement, optional, and self-regulating, and Butler said that they were better than anything the administration had to offer.[15] Nixon feared that Congress might find HMOs objectionable, so he made no mention of them in his 1970 health message to Congress. However, a few months later he appointed Elliot L. Richardson, an acknowledged HMO advocate, to replace Finch as HEW secretary. Richardson immediately established an HMO project office under provisions in the Public Health Service Act that allowed him to experiment with "alternate delivery mechanisms." Soon that office was preparing plans to distribute grants and federally guaranteed loans to would-be HMO sponsors.[16]

Richardson's activities cleared the way for Nixon to unveil his National Health Strategy to Congress in February 1971. Nixon declared that a proliferation of HMOs would ensure access to a "decent standard of medical care" for all citizens. The union of prepayment and group practice in one organization would produce meaningful efficiencies and competition, which in turn would regulate HMOs and generally improve the quality of medical care.[17] Although Nixon was most eager for prepaid plans to control rising health care costs, especially in the public sector, he emphasized their ability to improve quality of care and access to services, particularly for the poor in medically underserved areas.[18]

Richardson subsequently delivered to Congress a white paper entitled "Toward a Comprehensive Health Policy for the 1970s," in which he added details to Nixon's proposal. The administration hoped to develop 450 HMOs by the end of fiscal 1973, with one hundred in medically underserved areas. Richardson predicted that within another three years seventeen hundred plans could enroll forty million Americans, including ten million with family incomes below federal poverty levels. By the end of the decade the number of HMOs would be sufficient to enroll 90 percent of the population.[19] Many conservatives liked Nixon's new strategy because it was flexible and inexpensive, encouraged private investment in profit-making organizations, and imposed few mandates or regulations.[20]

The American Medical Association (AMA) immediately rejected Nixon's plan, labeling prepaid care unproven and experimental, even though an AMA-sponsored study in the late 1950s had found that care administered by doctors in prepaid group practices was as good as or better than traditional forms of care in the same community.[21] Even as the Marshfield Clinic's doctors were embarking on an experiment to test the promises of prepaid health care at their own expense, the AMA's House of Delegates was unanimously adopting a resolution opposing "federal government support of 'this mechanism' prior to its evaluation and valid proof of its effectiveness." Instead, the AMA lobbied Congress to enact its "Medicredit" program, which would provide tax credits to low-income individuals and families to purchase health insurance that would provide a basic level of care.[22] The clinic doctors, like many congressional Democrats, thought that the AMA's proposal for a multitiered health care system was distasteful and regressive.

AMA Opposition to Health Care Reforms

When Kennedy introduced his bill to provide a single standard of health care for all Americans in 1970, he observed that "there is perhaps no institution more resistant to change than the organized medical profession."[23] In fact, the tendency of the AMA to be more reactive than proactive about health care reforms had diminished its standing within the profession. Since the 1950s increasing numbers of young physicians had refused to join an organization that they considered regressive and self-serving. AMA members accounted for only half of the nation's practicing physicians in the late 1960s, and they tended to be more conservative than the profession as a whole. Surveys from that time found a growing acceptance of new delivery systems among senior medical students, interns, and residents and more physicians who believed that "working in a prepaid group practice setting was a good way for doctors to practice medicine."[24]

Organized medicine has a long history of animosity toward prepaid health care.[25] In the 1930s and 1940s medical societies routinely expelled physicians who worked in prepaid programs operated by consumer cooperatives and labor unions. Such practices forced many programs to close because doctors needed medical society membership in order to keep their license and hospital privileges.[26] The AMA allowed only local medical societies to operate prepaid health plans. During the Great Depression some societies formed "medical service bureaus" to help patients budget for a serious illness and ensure that their members had a steady income. While those plans attracted few subscribers and were short lived, they served as a model for the San Joaquin County Medical Society's Foundation for Medical Care in 1954 and later for the independent practice associations.[27] The AMA refused to relax its guard in the early 1970s when HMO legislation threatened to undermine traditional medical practice. According to one AMA leader, who spoke to a *National Journal* reporter only on condition of anonymity, "This organization will scream its head off if the federal government attempts to force the evolution of HMOs through the use of federal funds."[28]

The Rocky Road to Enactment

Nixon's national health strategy and the introduction of his HMO legislation by Sen. Jacob Javitts, R-N.Y., in March 1971 stole the thunder of proponents of nationalized health care.[29] Kennedy immediately shelved his health security bill and set out to reshape Nixon's proposal. If the country was not yet ready to embrace universal health care, Kennedy wanted to make sure government-funded HMOs would do a better job of financing and delivering medical care than the fee-for-service system.

Richardson and the Democrats agreed that the funding provisions in the administration's bill were inadequate to stimulate widespread HMO development, but their views on the federal government's role and reasons for promoting HMOs were widely divergent. These philosophical incompatibilities, reflecting idealism on one hand and pragmatism on the other, reverberated throughout Congress for the next two-and-a-half years.

As debate began, Nixon feared that inflation and slow recovery from an economic recession in 1969 and 1970 might help the Democrats win the 1972 presidential election. To slow inflation he imposed temporary wage-and-price controls on all sectors of the economy in August 1971.[30] His Economic Stabilization Program showed early promise but proved largely ineffective in the end, especially in the health care industry. The program limited physicians' annual fee raises to 2.5 percent and hospital revenue derived from price increases to no more than 6 percent. Sixteen months after Nixon lifted health sector controls, the consumer price index for medical care increased at an annual rate of 13.1 percent—three times faster than during the control period and nearly twice as fast as before the freeze.[31]

Despite skyrocketing health care costs, Kennedy's legislation reflected a prevailing conviction among Democrats that government had an obligation to provide all Americans with an adequate standard of medical care. Party members generally favored federal support for HMO development because they thought that it would hasten progress toward nationalized health care.[32] Kennedy therefore sought to include many components of universal insurance in his HMO bill. Rep. William R. Roy, a physician and Kansas Democrat who called for generous federal support of HMOs, was Kennedy's counterpart in the House. Both men disliked the idea of stockholders' profiting from sickness and therefore argued against administration proposals to permit and fund for-profit health maintenance organizations.[33]

Republicans supported federal promotion of HMOs in order to reduce private and public health care costs. Their legislative proposals sought to stimulate widespread development of economically viable HMOs, even when those organizations failed to address the needs of all citizens. To that end, GOP bills encouraged private investment in for-profit ventures and competition to promote cost efficiency, self-regulation, and quality.

Rep. Martha W. Griffiths, D-Mich., was Kennedy's coauthor of the health security bill and criticized Republicans for entrusting prepaid health care to private insurance carriers that "have already proved they simply can't handle the problem" of provider reimbursement in a cost-effective manner.[34] Walter J. McNerney, president of the Blue Cross Plans Association, disagreed. He told a Senate hearing, "The government can best set national goals and service priorities, and monitor overall performance, but much of the federal financing of health care can best be accomplished through contractual agreements with the private sector.[35] The next day Kennedy released a confidential memo from an undisclosed source showing McNerney clearly intended for the "private sector" to mean Blue Cross. The memo, sent to all seventy-four Blue Cross affiliates, announced formation of a "communications network" to convince congressional leaders that "only through Blue Cross can truly effective and efficient provisions be made for financing the health care of the nation.[36] In order to protect its policyholders and lucrative Medicare contracts from the threat of nationalized health care, Blue Cross budgeted $556,000, slightly more than $2.5 million in 2004 dollars, for public relations and lobbying in 1971 alone.[37]

Clark C. Havighurst, a Duke University law professor, also criticized insurance company involvement in HMOs because he "wanted to avoid domination of the market by Blue Cross and Blue Shield." Havighurst directed the Committee on Legal Issues in Health Care, which held a contract with HEW's National Center for Health Services Research and Development. Although excluding health insurers from HMO formation would sacrifice important sources of expertise and capital, such a policy would attract a much larger pool of HMO investors, he believed.[38] Havighurst favored for-profit HMOs because he believed that private investment would encourage the development of more facilities, competition, and consumer choice. Conversely, he thought that physician-controlled HMOs were ill advised because doctors lacked the management skills and motivation necessary to cut costs. He also advised universities to use their resources to expand medical school capacity rather than develop prepaid plans.[39] Havighurst often criticized organized medicine, perhaps deservedly so, but he ought to have recognized that many groups of physicians—like those associated with Kaiser Permanente, Harvard Community Health Program, and GMCHP—were spearheading innovation while improving the quality and cost efficiency of the care that they provided. Moreover, such plans were giving consumers more health care choices and increasing competition among providers and insurers in their respective communities.

Dr. Count D. Gibson Jr., chair of Stanford University Medical Center's Department of Community and Preventive Medicine, took issue with Havighurst's support of for-profit health care because he believed that HMOs should be exclusively nonprofit. Gibson's testimony was prophetic: He warned senators that proprietary HMOs would "cream off" desirable patients while dumping the poor, minorities, and elderly on public hospitals. There was also a danger in "absent landlord" ownership of HMOs, he said. "We can foresee the buying and selling of stocks in HMOs and the rapid development of large interstate corporations whose corporate standards bear no relationship to local needs.[40]

Despite mounting pressure from the AMA, Nixon reaffirmed his support of HMOs in a March 1972 health message to Congress. He also announced new initiatives that increased funding and technical assistance for new and existing HMOs and provided special financial incentives for HMOs serving Native Americans, Medicare beneficiaries and the poor. Perhaps as a concession to organized medicine, he backed away from his reliance on market competition and promised rigorous oversight of HMOs to ensure that their care conformed to professional standards.[41]

The administration, Kennedy, and Roy introduced three new HMO bills at the beginning of 1972. Although the bills contained major differences, lawmakers seemed ready to compromise and predicted passage of health care legislation by the end of the year. Seven key issues related to funding, profit status, structure, benefits, open enrollment, community rating, and quality of care occupied their attention. The White House counted on private capital to finance HMO development, but HEW estimated that 75 percent of nascent HMOs would require federal assistance—about $1.1 billion in grants and $2.8 billion more in guaranteed loans by 1980. The Roy and Kennedy proposals required more federal spending, with outright grants for development of clinical facilities. Kennedy remained adamantly opposed to public funding for profit-making HMOs, but Roy was willing to consider exceptions when such plans served medically deprived populations.[42]

The administration's bill was flexible about HMO structure and supported the independent practice associations (IPAs) favored by the AMA.[43] Dr. Ernest W. Saward of Kaiser Permanente in Portland, Oregon, opposed the provisions for flexibility. The Kaiser model was cost effective, he said, because it had full-time physicians working in autonomous, self-governing group practices; fully integrated clinical, hospital, and laboratory facilities; and a capitated reimbursement system. Saward noted that IPAs, by their very nature, lacked these organizational elements.[44] Havighurst wanted medical societies barred from forming IPAs because he believed that their existence tended to block the development of competing HMOs.[45] The Kennedy and Roy bills contained provisions that would make it difficult for new IPAs to qualify for federal support. Because of his friendship with Dr. Ben Lawton and familiarity with GMCHP, Kennedy's bill limited federal funding primarily to highly organized group practices that employed physicians but granted exceptions in rural areas where staffing and facility shortages required HMOs to affiliate with independent practitioners willing to engage in prepaid care.[46]

The three major bills before Congress in 1972 also varied widely in the range of medical services that federally funded HMOs would be required to provide. The differences reflected profound disagreements about the reasons for federal support. The administration, intent on reducing federal health care costs, required only that HMOs provide basic levels of clinical and hospital service. Kennedy, seeking something akin to national health insurance, sought a broad range of benefits and creation of a trust fund to finance prepaid care for the poor. Richardson estimated that Kennedy's proposal would cost $600 per person each year, compared to $300 for Roy's bill and $240 for the administration's bill.[47]

Democrats and the White House were also at odds over open enrollment and community rating, the two most important principles in Marshfield's health plan. Like Lawton, Kennedy insisted that HMOs open their enrollment to all willing subscribers, regardless of the financial risk involved in accepting people in poor health. The administration had called for open enrollment in earlier legislation but reversed its position when Richardson and others testified that such a practice would place HMOs at a competitive disadvantage with regular insurers who routinely rejected people with significant medical needs. The Kennedy and Roy bills required HMOs to use community rating in order to distribute risks throughout a population, but Richardson believed that such a requirement would give an unfair advantage to health insurance companies because they used actuarial rating systems.[48]

The Group Health Association of America (GHAA) agreed with the administration that HMOs ought to offer a basic level of benefits, or more if they chose, but that they need not offer open enrollment periods or community rating. Greater Marshfield's policies contrasted sharply with those of GHAA's member organizations. All but two members marketed exclusively to groups; although the Group Health Cooperative of Puget Sound in Seattle, and the Group Health Association in Washington, D.C., accepted direct-pay applicants, both screened for significant health problems. According to one Kaiser Foundation official, a premium involving provisions for open enrollment and direct-pay subscribers "would take us out of the market."[49] Furthermore, none of GHAA's members used a rate-setting system that spread risks throughout an entire community, as the Democrats proposed. Instead, GHAA members applied "community rates" to groups of workers with similar risks and administrative costs.[50] If Congress required HMOs to broaden their benefits and enrollments,

GHAA said that the legislation ought to apply those mandates to all providers and insurance carriers.[51] That was something that other providers and insurers would never allow to happen.

Congressional concerns about the quality of care in HMOs reflected a pervasive fear that incentives for reducing costs would adversely affect patient welfare. Kennedy's bill therefore called for a commission on quality health care, which would be independent of HEW, to develop quality control standards, monitor quality in federally funded HMOs, and regulate consumer protection.[52] The White House had rejected Paul Ellwood's proposal for such a commission in 1971, preferring to rely on competition among health providers to compel high-quality performance. Rather than see a commission established, Richardson hoped that pending legislation to establish professional standards review organizations would ensure quality in all federally funded health care programs.[53]

For all their differences, Congress and the administration generally agreed on the need to provide federal funding for health services to the poor.[54] Both Congress and the administration believed that preempting state laws incompatible with HMO development was essential despite resistance from medical societies.[55] Although the AMA had lost several court battles in its efforts to restrict prepaid care, Rick J. Carlson, a legal adviser with the Health Services Research Center, told Congress that nearly half the states still had legal barriers to HMO development. The greatest obstacle to the establishment of HMOs was the requirement that they operate with substantial reserves, just as traditional insurance carriers were required to, he said. Other major impediments to HMO formation and operation included common law rules against the corporate practice of medicine; medical ethics restrictions on advertising and soliciting business that limited HMO access to markets; and licensure laws that restricted an HMO's ability to assign certain medical tasks to paraprofessionals.[56] Ignoring objections from organized medicine, well-established health plans often used various types of employees to assist physicians with routine tasks. (The next chapter describes the Marshfield Clinic's successful efforts to train and obtain Wisconsin licensing for physician's assistants in order to alleviate doctor shortages in rural areas of the state.)

AMA lobbying in 1972 convinced Congress and the White House to halt Richardson's ad hoc funding of HMOs until Congress appropriated money for that purpose. Because Richardson's Office of HMOs had already distributed $16.5 million to nearly eighty potential health plan sponsors, lawmakers agreed to continue support of existing projects.[57] While not yet ready to enact HMO legislation, Congress approved amendments to the Social Security Act that would allow HMOs to enroll Medicare and Medicaid beneficiaries and authorized formation of professional standards review organizations (PSROs) to oversee hospital care for Medicare beneficiaries.[58] For all the Republican talk about letting competition control quality, PSROs were a big concession to those who favored regulation.

Enactment of the two amendments enraged the AMA and accelerated its campaign against HMO legislation. The association issued urgent calls to its members, asking them to contact or personally visit members of Congress and contribute money for lobbying efforts. During off-year elections in 1970 the AMA's national political action committee (PAC) gave more than $636,000, and local PACs contributed an estimated $2.5 million, to House and Senate candidates. Anticipating the need for even more money for the 1972 elections, an AMA official said, "We're in the driver's seat now, but once the election is over, it will be a different story. Any commitment we get from the While House to curb HMOs must be made before November seventh." Dr. Malcolm C. Todd, chair of the Physicians' Committee to Reelect the President and Nixon's former personal physician, told a reporter, "We used all the force we could bring to bear against this legislation. As a result, there has been some backtracking on the part of the White House, [which] directed the [HEW] Secretary to slow down on this thing.[59]

The AMA's success at persuading Nixon to withdraw his commitment to HMOs was evident when the Republican Party's 1972 platform mentioned HMOs only as a "worthwhile experiment." By the start of Nixon's second term most supporters of prepaid health care, including Richardson, had left the administration. The new HEW secretary, Caspar W. Weinberger, lacked enthusiasm for HMOs, and his attitude was evident in the legislation that the administration sought in 1973. Whereas Nixon's original bill had called for 150 plans within two years, his new bill called for only a short-term demonstration project with limited goals.[60]

AMA lobbyists succeeded in changing Democratic minds as well. Paul G. Rogers, the Florida Democrat who chaired the key House Interstate and Foreign Commerce Subcommittee on Public Health and Environment, originally supported a strong federal role in promoting HMOs, particularly in medically deprived areas.[61] After he won reelection, he sought to restrict to forty the number of programs eligible for federal assistance in the first year.[62] Still not satisfied, the AMA demanded that Congress limit federal support of HMOs to funding the completion and evaluation of Richardson's projects.

Nixon's new HEW team invited medical writers from around the nation to Washington in July 1973 to learn about the government's new health initiatives. "In glittering generalities," Stuart Auerbach of the *Washington Post* wrote, "administrative big guns such as HEW Secretary Weinberger and Chief Presidential Domestic Adviser Melvin Laird described the high priority that health has among the inner circle at the White House." According to Auerbach, Weinberger said the priority of health issues "is so high, inherently so high, that proponents of sound health programs should have great confidence as to their ability to secure adequate funding." The administration's commitment to HMOs, Weinberger assured the reporter, "has not changed, has not weakened." Gordon MacLeod, whom Richardson had brought from Yale to head the Office of HMOs in 1971, disagreed. When he resigned from his post in early 1973, he said, "The Administration now has reversed its previous position. Subordination of HMO activity from a national program with one hundred people, to a desk function with five or six people, is not consistent with the priority formerly given to HMOs by the Administration."[63]

The Aftermath

The HMO act that Nixon signed in December 1973, was far less comprehensive than any of the other HMO bills that had circulated. It offered few subsidies but contained many mandates. Instead of the $3.9 billion appropriation that Nixon originally proposed for HMO development, the final bill allocated a mere $325 million, spread over five-years, to assist new HMOs with marketing, initial operating costs, and planning, construction, and renovation of facilities. Nonprofit plans were eligible for grants and loans, but profit-making organizations could receive only loan guarantees to finance HMO activities in medically underserved areas. Health plans that met the rigorous federal qualifications were protected from restrictive state laws and eligible to participate in duel choice. That provision required companies with twenty-five or more employees to offer both prepaid and standard insurance coverage when an HMO was available locally.[64] Kaiser Permanente developed the concept of dual choice in the late 1940s as a marketing tool to reconcile the issue of free choice of physician with the closed nature of prepaid group practice.[65] The availability of dual choice in collective bargaining increased marketing opportunities for HMOs; it also enabled workers to switch plans if they became dissatisfied with their first selection.

HEW's implementation of the new legislation was halfhearted at best. Before Congress passed the HMO Act, 150 full-time federal employees worked on HMO development in HEW's Washington and regional offices. A year later the Washington office staff of thirteen included four secretaries, and many regional offices had no HMO staff. HEW also assigned various provisions in the new legislation to seven different bureaus, making it unnecessarily difficult for staffers to prepare, coordinate, and implement regulations. As late as 1975, many rules were unclear in their intent and some were not yet available. The dual choice provision was supposed to offer federally qualified health plans a valuable marketing tool, but HEW aides were slow to establish standards for federal qualification and even slower to recognize plans that met those standards. Because the qualification process was very costly and time consuming, only three plans were qualified by June 1975.[66] Some observers thought that HEW's top administrators deliberately sabotaged the program by staffing it with individuals poorly equipped to evaluate grant applicants or advise grantees. If that was their intent, they succeeded. The General Accounting Office reported that through fiscal year 1977 HEW had disbursed only $70 million of the $250 million authorized for grants and contracts.[67]

Even as Congress was completing work on the HMO Act of 1973, the Institute of Medicine of the National Academy of Sciences began drafting a policy statement regarding conditions under which HMOs would be better able to compete in the marketplace. Participating in the institute's deliberations were representatives from several large prepaid plans, other health care providers, planners, economists, and legal scholars. Most participants agreed that HMOs had the capacity to stimulate positive changes and increase efficiency in the entire health care system if allowed to compete fairly in the marketplace. But HMOs would get a "fair market test" only if they were free to determine their structure and no more constrained than traditional delivery systems. The institute's final report, *Health Maintenance Organizations: Toward a Fair Market Test,* was published in May 1974. Although too late to influence the original legislation, it laid the groundwork for the 1976 amendments to the HMO Act.[68]

James Doherty, the GHAA's legislative counsel and lobbyist, assembled a committee to translate the institute's recommendations into amendments. The participants included representatives from HMOs, provider organizations, insurers, national health care organizations, businesses, and labor unions. The AMA chose not participate because it had no desire to promote amendments that would enable HMOs to succeed. Among the recommendations promulgated by Doherty's coalition were the elimination of open enrollment and certain mandated benefits, as well as the relaxation of requirements for community rating.[69]

Another issue that concerned Doherty and many potential HMO sponsors was a provision in the HMO Act that permitted only two types of organizational structure: group practices dedicated primarily to prepaid care and independent practice associations. Most observers considered unreasonable and fiscally unsound HEW's insistence that group practice HMOs achieve a 50 percent level of prepaid care within three years. One legal analyst believed that the difficulties of meeting this requirement could be understood by looking at the Marshfield Clinic's health plan, which was "highly regarded as one of the success stories in the HMO movement." He noted that GMCHP accounted for only 10 percent of the clinic's revenue and would not meet federal HMO standards until it was responsible for more than half of the clinic's business. When HEW aides suggested that such groups as the clinic be classified as individual practice associations, the analyst said that a fifty-eight-year-old group practice could not be considered an IPA by any stretch of the imagination and called their suggestion ludicrous.[70]

The Senate's Labor and Welfare Committee heard a great deal of opposition to open enrollment and community rating during its hearings on HMO Act amendments. Representatives of several HMOs testified that open enrollment subscribers consumed far more services than group contract subscribers did, even when direct-pay applicants with serious health problems were rejected and treatment of preexisting conditions was withheld for several months. An official of the Harvard Community Health Plan said that open enrollment attracted sick people. In Harvard's experience the utilization rates by ambulatory patients were 145 percent higher and hospital utilization rates were five times greater for direct-pay subscribers than for group contract members.[71]

The Chamber of Commerce and organized labor also favored removing open enrollment mandates, arguing that direct-pay enrollees raised the price of premiums, cost employers more money, and reduced workers' take-home pay. Sen. Gaylord Nelson, the Wisconsin Democrat who was a close friend of Ben Lawton's, disagreed. "If we eliminate the open enrollment requirement, we won't be able to take care of sick people," he said. "We ought to be looking at what a successful open enrollment HMO [in Marshfield] has been doing rather than saying, 'We're scared of open enrollment and therefore should remove that provision in the law.'"[72]

Lawton had served on Doherty's committee but disagreed with nearly all its recommendations. In his "minority report," which he presented at a Senate hearing, he said, "The amendments supported by the other speakers this morning will maintain the health of the insurance companies, physicians and other providers. They will not have much to do with the health of the American people." Lawton told the committee that he favored open enrollment and community rating because the first provision gave sick people access to health care and the second enabled communities to share the cost of caring for those who were ill at any given time.[73]

Gregory Nycz, a Marshfield Medical Research and Education Foundation staffer who accompanied Lawton to the hearings, testified that while GMCHP's liberal open enrollment policy and community-wide rating system had raised monthly premiums $1 per subscriber, its premiums were still competitive with indemnity insurance policies requiring out-of-pocket payments.[74] A Kaiser representative noted that rural Wisconsin was not Los Angeles or San Francisco. Rural areas had a limited supply of "basket cases," whereas open enrollment in large cities would attract "vast numbers" of very expensive subscribers. (The speaker was apparently unfamiliar with the conditions of rural poverty that I address in chapter 4.) At Kaiser, he said, "we don't know what open enrollment would have cost us. We want to know a group's characteristics before offering it a contract." As one observer commented, no amount of evidence from Marshfield would have changed the minds of the HMO industry.[75]

Kennedy suddenly found himself aligned with the AMA in opposing the HMO amendments. Despite pressure from organized labor, Kennedy wanted to keep open enrollment and community rating in the law in order to provide coverage for people too sick to purchase conventional insurance policies. The AMA had waged an all-out effort to defeat HMO legislation a few years earlier. Now it opposed any amendments, Dr. Edgar Beddinfield Jr., the AMA vice president, told a Senate heating, lest the changes would "gut the HMO concept and subvert the original intent of the legislation." If HMOs are a demonstration program, asked one AMA representative, "why at this point do they want to cut back their benefits and only take care of healthy people?" "Where was the AMA," Kennedy asked, "when this committee was attempting to deal with an open enrollment program which would have provided some direct federal subsidies [for sick people]?"[76]

The amendments proposed by Doherty's coalition emerged virtually intact from the congressional hearings. President Gerald Ford signed them into law in October 1976, nearly three years after enactment of the original legislation.[77] These amendments eased requirements for federal qualification of HMOs and eliminated mandates for preventive dental care for children. They also allowed other previously mandated services, such as intermediate and long-term care, prescription drugs, rehabilitation services, vision care, and certain mental health treatments, to be offered as optional benefits. Requirements for open enrollment and community rating were waived until HMOs were well established. Other provisions allowed greater flexibility in HMO structure and reduced (from 50 percent to 35 percent) the time that physicians in federally qualified organizations needed to devote to prepaid care.[78]

George B. Strumpf, deputy director of the Division of HMOs at HEW, reviewed the problems confronting new health plans at an American Public Health Association meeting in 1976, shortly after passage of the new amendments. He reported that fewer than half the seventy-nine HMOs funded by Richardson's Office of HMOs before enactment of the federal legislation had survived. Of 108 projects funded by HEW since the 1973 legislation, sixty-seven were in feasibility or planning phases, and forty-one had been terminated, leaving none in operation. Strumpf said that two major reasons for HMO termination before and after passage of the HMO Act were insufficient commitment by sponsors and inadequate management capability. Two new reasons for termination among health plans after passage of the act were failure to understand the legislation's objectives and to conduct feasibility studies. More significant was that 62 percent of the terminations among Richardson's original group of HMOs and those started after enactment of the HMO Act resulted from an insufficient number of physicians who were willing to participate in those plans. Strumpf believed that many doctors were reluctant to participate in federally funded HMOs because they were supposed to dedicate large portions of their practice to prepaid care.[79]

According to Strumpf, the greatest financial barrier to HMO development was inadequate access to private capital. Lack of capital was a particularly serious problem in underserved areas, even though guaranteed federal loans were available. Twenty percent of the HMO Act's appropriation was set aside for rural areas, but HEW had awarded only 12 percent of the money in that category in the three years after passage of the act. Of thirty-nine plans approved, only seventeen programs remained active, and most were still in the planning stage.

Strumpf noted that the newly adopted amendments contained none of the recommendations prepared by a federally funded research panel for rural HMO development.[80] Nor did the amendments address the need for management training, which was even more pressing than the need for capital. Strumpf disagreed with members of the Senate Labor and Welfare Committee who recognized that financial problems were associated with open enrollment but apparently thought that the marketing benefits of dual choice would offset those disadvantages. "Available information indicates that the substantial costs of open enrollment cannot be met by marketing advantage," he said. "It is more reasonable and fair to impose the requirements on all sectors of the health care industry instead of on HMOs that enroll less than 5 percent of the U. S. population.[81]

The intent of the strategy developed by Paul Ellwood and enthusiastically endorsed by the Nixon White House in 1971 was that market forces would regulate prepaid health care. Instead, the 1973 law and its subsequent amendments made HMOs one of the most heavily regulated segments of the health care industry and placed federally funded HMOs at a competitive disadvantage with conventional health insurance carriers.[82] The HMO Act of 1973 clearly inhibited HMO development. Although 124 prepaid plans were begun in 1970–1974, only forty plans were organized in 1974–1978, when the legislation was significantly altered by a second round of amendments.[83] Early in the 1970s a perceived need for health care reform, some private capital, and small HEW grants had stimulated HMO formation in states where legal restrictions against such programs were lax or nonexistent. But subsequent federal and state legislation, ostensibly enacted to facilitate prepaid health care development, often had the reverse effect.[84]

Some health care reformers blamed Kennedy for saddling HMOs with too many regulations and social goals. They believed that he should have allowed competition to winnow out poorly administered plans that cost too much or gave poor care and that he should have been more real-istic about what HMOs could accomplish.[85] Other observers thought that Kennedy's ideas about open enrollment, community rating, and compre-hensive health care benefits would have had great merit if applied to all health insurers, but such changes were probably impossible, given the political strength of various interest groups. And few policymakers were willing to acknowledge that Marshfield's experience might have broad application.

Unlike the Marshfield Clinic, where the staff was trying to do every-thing for everyone, the folks at Kaiser Permanente believed that many reformers expected too much from HMOs. In a 1971 article Dr. Cecil C. Cutting, executive director of the Permanente Medical Group in Oak-land, California, wrote, "To blindly jump on the bandwagon of prepaid group practice to the exclusion of all other systems, and hail it as the solu-tion to the ills of national health care—as many are wont to do—is not only intellectually dishonest. . . . [It is] a detriment to those who are hon-estly seeking answers to questions of how we can improve the accessibil-ity and delivery of medical care. Every system has advantages and disad-vantages.[86] James Vohs, another Kaiser Permanente officer, noted that proponents of HMO legislation expected "organized health care delivery programs to solve all the problems of costs, manpower scarcity, inaccessi-bility, and uneven quality of medical care. . . . The mere establishment of HMOs will not guarantee the solution of certain problems related to the inflation of medical care costs. It will not necessarily solve problems re-lated to fragmentation of services. Nor is there any assurance that HMOs can correct the maldistribution of services in underprivileged or rural areas.[87]

The HMO Act of 1973 and its subsequent amendments failed to pro-mote prepaid care or reduce health care costs in the United States. The enticement of public funding was simply no match for the legislative and regulatory requirements that accompanied federal largesse. Instead, wide-spread development of HMOs erupted without any help from the gov-ernment during an economic recession in the early 1980s, when the na-tion's business community demanded more cost-efficient medical services and competition among providers began to transform health care into a corporate industry.

Chapter 3

Health Care in Rural America

A great many rural communities . . . cannot adopt the insurance method un-til they solve a more fundamental problem—how to attract and hold in their midst a sufficient number of practitioners to supply even the minimum med-ical demands of the population.

Pierce Williams, 1932

Nearly all HMOs that were developed during the 1970s were urban, even though one-quarter of the nation's population lived in rural and often medically underserved areas. The lack of services mattered little to rural residents until the early twentieth century, when physicians acquired tools to prevent and cure disease. As medical science improved, the urban-rural disparity in the quality of medical care grew into a serious problem. Recognizing that the needs of rural residents were going unmet, Congress reserved 20 percent of the five-year appropriation of $375 million to fund the 1973 HMO legislation for the development of prepaid health care plans in medically underserved areas.[1]

Proponents anticipated that new federally funded HMOs would draw doctors and other health professionals to the countryside, but skeptics thought that the mere availability of money would not overcome the tremendous obstacles to attracting physicians to small, poor communities to work by themselves or in small groups.[2] The pessimists were right. The U.S. Department of Health, Education and Welfare (HEW) received few applications for rural health plans and each year between 1974 and 1979 spent less than 14 percent of the funding earmarked for rural HMO development. Half of forty-two projects financed during that period failed to develop, often because their sponsors were unable to recruit doctors. As

58

a result the HMO legislation and health care revolution affected very few rural residents during the 1970s.[3]

The difficulties involved in establishing rural medical services were such that in 1975 the U.S. Public Health Service (USPHS) recommended preference for federal funding be given to organizations with previous experience in rural communities. Using the Marshfield Clinic's health plan as one model, USPHS officials urged the government to support medical facilities that were located in population centers with sufficient density to be financially viable and capable of offering primary care to outlying areas. Wherever adequate rural services were available, the agency encouraged government subsidies for low-income residents who failed to qualify for Medicaid or Medicare "until a national health insurance program is enacted."[4] Marshfield's efforts to improve rural health services during the 1970s show why it became a USPHS model.

Hard Times and Poor Health

In central Wisconsin and elsewhere rural residents are often uninsured or underinsured. Opportunities for good-paying industrial jobs are scarce, so most workers are self-employed or engaged in low-paying service jobs that offer no health benefits. Policies for farmers are especially expensive because they have the highest accident rate of any occupational group, yet because they are self-employed, they are ineligible for workers' compensation coverage. Farmers also suffer from a wide variety of chronic health problems related to their working conditions. Individual policies are well beyond their means, and farmers usually lack affiliation with an organization through which to purchase insurance at group rates.[5] Many older rural residents lack sufficient income to purchase either the voluntary component of Medicare covering physician and other outpatient services or supplemental policies for other health care services not insured by Medicare.[6]

The healthy rural life is a cruel myth. American farm families have higher infant and maternal mortality rates than urban residents. Their children often lack immunizations, dental care, and treatment for serious illnesses.[7] Historically, their military rejection rates have been nearly twice as high as those for people living in more populated areas, and rural residents have appreciably more debilitating diseases, especially after the age of forty-five. Compared with city dwellers, farmers and their rural neighbors also have higher rates of chronic depression, alcoholism, divorce, spouse and child abuse, and suicide.[8]

People who live in rural areas are not just poorer, older, and less healthy than their urban counterparts; the degree of rural poverty and chronic illness increases as population density declines.[9] Rural residents lack appropriate and timely health care services because they cannot afford to pay for care, live too far from doctors and hospitals, or both. Because they often wait until they are seriously ill to seek medical attention, they use relatively more emergency room and inpatient hospital services than any other population group.[10]

The proportion of rural physicians began to decline dramatically after World War II as older doctors retired and as new medical school graduates entered specialties that required the sort of professional facilities found only in urban settings. Nearly 5 percent of the nation's counties had no physicians by the mid-1970s, and hundreds of others had too few doctors to meet patient demand.[11] The Hill-Burton Act of 1946 had encouraged hospital construction in underserved areas for more than two decades, but rural hospitals in the 1970s were still widely scattered, ill equipped, and poorly staffed.[12]

Efforts to Improve Health Care Resources

Many reformers believed that the use of paraprofessional health care personnel in staff model HMOs would help relieve the nation's shortage of doctors. The concept was equally valid in rural areas, where such personnel could enhance a solo practitioner's productivity. Organized medicine was opposed to letting anyone perform duties normally assigned to physicians, even when those duties were routine, easily learned, and conducted under a doctor's supervision. To that end, medical societies lobbied for state laws that would prevent the training, hiring, or licensing of paraprofessional workers or their use in HMOs.

The Marshfield Clinic took a broader view. In response to physician shortages at the clinic and throughout central and northern Wisconsin, its Marshfield Medical Research and Education Foundation hosted a statewide seminar in 1967 to show doctors how specially trained physician's assistants could relieve their workload and contribute to better patient care. Eighteen months later Secretary of Defense Melvin Laird and HEW secretary Robert Finch visited Marshfield to announce their plans for increasing the nation's supply of health care workers. Laird said that his department was working closely with HEW to "channel military personnel with medical skills into civilian jobs."[13] Soon hundreds of former members of the military medical corps and nurses were seeking additional training so that they could assist doctors in their work.

Dr. Charles Hudson, an AMA president during the mid-1960s, first proposed using physician's assistants (he called them "externes") in a 1961 issue of the *Journal of the American Medical Association.* Duke University established the nation's first formal training program for physician's assistants in 1965.[14] The Marshfield Clinic hired and trained its first surgical assistant that same year and had ten physician's assistants working in various departments five years later. Most were nurses or former military medical corps aides who had received additional on-the-job training from the doctors with whom they were partnered. Seven physician's assistants worked with surgeons, while the other three were involved with kidney dialysis, home visits to new mothers and their infants, and oncology care.[15]

After the Comprehensive Health Manpower Training Act of 1971 authorized funding for programs to train physician's and dental assistants, the Marshfield foundation was one of forty sites selected to receive a five-year grant from the Bureau of Health Manpower and the first in Wisconsin to offer a formal training program for physician's assistants. The foundation had on file three thousand trainee applications and 175 requests from doctors who wanted to hire physician's assistants for their practice when Marshfield's Primary Care Physician Assistant Training Program began in 1972. The program's two-year curriculum was jointly sponsored by the clinic, Saint Joseph's Hospital, the University of Wisconsin's Wood County Center in Marshfield, and a local district of the Wisconsin Vocational Technical Adult Education program. Working closely with Wisconsin legislators, the foundation secured licensing for physician's assistants months before Marshfield's first class graduated in June 1974.[16]

A national committee formed in 1971 to develop minimum educational standards for primary care physician's assistants took nearly six years to complete its task because several panel members continued to question whether nonphysicians could perform tasks traditionally assigned to doctors. In 1977 nearly fifty training programs met newly approved standards or were in the process of gaining approval, and thirty-seven states offered certification or licenses for physician's assistants.[17]

Despite concerns in the medical community, several studies conducted between 1967 and 1978 found no quantifiable differences between physicians and physician-supervised physician's assistants, nurses, and nurse-practitioners with regard to quality of care or outcome of illness.[18] A national survey conducted by the University of Chicago's Center for Health Administration Studies found that consumers were generally content with the type and quality of services that they received from physician's assistants and nurse-practitioners.[19] Although consumers seldom are qualified to judge the technical quality of health care, patient satisfaction is an important element of good care.

Group practice HMOs seemed especially well positioned to relieve physician shortages by using physician's assistants, nurse-practitioners, and paraprofessional aides. In order to test the financial benefits of such helpers, researchers at Johns Hopkins and its Columbia Medical Plan in Maryland identified and reassigned approximately nine hundred primary outpatient care tasks among physicians, nurse-practitioners, physician's assistants, and health aides based on the skill requirements of each task. The realignment of duties resulted in considerable cost savings. Eight physicians usually were required to provide ten thousand patients with about fifty thousand visits a year. Under a revised staffing plan two physicians, four physician's assistants, and eight aides performed the same amount of service with comparable quality for a savings of $100,000. Nonphysicians managed 30 percent of all visits at Columbia in 1973. According to researchers, such staffing patterns required physicians who were willing and able to delegate responsibility and assistants who were skilled communicators. The researchers concluded that appropriately assigned nurse-practitioners and physician's assistants could markedly improve care because they usually had more time than physicians did to answer patients' questions and explain treatments.[20]

A survey of graduates from Marshfield's first two classes found most of them were still in Wisconsin or Upper Michigan a few years later. Eighty-five percent were in primary care settings, and 75 percent were in communities with fewer than ten thousand residents. A nationwide survey of physician's assistant programs reported that most graduates were in primary care, and half were working in communities with fewer than twenty thousand people.[21] Marshfield's administrators closed their program for physician's assistants in the early 1980s after hearing reports that medical schools were producing too many doctors.[22] Rural areas continued to experience physician shortages, however, because most new graduates chose to specialize and practice in large cities. Lewis thought that the decision to terminate Marshfield's physician's assistant program was premature and "one of the biggest mistakes we made." He said the physician's assistants who settled in rural Wisconsin and Michigan were "extremely valuable to small town doctors and a good source of referrals for Marshfield Clinic."[23]

The Marshfield Medical Research and Education Foundation also obtained grants in the 1970s for two other programs that improved health care services in rural communities. A Wisconsin Regional Medical Planning Grant in 1972 enabled the clinic to expand diagnostic and technological outreach services to outlying physicians. The clinic's cardiologists had begun providing long-distance interpretation of electrocardiograms (ECGs) in the late 1960s. Initially, rural practitioners attached ECG monitors to patients suspected of having cardiac problems, transmitted the heart signals to the Marshfield Clinic by telephone, and waited about three days for a cardiologist to call back with the results. State funding, together with the development of the computer and software programs to interpret ECGs, soon enabled the Marshfield Clinic to process and respond with teletyped reports within ten minutes. In 1979 the clinic interpreted and provided free consultation on more than twenty-four thousand ECGs from fifty-one hospitals and numerous clinics and private practice sites in Wisconsin and Upper Michigan.[24]

The Marshfield Clinic started regional laboratory services in 1973 after moving into new facilities adjacent to Saint Joseph's Hospital, where the two institutions shared a state-of-the-art laboratory. Each weekday a fleet of clinic vehicles collected laboratory samples from doctors throughout central and northern Wisconsin and delivered them to the Marshfield Medical Center laboratory, where they were processed by second-shift technicians. Laboratory staffers telephoned doctors if test results warranted immediate action; otherwise, drivers distributed printed test reports to doctors the following day. By 1979 the Marshfield laboratory was performing approximately eleven thousand tests a month for physicians and hospitals throughout Wisconsin. Laboratory couriers, who collectively traveled about two thousand miles each workday, transported most specimens. A prepaid mailing system was also available for sites lacking courier service. Computerized patient reports collated all procedures, results, and normal values for each patient, and the laboratory could print results at referral sites immediately. Before such outreach services were available, rural doctors, clinics, and hospitals often waited a week or more for ECG interpretations and diagnostic test results.[25]

A federal Rural Health Initiative (RHI) grant to the Marshfield Medical Research and Education Foundation financed the Northcentral Wisconsin Rural Health Network, a three-and-one-half year project designed to improve health care services for approximately 650,000 people living in twenty-five central and northern Wisconsin counties. Many rural Wisconsin communities had problems recruiting and retaining new physicians when elderly practitioners died or retired. Funding for that project, more than $140,000, enabled eleven communities to establish or enhance medical practices and develop services linked to medical resource centers such as the Marshfield Clinic. Project administrators helped design facilities, recruit and train support personnel, set up business procedures and medical records, and purchase equipment and supplies. Facilities that became Marshfield Clinic satellites used the clinic's daily courier service to send their paperwork to Marshfield for processing.[26]

Continuing professional education at Marshfield and its outreach sites also helped rural Wisconsin communities attract and retain doctors. The clinic, its research and education foundation, and Saint Joseph's Hospital sponsored more than a dozen weekly teaching conferences in Marshfield, as well as frequent seminars for physicians and other health professionals at locations throughout central and northern Wisconsin and Upper Michigan. As the technology became available, many of these programs were videotaped for distribution to outlying practitioners. Individualized teaching rounds allowed area rural doctors to spend time with Marshfield Clinic specialists for intensive study in the field of their choice. Several clinic specialists routinely traveled to sites as far as one hundred miles away to see patients and consult with local physicians. These outreach programs improved patient access to specialized care and provided opportunities for primary care doctors to learn new skills. Area doctors and hospitals were also encouraged to use free telephone lines to request reference services, searches, and photocopies from the clinic library; requested materials were dispatched via the couriers or through the mail until fax machines became available.[27] The goodwill that these programs engendered was largely responsible for the willingness of many small town doctors to affiliate with the Greater Marshfield Community Health Plan (GMCHP) as it expanded.[28]

The Marshfield Clinic's recruitment materials appealed to the "one doctor in four" who was attracted by "an uncommon clinic" where it was possible to practice with all the professional benefits and services of a major medical center yet live in a rural setting.[29] As the clinic developed new satellites and independent facilities in the 1970s, dozens of young doctors moved into central and northern Wisconsin. These facilities greatly improved access to health care but rarely showed a profit.[30] Despite an influx of physicians, the shortage of health care workers remained acute. Wisconsin's distribution of physicians in the early 1970s ranged from one doctor for every 378 residents in Dane County, where the University of Wisconsin Medical School was located, to one doctor for 5,625 residents in one northern county and none in two others.[31] In the late 1970s, 33 percent of the state's primary care physicians were sixty or older and 11 percent were seventy or older. Beyond the continuing shortage of health care personnel, thousands of people still lacked access to medical care because they were poor.[32]

Community Health Centers for the Poor

As part of President Lyndon B. Johnson's "War on Poverty" in the mid-1960s, the Office of Economic Opportunity (OEO) established a number of neighborhood health centers for low- income people in medically underserved inner cities.[33] These centers were unique on several counts. Unlike traditional public health clinics, which delivered services to passive recipients, these centers involved their target populations in the design and management of their own health care.[34] The centers also shifted services to local neighborhoods, where the emphasis was on primary and preventive care rather than emergency room care and hospitalization. The staff included people from the neighborhood who were recruited and trained as paraprofessional aides. Multidisciplinary teams broadened the notion of "medical care" to include such services as transportation, education, and counseling. Mainstream health care providers later adopted many of these concepts. OEO was operating about one hundred neighborhood health centers in 1968 when HEW began to fund the development of family health centers and medical service networks in medically underserved rural areas.[35] HEW's health centers replicated the extensive outpatient medical and support services of the urban centers, but neither of those programs offered inpatient care. Instead, the centers referred seriously ill patients to public, university, or nonprofit community hospitals for charity care.[36]

Leaders of the Marshfield Clinic had tried to obtain federal health care subsidies for low-income residents in 1968 when an OEO survey found high levels of poverty in five central Wisconsin counties. After failing to make progress on their own, the Marshfield Clinic officials hired a consultant in 1971 to prepare a grant proposal for submission to OEO. Frederick (Fritz) J. Wenzel, director of the Marshfield Medical Research and Education Foundation, which planned to administer the OEO program, had testified at a U.S. Senate hearing earlier that year. "Ghettos do not exist only in large metropolitan areas," he said. "The Greater Marshfield area comprises forty-four thousand people and we find twenty-two thousand who fall into the category of economically disadvantaged at one level or another. Approximately four thousand are eligible for assistance under OEO guidelines."[37]

While waiting to hear from the OEO, Lewis and Wenzel learned of new funding from HEW to serve low-income populations and quickly submitted a second proposal. A month after the OEO denied Marshfield's application in May 1972, HEW awarded the foundation a planning grant of more than $500,000 to establish a subsidized family health center in conjunction with GMCHP.[38] The clinic's jubilant press release reported that the new program would "provide totally comprehensive services to families with annual incomes of less than seven thousand dollars, thus placing the health plan well within the range of all economic groups" in the immediate area.[39]

Marshfield's administrators were eager to start the Family Health Center of Marshfield (FHC), but they wanted to offer low-income enrollees the same benefits that other health plan subscribers received. Lewis therefore wrote to Dr. Hazel Swann, chief of HEW's Family Health Center Branch, requesting waivers to avoid making FHC enrollees "second-class citizens." Lewis advised Swann that incorporating FHC into GMCHP would reduce the center's administrative costs and help to produce more meaningful data for the federal government regarding use of medical services by low-income families.[40] Shortly after receiving the waiver requests, Swann visited the clinic and told a Milwaukee reporter that she was amazed by what was happening in Marshfield. "I'm going back to Washington and demand extensive study of Wisconsin's services so that the rest of the nation can benefit" from the clinic's experience.[41] Despite Swann's enthusiasm, Marshfield waited another eighteen months to get the waivers. When the FHC finally opened in March 1974, it was the first federally subsidized health center in the nation to provide inpatient hospital care.[42] GMCHP's monthly family premium that year was $59.60, but FHC enrollees paid between $1.19 and $14.49, based on family size and income. In order to ease the burden of payments for farmers, the foundation arranged for dairies to deduct monthly premiums from the money that the dairies paid to farmers for their milk each week or month.[43]

Identifying and marketing to eligible families required a considerable outreach effort, but within eight months Marshfield's FHC was serving 245 families with nearly fourteen hundred individuals in a three-county area. Two-thirds of the subscribers were farm families, and another one-fifth were unemployed or retired. FHC families tended to be larger and younger than those in GMCHP, and 42 percent had no history of previous health insurance coverage. Because of their long-standing habits of self-reliance, FHC members used relatively few medical services until the program put additional outreach services in place.[44]

Soon after the Marshfield FHC started, its administrators began to request waivers from federal agencies that would allow Marshfield to evaluate additional benefits for inclusion in its own and other health center programs. Greg Nycz, who became FHC's director shortly after joining the Marshfield Medical Research and Education Foundation as a biostatistician in 1972, was extensively involved in many of these proposals. He and Wenzel first asked the Bureau of Community Health Services (BCHS), which was responsible for the oversight of health center programs, for waivers to provide dental care and drug benefits for children younger than thirteen.[45] The intent of the dental care benefit was to combat high rates of caries because private well water was not fluoridated. The purpose of the drug waiver was to ensure that children received medication prescribed by their doctor.[46] BCHS ignored the request for a dental waiver but asked the foundation for a proposal that would provide outpatient prescription drugs to all Marshfield FHC members. That benefit enhancement, which began in March 1975, paid the full cost of all prescription drugs, including contraceptives, when members obtained them from participating pharmacies in GMCHP's service area.[47]

The second time that Wenzel requested a waiver to offer dental care to FHC children, Dr. Norbert M. Sabin, the chair of the Wisconsin Dental Association's Program Committee, heard about the project and sent out a strongly worded letter to all central Wisconsin dentists. Sabin reminded them that the American Dental Association's House of Delegates opposed "HMOs and programs that deny the concept of freedom of choice, and any other legislation that would subsidize programs in such a way as to compete unfairly with the private practice of dentistry." He said that local dentists should boycott the project because "the Marshfield Clinic Foundation is providing services supported by the Health Services Administration, which is interested in accumulating information that might be useful when they get into serious discussions about National Health Insurance."[48]

When FHC received funding for its dental program, all but four of the thirty-five dentists in GMCHP's service area agreed to participate on a fee-for-service basis.[49] During the program's first year in 1975, Nycz reported that 70 percent of FHC's children in the four-to-twelve age group saw a dentist, many for the first time. Each child averaged about 3.15 visits, reflecting a high level of unmet need. The frequency of their visits fell to maintenance levels, and costs per child diminished substantially as children remained in the program.[50] FHC subsequently received permission to provide preventive dental services to older children and then to adults. Based on Marshfield's evidence, BCHS subsequently required the nation's other health centers to furnish their patients with drug benefits and preventive dental services.

Another waiver and more supplemental funding allowed FHC to hire a patient educator in 1975. The educator explained FHC's program to new enrollees and encouraged them to use its health screening, immunization, and dental programs. She also collected and prepared educational materials for distribution in newsletters, radio broadcasts, and pamphlets. After four years FHC's five thousand enrollees were using outpatient and hospital services at rates very similar to those of other GMCHP subscribers. Administrators believed that the normalization of FHC utilization patterns was the result of enrollees' learning to seek early intervention and prevention services. The Marshfield Clinic assumed financial responsibility for patient education in 1978 when federal funding ceased and subsequently hired a physician who specialized in preventive medicine to plan and implement additional health maintenance measures. As a result the clinic soon began to offer immunization and cancer-screening services to all residents in the four-thousand-square-mile area served by FHC and GMCHP,[51] and it bore the costs of services to people not enrolled in its health plans.[52]

Supplemental funding from BCHS also allowed the Family Health Center to increase outpatient mental health benefits and to use nursing home services without the usual requirement of hospitalization first.[53] Wenzel repeatedly asked BCHS for permission to enroll individuals in the Family Health Center, reasoning that individuals without family connections were just as deserving of subsidized medical care as family members. The bureau's Richard Bohrer said, "We agreed with Wenzel's concept, but Marshfield's FHC received its initial funding under a demonstration program designated to evaluate prepaid care for low income families, not individuals. After the demonstration phase was completed, we redesigned the program and accepted Wenzel's proposal so that qualified individuals could enroll in FHCs nationwide."[54]

Marshfield was one of about forty prepaid demonstration projects funded by BCHS in the mid-1970s. Ten percent of the programs failed in their first year, and only one-third were still in business twenty years later. Bohrer, who joined the U.S. Public Health Service in 1969 and began working with FHCs in 1971, said that Marshfield's plan was unique because it incorporated family health services into an existing HMO sponsored by a well-established medical facility. Financial and technical support from the clinic and its medical research foundation allowed his bureau to experiment with many benefit options. For example, he said, "Marshfield documented better than any other program that FHC's inpatient benefit killed them financially because people had a lot of health needs. For two or three years after people entered their program, they overused hospital services but then dropped down to normal utilization patterns."[55]

Bohrer called Wenzel and Nycz "living legends in the health center movement" and credited them with helping him to create an informal network for FHC administrators. "The network was a tremendous success for those programs that were starting from scratch," he said. After Congress placed all publicly funded health centers, including those of the Office of Economic Opportunity, under the Bureau of Community Health Services in 1975, the family health centers joined the National Association of Community Health Centers.[56] In 1977 that association included 127 neighborhood health centers, twenty-seven family health centers, and ten community health networks, which together served fewer than two million Americans. Because of funding restrictions, only a small fraction of those eligible for federally subsidized care actually received it.[57]

Central Wisconsin residents participating in Marshfield's FHC often expressed their gratitude in letters to program staff. One husband wrote:

I am 57 years old and a small dairy farmer, a veteran of WW2. My wife has a chronic lung condition which requires continuous medical attention. She is now on Oxigen therapy 12 hours per day, which the Marshfield Health Plan pays for (approximately $150 per mo. plus much medication.) Her hospital and medical bills were in the area of $6,000 last year. I am a dsiabetic, which at present I am controling with diet. . . . Much of our married life we were not able to afford Health or Medical Insurance. I would have had to sell my $20,000 farm and Homestead to pay last years medical bills. As things are now we are able to get along with a large garden and our own milk, poultry and rabbits. We don't need other help but your medical assistance is sorely needed.[58]

A mother whose family recently enrolled in FHC wrote:

This insurance has been a God send. It's the first year that we've been able to take our kids to the doctor when there sick right away instead of waiting till there really bad. The year before my son was sick, no insurance. We waited around before taking him to hospital till he had Pneumonia then lay in oxygen tent 3 days. This year because of our insurance we caught it in time and he was able to get well at home. This insurance is the best way for low income family. You feel proud because your paying your own premium . . . your paying what you can. We are hard working people who need a little help over the rough spots. If you've never sat helplessly by your child at night who coughs till there sick or up all night with a earache or tooth ache because you can't afford it, you wouldn't no how we feel.[59]

Consumer Participation

Consumer participation in federally subsidized health centers dated from development of OEO's neighborhood health centers in the 1960s. Consumer participation continued to be a requirement for other federally funded health centers and eventually for all federally funded HMOs. The Group Health Association of America, which represented the interests of many consumer-operated health plans, had lobbied for inclusion of such a mandate in OEO's legislation and the HMO Act of 1973.

When it was organized in 1974, the Family Health Center of Marshfield was required to provide opportunities for its members to participate in its governance. GMCHP was under no such obligation because it began without federal funding and before passage of the HMO Act. Nevertheless, GMCHP formed a consumer advisory committee, hoping that its members would help sell the plan to the community and provide feedback from its subscribers. Such committees had merit, but members often misunderstood their role. Marshfield's experience was typical.

The GMCHP advisory committee, composed of seven Marshfield community leaders representing a cross-section of local interests, convened for the first time on 1 April 1971, when the health plan was one month old. After the initial meeting, Lewis reported that the members had decided to call themselves the "Community Committee," rather than "Community Advisory Committee," because they did not intend to be a "rubber stamp."[60] Furthermore, he said that the chair wanted the committee have authority to "review, recommend and approve" all financial matters related to the health plan, including rates.

Unhappy in his advisory role, the chair demanded at subsequent meetings that his committee be accorded equal status with the three partners in formulating health plan policy and negotiating rates. He asked the partners to add prescription drugs and dental care to their benefit package and to include committee members in negotiations with local pharmacists and dentists. And he directed a Blue Cross executive to draw up documents enabling the committee to play a decision-making role in the health plan, and to provide someone qualified to speak about prescription drugs and dental benefits at the committee's next meeting.[61] Lewis told the chair that he welcomed committee participation in negotiations with local dentists and pharmacists. Neither he nor hospital officials objected to committee representatives' attending meetings at which the partners set their rates. However, Lewis said that the partners conducted rate setting and other business matters during normal working hours when committee members might find it difficult to attend because of their own work commitments.[62]

When the chair addressed a Marshfield Rotary meeting on the Community Committee's first anniversary, he left his audience with the impression that he distrusted clinic physicians and thought that they earned too much money. No one could blame GMCHP's problems on the Community Committee, he said, because the health plan had started before the committee was organized. While health plan members were entitled to quality medical care, the chair said that the clinic's "Cadillac-type of service" was excessive when "Ford or Chevrolet-type care would do." He said that premiums were too costly and that because of that he thought that his committee should have a role in determining rates. Furthermore, he said that the clinic's fee-for-service arrangement with the health plan gave doctors no incentive to prevent disease or lower health care costs. Instead, they made more money when their patients were sick. Medicine as practiced by the clinic and hospital in Marshfield was a monopoly, he warned, and all monopolies needed regulatory agencies to keep their rates in line. In order for the Community Committee to carry out its functions, the chair said that he wanted the authority to hire an independent consultant to represent consumers.[63]

Lewis ignored most of the chair's remarks, except for those relating to the clinic's reimbursement arrangement, which had initially called for GMCHP to pay the clinic on a fee-for-service basis. Lewis told the chair that his call for the clinic to accept capitation "has in my mind established the value of your committee. While we've been talking about it on and off, your rather dramatic feeling on this issue has forced us to reevaluate our whole position."[64] The clinic's board of directors voted less than a week later to accept capitation-based reimbursement from the health plan. When the Community Committee voted soon afterward to approve a second-year rate increase, the chair abstained from the vote. He thought that the rates were already too high, especially when they did not include his proposed drug and dental benefits.[65]

Community Committee members spent most of their first few years reviewing GMCHP's financial and enrollment reports and trying to draft bylaws that would formalize their role. They also reviewed educational materials and grant proposals, conferred with dentists and pharmacists, and attended meetings where health plan partners discussed rates and other policy issues. During the summer of 1972 the committee helped develop questions for a subscriber survey. Although 53 percent of the respondents rated the health plan as excellent, and 45 percent more reported that it was very good or good, the chair continued to distribute information about other health plans that he felt cast GMCHP in a bad light.[66]

The chair clearly expected the Community Committee to play an administrative role in GMCHP's operation and was frustrated by the partners' failure to supply him with the resources that he believed were necessary to perform his job.[67] Other committee members did not want to participate in the plan's management and thought that they received sufficient information for their role as advisers. Indeed, when committee members finally approved their bylaws, their duties were entirely advisory.[68]

GMCHP's Community Committee added a few FHC enrollees after

that program started in order to meet the federal consumer participation requirements. The committee remained advisory until the Health Revenue Sharing and Health Services Act of 1975 mandated consumer governance for federally funded health centers.[69] At that point the committee reorganized, added several more FHC enrollees, and became the Family Health Center Governing Board. The new board was responsible for setting FHC policies, benefits, and services, but the Marshfield Medical Research and Education Foundation continued to administer the program.[70]

The Consumer Council for the Columbia Medical Plan, organized by Johns Hopkins Medical Institutions in 1969, was one of many other advisory panels with a similar history. The council found itself increasingly embroiled in a number of sensitive and complex issues as it tried to clarify its relationship with health plan managers and policy makers. In the case of the Columbia panel its nine members were relatively knowledgeable about health matters because of their vocational or personal interests. Nevertheless, plan administrators denied the council's requests to increase its representation from one to three members on the Columbia Hospital and Clinics Foundation's board of trustees and to participate in the budget review process. Although Columbia's council adopted bylaws in 1971 that defined its functions as activist, its members received a growing number of requests to react to policies already adopted and to offer advice on seemingly insignificant matters. As membership changed, the Columbia council abandoned its efforts to influence policy making and financial matters and focused instead on improving communication between Columbia's managers and consumers.[71]

Advocates for consumer participation argued that advisory and governing boards with enrollee representation assured members access to quality medical care as well as mechanisms for lodging and resolving complaints. In addition, consumer committees could help subscribers use their plans effectively and encourage healthy lifestyles.[72] Opinions about the optimum level of authority for such bodies varied widely, however. Although some observers felt that subscribers were entitled to participate in all policy decisions, most consumer representatives seemed more interested in membership recruitment, patient education, benefits, and access to services.[73] Two studies from the 1960s yielded conflicting results regarding subscriber involvement. One reported that consumer sponsorship of and participation in the governance of prepaid health care organizations had a favorable influence.[74] The other found that the nation's two largest cooperatives, the Health Insurance Plan of Greater New York and the Group Health Association in Washington, D.C., had chronic problems because their governing boards lacked sufficient skills to manage their plans themselves.[75]

Consumer advocacy for improved rural health care services became extremely effective after Marshfield's Family Health Center Governing Board reorganized to give low-income members a greater voice. When FHC celebrated its twenty-fifth birthday in the 1990s, clinic administrators credited some long-time board members for their leadership and guidance in making FHC an award-winning program for all residents in eleven central and northern Wisconsin counties.[76] However, FHC's very existence and its many outreach services would not have been possible without the clinic's strong commitment to improving rural health care.

The Marshfield Clinic's aggressive pursuit of federal and state funding enabled it to train physician's assistants; provide outreach laboratory, electrocardiogram, consultation, and education services; create new medical facilities and resource networks for rural communities; develop a multi-county health center program for low-income families; and supply free screening services in every county where its health plan was operating. Those who see self-interest in the clinic's beneficence would argue that the clinic and GMCHP benefited directly from the outreach activities because these services increased referrals, made communities more receptive to the health plan's expansion, and improved the health of its subscribers. All those consequences strengthened Marshfield's influence in northern Wisconsin, but they also carried an increasing need to cooperate with local providers.

Others might say that the clinic could afford to be altruistic because it was a major health care force in a rural setting. I would argue that other providers in Wisconsin cities to the east and west of Marshfield had equal opportunities but never developed their potential for meeting the needs of rural people living within their reach. The clinic's physicians acknowledged that many of their outreach programs benefited competing providers and insurers, but northern Wisconsin's levels of poverty and medical need, far higher than in many cities, compelled them to share their professional outreach services with all residents and health care providers.

Marshfield's experience with grants reveals how government programs deal with health care problems in a patchwork fashion that increases bureaucracy but never quite solves the problems—personnel and facilities shortages, uninsured populations, and various diseases, for example. More often than not, public programs operate at cross-purposes with one another, protected by administrators intent on guarding their own turf. Is it any wonder that programs never have enough money to meet the needs of their target populations?

Chapter 4

Affiliated Providers and
Necessary Compromises

We tried to keep everyone happy. We wanted our health plan subscribers to use their regular doctors, and we wanted those doctors to send us their referrals.

Russell Lewis, M.D.

The Greater Marshfield Community Health Plan was conceived as a prepaid group practice health plan similar to the Ross-Loos plan in Los Angeles and several Kaiser-Permanente plans on the West Coast. Instead of growing out of established group practices, an increasing number of new HMOs in the 1970s were independent practice associations, networks of loosely organized physicians who worked out of their own offices. In reality, many plans became hybrids: IPAs often included small groups of specialists, and staff model HMOs sometimes needed to supplement the services of their own physicians with those of independent practitioners who were engaged in particular specialties or located closer to subscribers.

GMCHP quickly evolved into a hybrid because its founders wanted to accommodate patients who lived in or used physicians practicing in nearby communities. With each expansion into a new area the health plan invariably signed affiliation agreements with local providers so that new subscribers could continue to use them for routine care. The clinic accepted a monthly capitation from GMCHP for outpatient services, as many group practice HMOs did, but it used a portion of its reimbursement to pay physicians who were affiliated with the health plan on a fee-for-service basis, which was similar to most IPAs.

Because of its rural setting GMCHP faced two particularly difficult challenges with regard to affiliated providers. First, it had to affiliate with nearly every available medical practitioner, hospital, dentist, and mental health counselor in its coverage area because practitioners and facilities were in such short supply. Second, the clinic's role as a tertiary care provider in central and northern Wisconsin required that its health plan maintain good relations with the affiliates upon whom it depended for referrals. The clinic and its health plan were seriously compromised by GMCHP's inability to select from an assortment of providers and facilities, as urban HMOs could do, or to control the affiliates' utilization rates, costs, and quality of care without alienating them. These issues created a great deal of conflict within the clinic and the broader provider community. They became particularly troublesome in the 1980s when rising health care costs and market competition necessitated cost-efficient care. (For further discussion of the difficulties of the 1980s, see chapter 8.)

Beyond the problems peculiar to HMOs in medically underserved rural areas, Marshfield's experiences with affiliated providers illustrate the difficulties that all types of health plans, especially IPAs, encountered when trying to ensure that their independent affiliates practiced cost-efficient, high-quality care. Marshfield's encounters with affiliates also show how the HMO-induced health care revolution forced doctors to change the way that they practiced medicine and dealt with their peers. There was no place for unquestioning cordiality among traditional practitioners in the prepaid setting, where physician-administrators had to demand certain standards of care so that their plans would be financially viable and valued by consumers.

Problems with Affiliated Physicians

The administrators of the Marshfield Clinic believed that doctors who affiliated with their plan got a good deal. The office expenses that affiliates incurred for subscribers were 10 to 15 percent less than for fee-for-service patients because the affiliated physicians did not have to send out bills, collect payments, or write off bad debts. And, unlike reimbursements from insurance company and government programs, which often arrived months late, GMCHP paid its affiliates promptly, sending checks for 92 percent of their customary fee-for-service charges each month. The affiliates received the remaining 8 percent as an end-of-year bonus if sufficient funds were available. In six of GMCHP's first eight years the affiliates received 100 percent of their invoiced charges. Most health plans withheld some portion of physician reimbursements until their fiscal year ended, but some also recalled monies that they had already paid to providers when cost overruns occurred. GMCHP never asked affiliates to assume financial responsibility for its deficits, but it eventually changed to a 90/10 percent reimbursement formula, like other Wisconsin HMOs, in order to have a greater reserve in case of a shortfall.

Members of the clinic's executive committee initially insisted on reviewing the qualifications of all providers seeking affiliation with the health plan so that they could ensure that the care provided by the affiliates would reflect well on the clinic and its health plan. Rather than complicitly sanction lower standards when GMCHP moved into areas with few, if any, qualified medical doctors, the executive committee created a GMCHP "credentials committee," composed of four clinic and three affiliated physicians, to review the qualifications of new applicants. Although several providers who applied for affiliation had poor credentials or were known to provide substandard care, the credentials committee accepted them so that the health plan could serve their patients. As one mayor, who petitioned GMCHP to affiliate with his village's only doctor, explained, "'We'd rather have a bad doctor than no doctor at all.'"[1]

The activities of some affiliated physicians caused great concern. One, a "circuit-riding" surgeon, was rarely available to deal with his patients' postoperative complications. When a clinic surgeon tried to have the circuit rider censured for professional irresponsibility, the State Medical Society of Wisconsin and the Wisconsin Medical Licensing Board gently admonished the surgeon in question and allowed him to keep his license.[2] (I will return to this issue—the medical profession's failure to use its state-vested authority to control wayward physicians—in chapter 8.)

GMCHP paid whatever its affiliates charged until some raised their fees beyond what the clinic's highly trained specialists were charging for similar procedures.[3] Because the clinic was reluctant to control doctors' fees for fear of incurring an antitrust investigation, GMCHP asked affiliates to submit their fee schedules before each fiscal year so that it could factor their charges into its rate calculations. The health plan also asked affiliates to honor their fee schedules for an entire year, but many raised their fees whenever they learned of others' charging more than they did.

GMCHP finally turned to its credentials committee, by then renamed the insurance committee, for help in reviewing all professional fees and recommending maximum reimbursement levels for each service or procedure. Starting in 1979, the health plan refused to recognize fee increases made during the fiscal year or to pay more than the maximum reimbursement for any service.[4] Several doctors vigorously protested the new policy but nevertheless remained in the plan.

GMCHP based reimbursements to Saint Joseph's Hospital in Marshfield and its two affiliated hospitals in outlying communities on their daily rates for the preceding fiscal year. This formula assumed that rates would rise about 10 to 15 percent each year, an amount equal to what hospitals would save in administrative costs when caring for prepaid patients. The hospitals seldom encountered financial risk, but the health plan lost money whenever inpatient utilization rates were higher than anticipated. GMCHP staff members were able to monitor how much clinic physicians used Saint Joseph's Hospital and asked those showing inappropriately high utilization rates to modify their behavior.

GMCHP's widely scattered affiliates were a different story. They routinely admitted patients to their local hospital for inappropriate reasons and allowed unjustifiably long stays without regard for cost. For example, patients belonging to one group of affiliated doctors spent 41 percent more days in a local hospital than a similar group of patients under the care of Marshfield Clinic physicians at Saint Joseph's Hospital.[5] When GMCHP finally assigned staffers to monitor hospital admissions and lengths of stay at affiliated hospitals, the hospital administrators and physicians complained that such interference greatly reduced their revenue. This reaction was apparently quite common. The federal Office of HMOs reported in 1985 that rural HMOs had particularly difficult problems tracking and controlling hospital utilization. Physicians who practiced in such plans were unaccustomed to peer review and had ingrained practice patterns that were often inappropriate for participation in prepaid health organizations.[6]

Marshfield Clinic doctors involved in monitoring the affiliates thought that some had appalling treatment practices and fees that were grossly incompatible with their training and credentials. Dr. Nelson Moffat, a former clinic president, said, "We wanted to include as many doctors possible. We didn't want to appear too exclusive, but we felt we had to uphold some standards of practice. There were some terrible doctors. We knew who they were, but we accepted them because their patients thought they were good."[7] Dr. Dean Emanuel, another clinic physician, believed that GMCHP ought to demand a certain standard of care from its affiliates. He reported that "the Nicolet Group in Minneapolis had no compunction about kicking out doctors who were incompetent, greedy, or failed to perform." Had he been responsible for dealing with doctors who charged too much for substandard care, he said, "I would not have criticized the way they practiced medicine. Instead, I would have told them that they were too expensive for our plan, that we couldn't afford them. That's what Nicolet did."[8] However, Nicolet had the luxury of being able to choose other doctors. Some clinic physicians thought that Lewis was much too lenient with affiliates, but few of them wanted his job as the health plan's medical director. Emanuel, who served for a brief spell as assistant medical director some time later, found that the frustrations of the position far outnumbered its rewards.

Problems with Other Affiliated Providers

In addition to physicians, GMCHP was affiliated with optometrists, pharmacists, dentists, mental health counselors, and other health care providers so that they too could offer convenient service to subscribers who lived beyond Marshfield. In order to be fair to Marshfield's independent providers, GMCHP offered them the same opportunities for affiliation as their counterparts in other communities. Clinic specialty departments invariably resisted the affiliation of independent providers because they were concerned about controlling quality, unwilling to share GMCHP's income with outsiders, or both. A few examples show that reactions varied widely, with some departments more willing to compromise than others.

The Marshfield Clinic's ophthalmology department initially refused to allow independent optometrists to perform eye examinations on GMCHP subscribers because it would not be able to monitor the quality of their services. However, clinic ophthalmologists consented to affiliation in 1975, once the independents agreed to participate in peer review. Concerns about examination standards, meaningful peer review, unnecessary utilization, and excessive charges surfaced from time to time, but relations between GMCHP and the affiliated optometrists were generally congenial.[9]

Negotiations with pharmacists were somewhat more difficult. Early in GMCHP's operation, Blue Cross and the Community (Advisory) Committee promoted a prescription drug benefit similar to what other HMOs offered. Lewis was afraid that such a benefit would increase tensions between the independent pharmacists who operated a pharmacy in the clinic building and those who owned drugstores in the community. However, he liked the concept and eventually agreed to discuss the issue with area pharmacists.[10] Negotiations progressed smoothly until Blue Cross suggested charging subscribers a small fee for each prescription purchase, as other HMOs did. At that point the pharmacists objected to having their services singled out for copayments. GMCHP decided to add a drug benefit anyway but had to drop the idea when Blue Cross actuaries calculated that the cost, even with a copayment, would increase monthly premiums beyond the $60 ceiling set for the coming year.[11] GMCHP subsequently added an optional prescription drug benefit for group contracts.

GMCHP's problems with area dentists began in 1971 when it was trying to find federal money to subsidize care for low-income residents. Upon learning from a consultant that the Office of Economic Opportunity would require dental coverage for Family Health Center participants, Blue Cross suggested that GMCHP offer a similar benefit to regular subscribers as well.[12] Although the OEO subsidy failed to materialize, preliminary discussions with some local dentists about dental coverage for GMCHP subscribers immediately exposed four thorny issues.

The local dentists were losing money and angry because their patients who belonged to GMCHP were having certain types of x-rays and minor surgical procedures performed at the clinic's oral surgery department. GMCHP covered procedures done in-house but not by other local dentists.

But in addition to the rift between local dentists and the clinic's oral surgeons, the local dentists were themselves divided into two camps—the independent practitioners and those who worked at the Marshfield Dental Clinic (which was not associated with the Marshfield Clinic). In addition, Blue Cross marketed a dental plan in direct competition with Wisconsin Dental Service, which was owned by the Wisconsin Dental Association. Last, Blue Cross wanted GMCHP to offer an exclusive dental service contract to the Marshfield Dental Clinic.

The independent dentists, fearful of losing all their patients with GMCHP coverage if such a contract was signed, demanded that the health plan make arrangements with the Wisconsin Dental Service instead.[13] The Marshfield Clinic's oral surgeons preferred to have only GMCHP cover their procedures, but the Marshfield Dental Clinic claimed that such a policy was unethical because it would deny patients free choice of dentists.[14] When GMCHP agreed to affiliate with local dentists and reimburse them for performing certain surgical procedures on its health plan subscribers, the Wisconsin Dental Service initially approved of the arrangement. The deal fell through, however, when some local dentists objected to the dental service's cooperating with GMCHP because of its ties to Blue Cross.[15]

Nearly all the area dentists agreed to participate in the Family Health Center dental program in 1974. And after another round of negotiations in 1975, the Marshfield Clinic agreed to their affiliation for certain services to GMCHP's regular subscribers as well. Despite widespread objections to participation in peer review, almost every dentist in the health plan's coverage area applied for affiliation.[16] The dentists were allowed to set their own fees and had the same reimbursement formula as physicians. Nevertheless, many dentists believed that they lost revenue by participating in the plan. Some tried to compensate by increasing their charges for GMCHP patients. Others billed GMCHP subscribers directly for the 10 percent that the plan withheld, just in case the health plan failed to make year-end bonus distributions.[17] Arrangements between GMCHP and area dentists regarding covered procedures and charges continued to be confrontational until 1985, when GMCHP limited its dental coverage to major procedures performed by clinic and affiliated oral surgeons.[18]

Massive resistance within the Clinic's psychiatry department delayed for several years GMCHP's efforts to affiliate with mental health providers. Marshfield had many mental health treatment resources during the 1970s. The clinic had six psychiatrists, four psychologists, and four medical social workers. Saint Joseph's Hospital offered acute short-term care, and Wood County's Norwood Health Center provided extended inpatient services. Elsewhere in GMCHP's coverage area mental health services were scarce or nonexistent. Indeed, many communities made do with well-meaning nonprofessionals who provided ad hoc counseling, usually for alcoholism and sometimes under the supervision of a medical doctor.

The staff of the psychiatry department initially insisted that GMCHP subscribers receive all their mental health services in Marshfield because staffers did not want "other people creaming off the health plan's profits." The department's refusal to affiliate with all but a few independent psychiatrists became progressively more unreasonable as the health plan expanded into distant counties.[19]

GMCHP was more than seven years old when the psychiatry department chair agreed to a "memorandum of understanding" that allowed qualified mental health professionals to counsel health plan enrollees if a clinic or affiliated physician supervised the counselors' services.[20] Lewis quickly approved applications from care givers who had been waiting several years to serve GMCHP subscribers in their local communities and met the standards set forth in the memorandum. Fearing that the influx of affiliates "would indubitably drain the Marshfield Plan of its profits in the long run," the department revised the memorandum to require that psychiatrists supervise all mental health services.[21] Reed Hall, the clinic's legal counsel, found that those revisions were in violation of Wisconsin statutes and recommended that the clinic retain the memorandum's original language.[22]

After the clinic's executive committee accepted Hall's recommendation, the psychiatry department refused to check the credentials of various therapists who applied for affiliation, and GMCHP's insurance committee got the job. Thereafter, members of that committee usually agreed with Lewis that counselors with inadequate training could become affiliates "if a health plan physician deemed an individual's services to local residents more beneficial than no counseling at all."[23]

The psychiatry department's concerns about affiliates' "creaming the system" were validated in 1986 when Marshfield Medical Research and Education Foundation analyzed GMCHP's expenses for outpatient mental health care. It found that patients treated by affiliated providers averaged more visits and cost the health plan considerably more money than those treated by clinic staff.[24] After uncovering record-keeping and billing irregularities at one counseling office, GMCHP instituted random audits of all affiliated mental health providers.

The Marshfield Clinic would have experienced far fewer problems if it had restricted the health plan's growth or the affiliated providers had been less eager to enhance their income from the plan. Independent practitioners clearly derived considerable financial benefit from GMCHP affiliation in the 1970s. Their reimbursements were fair and timely, and the year-end distributions were a generous bonus. While GMCHP's monitoring of affiliates' performance and contact with patients in outlying communities improved patient care, its efforts to control utilization and costs were largely ineffective. Many affiliates found GMCHP's supervision of their conduct to be intrusive and excessive because they were unaccustomed to the peer review process, a normal activity in group practices where doctors share records and care for one another's patients. Despite its efforts to help affiliates improve their care, the Marshfield Clinic had to compromise its standards of excellence, and its health plan did not meet HMO industry standards for vigilance.

GMCHP at Five Years

Inspectors from the Group Health Association of America found GMCHP's oversight of affiliates inadequate in 1976 when they visited Marshfield to evaluate the health plan for membership in their national organization. The team noted that the five-year-old GMCHP and its subsidiary health plans served more than one-third of the nearly one hundred thousand residents in its four-county coverage area. The team found that GMCHP's twenty-eight affiliated doctors "did not meet the minimum GHAA standard" because they were not subjected to the same quality controls as doctors working under the close scrutiny of their peers in the clinic. The team therefore recommended that "Greater Marshfield Plan take steps to solve the problem of the participation of physicians in the outlying clinics and offices."[25]

The visitors were surprised to find a large medical center with 144 staff physicians and twenty-four hundred other employees in a community that had slightly more than sixteen thousand residents. The clinic had recently relocated to a new $8 million facility that was physically and, to some extent, functionally integrated with Saint Joseph's Hospital. The two institutions shared several operations, including a laboratory and patient records department. The hospital was just beginning a $27 million expansion project that would increase its capacity to more than five hundred beds.[26]

GHAA usually required member health plans to devote a substantial portion of their business to prepaid care. Although GMCHP accounted for only 17 percent of the clinic's revenue, the inspection team considered that amount acceptable, given the clinic's rural location and its role as a tertiary referral center. Dr. John Smillie, a reviewer from the Permanente Medical Group, found the Marshfield surgeons "very conservative in doing surgery." He said, "It is apparent from the surgical logs where the indications for surgery are recorded that the indications compelling surgery are perhaps as stringent as any prepaid group practice in the country. The stringency applies equally to health plan members and fee-for-service patients." Smillie also reported that the clinic's medical records were unusually clear, complete, and legible. The system for protecting and tracking the more than three thousand records used in patient care each day was, in his words, "the best I have ever seen."[27] The visitors, whose other comments were equally laudatory, said, "This is an outstanding plan. Commitment of . . . Marshfield Clinic to the aggressive support and development of the prepaid plan concept, as well as its commitment to consumers in Marshfield, appears to be complete."[28]

Among the nation's 175 HMOs, GMCHP stood out and attracted considerable attention in 1976 because of its rural location and unusually successful enrollment. Four million of the nation's 6.5 million prepaid subscribers belonged to a few older organizations like the Kaiser Permanente health plans. With thirty-six thousand subscribers Greater Marshfield was one of the largest of the plans organized since the late 1960s. It was also the fourth largest of fifty-two HMOs sponsored or operated by Blue Cross. The three larger plans were all in urban settings: the forty-four-year-old Group Health Association in Washington, D.C.; the six-year-old Harvard Community Health Plan in Boston; and the thirty-six-year-old Metro Health Plan in Detroit.[29]

GMCHP's success, which resulted from the clinic's efforts to develop medical resources and affiliated providers in outlying counties, enabled thousands of rural residents to lead healthier lives. Its affiliation agreements and satellite clinics also expanded the referral base that the clinic's rapidly growing staff of specialists needed, as many were trained to treat diseases that afflict relatively few patients in any population.[30] The clinic's disparate motivations of altruism and enterprise may seem incompatible, but both were based on the conviction that rural people deserve medical care of a breadth and quality usually available only to metropolitan residents.

Chapter 5

Emerging Problems with Medicare and Medicaid

I had severe reservations [about Marshfield's Medicare demonstration project]. The government will torment you to death with regulations. . . . The clinic wanted to cooperate with Washington and saw it as another opportunity to shine their star. We should forget those noble experiments.

Leo Suycott

The Greater Marshfield Community Health Plan was the first HMO in Wisconsin and one of the first rural plans in the nation to participate in a state-sponsored HMO-Medicaid contract. It was also one in a small group of HMOs to participate in the first Medicare risk-contracting demonstration with the federal Health Care Financing Administration (HCFA), created in 1977 to administer Medicaid and Medicare. In effect, GMCHP was doing what proponents had wanted HMOs to do in order to reduce government spending. But repeated failures of public policy and government agencies slowed the development of HMOs and discouraged their involvement in public programs that serve the poor and elderly. GMCHP's initial experiences with Medicaid and Medicare were short lived but worth studying because they show why so few HMOs enrolled public beneficiaries during the 1970s and 1980s, especially in rural areas.

The Marshfield Clinic lost millions of dollars while GMCHP participated in Medicaid and Medicare, but the clinic tried to stay with both programs because it wanted to help devise reimbursement formulas that would encourage HMOs to enroll those people who needed medical care.

However, inconsistent public policies, inflexible government staff and procedures, late reimbursements, and, worst of all, low compensation levels for rural providers made long-term participation impossible. Neither Wisconsin nor the federal government was willing to adjust reimbursement formulas so that the Marshfield plan could afford to enroll people with serious health problems. As a result both the state and federal governments lost valuable opportunities to demonstrate how prepaid care could meet the needs of all public beneficiaries—and the Marshfield Clinic lost its dream of a health care utopia.

Medicaid-HMO Contracting in the 1970s

GMCHP's adventure with Medicaid began in 1975, shortly after the Ford administration lifted cost controls on the health care industry. As health care costs began to rise faster than they did before the freeze, the U.S. Department of Health, Education and Welfare (HEW) estimated that Medicare and Medicaid expenditures would jump from $25 billion in fiscal 1976 to $30.4 billion in fiscal 1977.[1] Medicaid had become the most expensive social program in many states.

Congress created Medicaid in 1965 as a federally sponsored, state-administered program to provide health care services to low-income families receiving Aid to Families with Dependent Children (AFDC). Amendments to the Social Security Act in 1972 extended Medicaid coverage to blind, aged, and disabled individuals with low incomes who received Supplemental Security Income benefits. States administered their programs according to federal guidelines but were free to establish their own eligibility criteria. Some states served only their most needy residents, whereas others covered people who did not qualify for welfare but lacked sufficient income to purchase insurance or pay their medical bills. Congress had patterned Medicaid after the traditional private health care system in order to appease the special interest provider groups. Because the program incorporated few utilization or cost controls, insurance carriers hired by the states to administer claims simply reimbursed all charges submitted by doctors and hospitals.[2]

In an effort to reduce state and federal costs for Medicaid, other 1972 amendments to the Social Security Act enabled states to contract with HMOs to provide services for Medicaid beneficiaries. California was among the first states to take advantage of that option, and a year later it had more contracts than a dozen other states. Medi-Cal had about 250,000 enrollees in fifty-four HMOs in 1975 when a state auditor discovered that some HMOs were using less than half their payments for patient care. California and federal auditors eventually identified forty Medi-Cal plans that used improper marketing practices, had excessive administrative costs and profits, and provided poor quality care.[3] Congress reacted to these abuses by amending the HMO Act in 1976 to require federal certification of HMOs serving Medicaid and Medicare beneficiaries. The lawmakers also limited the enrollment of public beneficiaries in HMOs to no more than 50 percent of membership, reasoning that a significant presence of private subscribers would motivate health plans to provide better service. Because of the new requirements Medi-Cal lost all but eighteen HMOs.[4] A few other states encountered similar problems with prepaid Medicaid contracts, but the size of California's scandal stigmatized and delayed the progress of HMO-Medicaid enrollment nationwide.

The Marshfield Clinic's leaders had tried to incorporate Medicaid beneficiaries in their health plan from the beginning, but Wisconsin lacked statutory authority to contract for prepaid Medicaid services. The clinic finally convinced state lawmakers to approve Medicaid-HMO contracting in the spring of 1974. The Marshfield Medical Research and Education Foundation immediately organized a series of meetings with Wood County social workers and the staff of Wisconsin Health and Social Services to develop a contract for serving Medicaid beneficiaries in the Marshfield area. State agency staffers were unenthusiastic about the project because they had no experience with prepaid care. Negotiations broke down after several meetings and resumed in 1975 only after the state hired someone qualified to work on such contracts.

The Marshfield Medical Research Foundation had just submitted a contract application to the state's new employee when the U.S. Department of Health and Human Services (HHS, formerly HEW) invited Marshfield and Wisconsin to participate in a federal program called Health in Underserved Rural Areas (HURA). HURA had been developed in 1974 to fund and evaluate innovative rural health care projects. It offered an ideal opportunity for Wisconsin to experiment with prepaid Medicaid contracts. So Marshfield and the state agency submitted a joint proposal for a three-year study to evaluate the integration of Medicaid recipients into an established rural HMO.

When Wisconsin's Medicaid administrators received a HURA grant in June 1976, they wanted to use the program's model contract.[5] However, GMCHP insisted on drafting a document that would include Medicaid beneficiaries in its community risk pool and offer them the same benefits as other enrollees. The state eventually agreed to capitate GMCHP for all its usual services on a community-rated basis and to reimburse other providers directly for such services as eyeglasses and prescription drugs, which were not covered by the health plan.

The Marshfield Clinic soon encountered major difficulties with its Medicaid project. Wisconsin was in the process of terminating a contract with Electronic Data Systems (EDS), the Ross Perot company that processed Medicaid payments, and negotiating with a new processor.[6] Because many EDS files contained inadequate information or were inaccessible, HURA project staff members had to develop actuarial data manually from microfiche files. The state was also restructuring its Medicaid program, so Marshfield's HURA contract was a low priority. And to make matters even worse, implementation of the state's new computer system was causing massive confusion in claims processing.

GMCHP finally began enrolling eligible families in October 1977. The GMCHP sales staff had planned to market the HURA health plan by chatting with individuals in person, just as they had done with Marshfield's federally subsidized Family Health Center (FHC) program. Because privacy safeguards in the Social Security Act prevented the state from releasing the names of Medicaid recipients, GMCHP had to rely on media announcements, mailings distributed by the state, and county social service workers to inform people about the program. Despite those difficulties, the health plan managed to enroll 20 percent of eligible Medicaid beneficiaries within a few months.

Tracking the changing eligibility status of Medicaid beneficiaries created enormous problems because the program had to rely on at least four different electronic data-processing systems operated by the Marshfield Clinic, Blue Cross, the state of Wisconsin and its contractors, and files from four county offices, some of which were still using paper forms. In order to ensure that patients received uninterrupted care, Marshfield's FHC obtained state approval to hire a coordinator who worked with county case workers and FHC eligibility specialists to move patients between the HURA program and FHC as their financial circumstances changed.[7]

Late notification of newly eligible clients also hampered GMCHP's efforts to enroll Medicaid recipients. County case workers were supposed to offer qualified clients an opportunity to participate in HURA. But case workers' motivation to assist with enrollment was uneven, and no one monitored the information that clients received about the program. When patients lost their Medicaid eligibility, late notification of GMCHP caused a financial burden for its affiliated physicians, who were paid shortly after treating HURA patients, only to learn months later that some patients were ineligible for Medicaid at the time of treatment. The affiliates then had to reconcile inappropriate reimbursements with GMCHP and try to collect payments directly from their patients.

GMCHP also incurred financial losses because Wisconsin's data-processing system made no provisions for families in which only certain individuals involved in divorce settlements qualified for medical assistance. As a result the health plan unknowingly provided unreimbursable care for ineligible family members. State capitation payments to GMCHP were habitually late, and the state often failed to implement contractually required increases in the annual capitation for as long as six months. Marshfield also experienced heavy financial losses each year because its Medicaid enrollees were demonstrably sicker and required more services than their counterparts in the fee-for-service system.[8]

GMCHP terminated its Medicaid contract with Wisconsin at the end of the HURA grant period in September 1981 when the parties could not agree on new capitation rates.[9] At the time state Medicaid staffers were negotiating first-time contracts with HMOs in Wisconsin's two most populous counties. The reimbursement rates for those contracts were far higher than what the state was willing to pay Marshfield. GMCHP's administrators were eager to continue their Medicaid program, but its unreasonably low capitation had increased premium costs for all other subscribers. Lewis told the Wisconsin Health and Social Services secretary, "We can no longer expect our regular members to pay for the financial losses we have taken under the Medicaid program."[10]

After the HURA project ended, Wisconsin Health and Social Services and Marshfield Medical Research and Education Foundation staffers suggested in their final report that "perhaps the greatest value from this demonstration program lies not in the analysis of data it generated, but rather in the illustration of problems encountered by states substantially unprepared for, but attempting HMO contracts."[11] A joint HCFA and

U.S. Public Health Service task force that examined incentives for HMO-Medicaid contracting in 1980 confirmed the universality of Marshfield's experience. It also found that the two federal agencies had no coordination at their national or regional levels and no strategy for motivating states and HMOs to participate in Medicaid contracts.[12]

The federal task force cited several reasons why states had difficulty implementing Medicaid contracts. The states usually lacked the technical expertise and data needed to establish accurate capitation rates. They were reluctant to hire adequate staff to administer HMO contracts. Their procedures for determining eligibility and notifying HMOs of changes in status were inordinately complicated. Federal regulations prohibiting states from disclosing the names of eligible Medicaid recipients made marketing difficult. State administrators feared the high turnover rates in Medicaid eligibility would encourage HMOs to defer, and therefore avoid providing, preventive and palliative care. Last, many states questioned whether cost savings would be sufficient to justify the added trouble and expense of prepaid contracting.

HMO administrators told the task force that Medicaid negotiations were unduly complex and protracted. The resulting contracts often featured low capitation rates, overly generous benefit packages, high financial risks, and burdensome reporting requirements. Lack of direct access to eligible beneficiaries compounded the difficulties of marketing to a population that was not a cohesive group. Late capitation payments caused costly administrative problems. HMO administrators worried about unstable Medicaid eligibility and potentially high utilization rates. They also feared the possibility of acquiring a "welfare image," even though federal legislation in 1976 had limited enrollment of Medicaid and Medicare beneficiaries to 50 percent of an HMO's membership.[13]

The task force reported that Medicaid recipients had no incentive to enroll in HMOs because they usually lost their ability to seek care from any willing provider and received no additional benefits. Like many other consumers, they had little understanding of HMOs and were reluctant to switch from their usual sources of care, no matter how fragmented they might be.

The task force cited three studies showing the beneficial effects of HMO-Medicaid contracts. One study reported that Medicaid beneficiaries in prepaid group practice plans used 38 percent fewer hospital services than beneficiaries in the fee-for-service system.[14] Another study was unable to identify adverse effects when Medicaid beneficiaries in prepaid group practice plans experienced low utilization rates for physician visits, prescription drugs, and hospitalization.[15] And a third study found that prepaid care for AFDC beneficiaries in New York City cost at least 11 percent less in 1974 than fee-for-service care for a similar population in 1972.[16] Based on these and other findings, the task force recommended better planning and coordination at federal and regional levels, as well as improved technical assistance for states and HMOs. It also proposed several revisions in federal and state legislation, regulations, and administrative policies. Many of the task force recommendations were incorporated in the Omnibus Budget Reconciliation Act of 1981 (OBRA).

New Medicaid Initiatives in the 1980s

OBRA gave states wide latitude to experiment with reducing Medicaid costs and greater flexibility in contracting with HMOs and other types of prepaid health plans. The ensuing regulations allowed HMOs to limit a patient's choice of providers, control utilization, and offer incentives for enrollment.[17] During California governor Ronald Reagan's administration in the 1970s, Medi-Cal controlled usage by requiring enrollees to pay small fees for most services. The state's copayment experiment proved penny wise and pound foolish, however. Fewer women sought prenatal care and immunizations for their children, and many patients waited until they were desperately sick before seeking help. As a result Medi-Cal's hospital use and overall costs increased significantly. When the issue of copayments resurfaced in OBRA's Medicaid regulations during Reagan's presidential administration, the Academy of Pediatrics successfully lobbied to exempt children and pregnant women from such copayments.[18]

In the wake of OBRA's regulatory changes Wisconsin restructured its Medicaid program in 1983. The new "Wisconsin HMO Preferred Enrollment Initiative" required all AFDC beneficiaries in the state's two largest metropolitan counties, Dane and Milwaukee, to join an HMO if at least two plans were available in their area. AFDC beneficiaries with severe health problems and all Supplemental Security Income recipients were allowed to remain in the fee-for-service system with their usual doctors.

GMCHP contracted to serve AFDC Medicaid recipients in its entire coverage area for a fifteen-month trial period.[19] Because GMCHP was the only HMO in that area, the state gave Marshfield a waiver to enroll all AFDC beneficiaries. However, the beneficiaries could "disenroll" if they preferred to stay with their usual providers and receive care through the fee-for-service system. Although GMCHP covered all benefit costs for Medicaid enrollees, recipients opting for fee-for-service care had to pay small fees for certain services unrelated to prenatal or pediatric care. The start of Marshfield's project was delayed by several months of negotiations, so the trial period was severely attenuated. In November 1983, after only one month of operation, GMCHP enrolled more than four thousand Medicaid beneficiaries. Because the health plan had agreed to capitation payments substantially below its estimated costs, it flagged the charts of Medicaid enrollees to remind doctors to seek prior approval from health plan staffers for nonemergency hospital admissions. Clinic physicians were opposed to identifying payment methods on patient charts because they wanted everyone to receive equal care, but they compromised their policy in this instance because they anticipated enormous losses from the program.[20]

Marshfield's HMO Preferred Enrollment Initiative program had barely started when state administrators announced plans to reduce GMCHP's capitation rate for the next fiscal year. Although Medicaid's reimbursements to fee-for-service physicians around the state averaged 65 percent of their charges, GMCHP's capitation represented only 45 percent of its fee-for-service costs. Marshfield had agreed to accept a lower capitation than HMOs in the two metropolitan counties because its hospitalization rates were much lower than theirs were. But the clinic's leaders refused to accept a further reduction in their capitation because they believed that they were already operating at maximum efficiency.[21]

GMCHP offered to renew its contract with a capitation that represented 60 percent of the fee-for-service charges, but the state held out for 30 percent. Greg Nycz, the foundation staffer who represented the Marshfield Clinic during most of its Medicaid negotiations, said, "I'll never forget our meeting in Madison when we gave state administrators our final offer. One of them said to Doctor Lewis, 'Don't make any rash decisions. You just wait, go home, and think about it. If you don't take this contract, we'll give it to someone else.' And Doctor Lewis said, 'Who? We're the only ones there.'"[22] Clinic leaders told state health officials that they refused to be penalized for practicing efficient medicine and canceled their contract, effective September 1984.[23]

Ten years after becoming Wisconsin's first HMO to experiment with Medicaid contracting, GMCHP was the first to withdraw from the state's expanded HMO initiative. Twenty-one percent of Wisconsin's Medicaid population was enrolled in thirteen Dane and Milwaukee county HMOs by 1985, but Medicaid recipients in few other counties were involved in HMOs until the 1990s. Instead, the clinic and most Wisconsin physicians who accepted Medicaid beneficiaries continued to treat them on a fee-for-service basis. Doctors in the state and elsewhere who refused to treat Medicaid patients usually cited low reimbursement levels as their reason.

Other states fared no better than Wisconsin with HMO-Medicaid contracting under the 1981 legislation. Fourteen states took advantage of its Medicaid waivers, but only six states—California, Minnesota, Missouri, New Jersey, New York, and Florida—responded to HCFA's requests for Medicaid "managed care" demonstration projects in 1982. The results were dismal by all accounts. Florida's project never materialized and was terminated in the late 1980s. Programs in Minnesota and New York were not implemented until 1985. All encountered the same problems as their predecessors.[24]

A 1985 study, which questioned whether the 1981 legislation had reduced the barriers to HMO contracting, concluded that success was more closely related to particular administrative policies in some states than to changes in federal legislation. Another study produced more disturbing results: It reported that beneficiaries who had been in HMOs before they lost their Medicaid eligibility suffered serious health problems, sometimes much worse than their counterparts who had been in the fee-for-service system.[25] Because few states offered a supportive environment for prepaid contracting, only 11 percent of the nation's Medicaid population was covered by HMOs in the late 1980s.[26]

From the available evidence it seems to me that relatively few low-income families that participated in prepaid plans during the first two decades of the HMO movement benefited from the experience. Most were tossed back and forth between systems and providers, sometimes losing their usual sources of care in the process. (Medicaid patients enrolled in GMCHP were an exception: All the doctors in the coverage area were associated with the health plan so patients rarely had to change doctors.) Medicaid beneficiaries in the fee-for-service system often received marginal care, but they were probably better off during this phase of the health care revolution than most of those who were forced to join HMOs or were periodically shuffled between the traditional and prepaid systems.

Early Medicare-HMO Contracting Opportunities

The enrollment of Medicare beneficiaries in prepaid health care plans had an equally disappointing history until Congress allowed new types of contracts that were attractive to HMOs, especially those located in areas where health care costs and reimbursement levels were high. Efforts to enroll Medicare beneficiaries in rural areas progressed far more slowly. What happened in Marshfield explains why.

When Congress created Medicare in 1965, it allowed physicians to be reimbursed by fee for service or capitation. Capitated payments were subject to retrospective adjustments based on actual usage and costs. Hospital reimbursements were always based on daily rates, even when patients received their care in a prepaid system. Only twenty-three prepaid group practices accepted capitation during the late 1960s, usually to accommodate retired employees who wanted to remain in their health plan.[27] The 1972 amendments to the Social Security Act expanded Medicare coverage to patients with end-stage renal disease, permanently disabled workers, and dependents of workers who were eligible for old age, survivors, and disability insurance under Social Security. The amendments also authorized capitated payments to hospitals, but regulations released in 1975 retained the unpopular cost-based retrospective reimbursement arrangement.

HEW also offered a "risk-contract" option that would pay HMOs an annual capitation rate equal to the fee-for-service cost of caring for Medicare beneficiaries in their area, a formula commonly referred to as "adjusted average per capita cost," or AAPCC. HEW's risk-contracting agreement required participating HMOs to bear the losses if their costs exceeded capitation and allowed them to retain only 20 percent of any savings that they realized from keeping costs below their AAPCC. The challenge of enrolling individual Medicare beneficiaries and dealing with complicated reimbursement arrangements dissuaded HMOs from participating in such contracts.[28] HCFA had eighteen cost-based contracts and only one risk contract by January 1978; together, they covered less that 1 percent of Medicare's population.[29] The risk-contracting requirements were so unattractive that the Group Health Cooperative of Puget Sound was the first (in 1976) and only health plan to use that option. In fact, an administrator from that cooperative reported delays as long as five years in reconciling accounts with HCFA.[30]

Congress never intended for Medicare to pay all of a beneficiary's health care bills, no matter how providers were reimbursed. From the beginning, people with sufficient means purchased private supplemental insurance ("Medigap" policies) to pay deductibles, copayments, and services not covered by Medicare. Some states offered Medicaid supplements to assist low-income Medicare beneficiaries in meeting these costs. By 1977 Medicare covered only half the medical costs incurred by its noninstitutionalized beneficiaries. Most Medigap policies were inadequate: Only 60 percent of policies paid for benefits not covered by Medicare, such as outpatient physician visits, preventive and diagnostic services, mental health care, and skilled nursing home care. But what was more significant was that 75 percent of the policies provided clients insufficient protection against catastrophic expenses. The so-called Baucus amendment to the Social Security Act in 1980 required policies labeled "Medicare supplement" and sold after 1 July 1982 to meet certain minimum standards, but changes occurred slowly because of exemptions for existing policies.[31]

HMOs, especially those involving group practices, were thought to be particularly well suited for coordinating the care of seniors who had many chronic diseases. The prevention and early intervention services offered by such plans reduced the need for hospitalization and nursing home care. They also simplified claims procedures for beneficiaries and providers.[32] A comparison of standard and prepaid Medigap policies in 1976 concluded that HMOs were potentially better because they provided a broader range of services. However, HMOs varied widely in quality, and few plans accepted Medicare beneficiaries.[33]

Most central Wisconsin physicians accepted "Medicare assignment" when the federal program started, that is, they billed Medicare for 80 percent of what they were allowed to charge the federal program and billed their patients for the other 20 percent. As Medicare reimbursements dropped to unreasonably low levels, many doctors refused to take assignments of Medicare patients. (The clinic stopped taking Medicare assignment and began billing patients directly in January 1976 when losses from the program became unacceptable.) Elderly beneficiaries found the process of paying their doctor bills and then reclaiming some portion of their payments from Medicare extremely burdensome.[34]

Medicare Demonstrations in the Late 1970s and Early 1980s

The Marshfield Clinic also tried to serve Medicare beneficiaries through GMCHP when it began but was unable to make suitable arrangements with federal administrators. The thousands of central Wisconsin seniors who were too old to enroll in GMCHP when it was founded were joined each year by roughly four hundred who had lost their health plan membership when they became eligible for Medicare. Among older subscribers who responded to a GMCHP survey in the late 1970s, their greatest fear and often only complaint was having to leave the health plan as they turned sixty-five.[35]

Faced with mounting pressure from seniors, the administrators at the Marshfield Medical Research and Education Foundation submitted several proposals for Medicare risk contracting to HCFA in 1977 and learned that HCFA was considering similar concepts. HCFA announced its demonstration project, Alternative Models for Prepaid Capitation of Health Care Services of Medicare/Medicaid Recipients, in May 1978. The project was designed to test new incentives for increasing HMO-Medicare involvement and to study how health status influenced HCFA's adjusted average per capita cost (the AAPCC) reimbursement formula.[36]

Twenty-nine organizations responded to HCFA's request for proposals.[37] The Marshfield Medical Research and Education Foundation was one of seven organizations to receive a contract and one of five to start a program. Three of the other participants were Fallon Community Health Plan in Worcester, Massachusetts; Kaiser Permanente Health Plan in Portland, Oregon; and Health Central in Lansing, Michigan. The fifth participant was InterStudy, a research group founded by the HMO advocate Paul Ellwood, which sponsored four Twin City plans: HMO Minnesota, SHARE Health Plan, and MedCenters Health Plan in Minneapolis, and Group Health Cooperative in St. Paul. According to the terms of its contract, GMCHP accepted full financial risk for providing all necessary medical services under Medicare Parts A and B in return for a fixed capitation based on 99 percent of Marshfield's AAPCC.[38] HCFA estimated Marshfield's reimbursement rate by using area fee-for-service costs for treating the Medicare population and average statewide fee-for-service costs for treating people with end-stage renal disease.[39] The formula was adjusted for age, sex, and other demographic characteristics but not for health status.

To determine GMCHP's Medicare premium Blue Cross actuaries first estimated what it would cost the health plan to care for Medicare recipients. That estimate, expressed as a multiple of the health plan's community rate, was called the "adjusted community rate." Based on the clinic's experience in caring for elderly patients, GMCHP actuaries estimated that Medicare enrollees would cost 3.2 times as much as younger enrollees— or slightly less than the national adjusted community rate average of 3.4.[40] The difference between Marshfield's estimated adjusted community rate and what HCFA was willing to pay (99 percent of the AAPCC) established the monthly premium that Medicare participants would pay. For example, GMCHP's adjusted community rate for the first contract period was $96.09 per month, and HCFA's capitation was $74.42, so GMCHP Medicare enrollees paid a monthly premium of $21.67. Marshfield's and HCFA's estimated costs for treating Medicare patients in central Wisconsin were the lowest of any HMO in the demonstration, but the difference between the two estimates made GMCHP's premium the highest.[41]

Marshfield's Medicare program opened enrollment on 1 April 1980 and began operation on June 1. Before receiving final authorization from HCFA, the Marshfield Clinic experienced an unprecedented number of appointment cancellations from seniors who chose to wait until they had health plan coverage. Demand for the program was so great that GMCHP held the first four days of enrollment in the city's national guard armory in order to accommodate the crowd.[42] The health plan accepted all applicants, regardless of their health status, and gave them the same benefits as other subscribers, including many routine and preventive services not covered by Medicare. The plan required no copayments for service but did not cover prescription drugs, eyeglasses, hearing aids, custodial nursing home care, or most dental services.

More than 36 percent (7,139) of the area's Medicare population enrolled in GMCHP during the first contract period, which delays in Washington attenuated from one year to a mere three months. The first subscribers tended to be relatively young and healthy. Because they required less care than average Medicare beneficiaries did, GMCHP showed a slight profit for the program's first three months. HCFA therefore reduced Marshfield's capitation for the second contract year from 99 to 95 percent of AAPCC. A breakdown in Blue Cross computers hid significant and growing shortfalls until months after the second fiscal year ended in September 1981. Only then did GMCHP learn that losses of nearly $1.3 million had depleted its reserves and placed its entire health plan at risk. Direct and indirect losses during the second fiscal year totaled about $2.65 million for GMCHP's partners. In addition to those costs sustained by Blue Cross and Saint Joseph's Hospital, Medicare reimbursements to the Marshfield Clinic were approximately $1 million less than it would have received on a fee-for-service basis.[43]

GMCHP blamed the losses on high hospital utilization rates of the seriously ill people whom it attracted through its liberal open enrollment policy (known as adverse selection) and on the failure of HCFA's reimbursement formula to account for the extra cost of serving high-risk clients.[44] The health plan had expected to get by with 2,080 hospital days for each one thousand Medicare enrollees but used 2,593 days instead. (Outside Milwaukee, where hospital utilization rates were especially high, Wisconsin averaged 2,500 hospital days for each thousand Medicare fee-for-service beneficiaries.) GMCHP's higher-than-expected hospitalization rate was the result of its continuous open enrollment, which attracted many seriously ill beneficiaries. In addition, some residents moved their aged parents with chronic health problems to Marshfield so that they could join the health plan. When GMCHP became aware of its losses, it abandoned any effort to enroll institutionalized beneficiaries after capturing only 20 percent of that population.[45]

Marshfield's capitation was well below what other participating HMOs received. For example, in 1981 HCFA paid Marshfield a monthly capitation of $75, but Fallon Community Health Plan in Worcester, Massachusetts, received $120, and Kaiser Permanente's program in Portland, Oregon, received $114.[46] The capitation for four HMOs in the Twin Cities demonstration project was $148, nearly twice as high as Marshfield's, even though St. Louis Park's MedCenters Health Plan screened out 15 to 20 percent of its applicants, and HMO Minnesota, a Blue Cross participant in Minneapolis, rejected 90 percent of its applicants that year.[47] Because the capitation was based on service to a cross-section of an area-wide Medicare population, HCFA overpaid HMOs that enrolled only healthy seniors. Marshfield's Greg Nycz called HMO Minnesota's enrollment practices "a big scandal." He said that Ellwood's InterStudy research group wanted to have a demonstration project in the Twin Cities and that HMO Minnesota had agreed to accept the reimbursement formula only if it could "medically underwrite," that is, deny enrollment to patients with serious health problems. Although HCFA was aware of the situation, HMO Minnesota was still rejecting 50 percent of its applicants two years later, according to Nycz.[48]

Shortly after learning of GMCHP's mounting losses in 1981, Lewis and Nycz testified at congressional hearings on Medicare-HMO reimbursements. They and many others wanted HCFA to change its capitation methodology, especially so that HMOs would receive extra compensation when they enrolled beneficiaries with serious health problems.[49] Back home, Lewis tried to cut losses by closing enrollment to all but existing health plan members who turned sixty-five or otherwise became eligible for Medicare. After GMCHP initiated several measures to reduce hospital use, its most costly benefit, Medicare inpatient care fell by nearly 20 percent by the end of the contract period.[50] Despite these and other measures, GMCHP's losses in September 1981, after sixteen months of operation, totaled more than $3 million. GMCHP had 32 percent of the Medicare enrollees in HCFA's entire demonstration program, and it was the only health plan losing money.[51]

HCFA agreed to return GMCHP's reimbursement to 99 percent of its AAPCC and share any losses incurred during the final year of the risk-contracting demonstration, but it continued to give the other participating plans significantly higher capitations than Marshfield's.[52] When GMCHP lost another $500,000 and HCFA lost $1.75 million as a result of their 1982 cost-sharing agreement, the agency decided to close Marshfield's project. HCFA staffers refused to revise their AAPCC formula for Marshfield—even though the demonstration was supposed to study how health status influenced that formula—or to establish a precedent for paying more than the formula allowed.[53] Termination came as a surprise to GMCHP administrators, who had made considerable progress in reducing hospital usage and planned to pursue further economies. While still losing money, they assumed that their willingness to help HCFA improve its capitation formula would lead to an extension of their contract.

One HCFA staffer recommended keeping the Marshfield project for an additional year, but her supervisors decided that the research value of an extension was not worth the agency's losses from the cost-sharing agreement.[54] That attitude contrasted sharply with the clinic's willingness to lose more money if it could help HCFA with the formula. When terminated, GMCHP's demonstration had lasted twenty-eight months and enrolled nearly 40 percent of the Medicare beneficiaries in an eight-county area. The health plan's aggregate losses from involvement in the program exceeded $3 million, nearly 12 percent of its revenue. HCFA continued all the other participants at 95 percent of their AAPCCs.[55]

HCFA staffers considered the Marshfield demonstration project to be unique in several respects. GMCHP was the only HMO that had both affiliated and staff physicians, all of whom treated fee-for-service as well as prepaid patients. GMCHP was the only HMO that offered continuous open enrollment during its first two contract years and never denied admission to applicants, no matter how sick they were. Marshfield's penetration of its Medicare market was significantly higher than the other participating HMOs', which averaged only 10 percent penetration. GMCHP was the only HCFA project located in a medically underserved area, as defined by U.S. Public Health Service criteria. Marshfield's costs for serving Medicare beneficiaries were only about 60 percent of the national average, whereas costs at the other participants' locations were significantly higher than the national average. Finally, GMCHP was the only HMO in the demonstration group to experience adverse selection, high-risk patients attracted to the plan by open enrollment. According to one HCFA staffer, "Adverse selection is a serious issue that must be addressed in any discussion of proposed HMO reimbursement [legislation]."[56]

Marshfield's risk-contracting experiment with Medicare led to long-term cost savings in central Wisconsin. When GMCHP lost money, the clinic's physicians adopted more efficient measures in all areas of patient care. When the average length of stay for all patients at Saint Joseph's Hospital in Marshfield declined significantly between 1981 and 1982, nine thousand fewer hospital days resulted in a savings of $2.8 million for patients and their insurers.[57]

After HCFA terminated its demonstration project, GMCHP created the Senior Security Health Plan, a new prepaid Medicare program with identical benefits. Although monthly premiums increased by $15.50, more than 98 percent of the Medicare enrollees transferred to Senior Security.[58] The program proved so popular that more than two thousand applicants had to be placed on a waiting list until the health plan restored its reserves and could once more offer enrollment to any beneficiaries who wanted to join.[59] GMCHP recovered its losses from the HCFA experiment and finally showed a profit in 1985. Elsewhere in Wisconsin, more than two-thirds of the state's licensed practitioners refused to accept Medicare's low reimbursement levels and billed their elderly patients directly.[60]

Only one published government report was critical of Marshfield's role in the HCFA demonstration. The authors observed that Fallon's Medicare enrollees in Massachusetts cost 31 percent less to treat in the second year than they did before they enrolled in the program, whereas Marshfield's participants continued to cost more than the unenrolled group. The authors failed to consider GMCHP's adverse selection because of liberal enrollment policies. Instead, they blamed the health plan for failure to reduce its costs. They said that the affiliated physicians had no financial risk and therefore no incentives to reduce their patients' use of hospital services. Moreover, the authors said that they clinic physicians had not economized because they were unaware of their patients' payment methods.[61] In fact, the affiliated physicians risked losing their year-end bonus distributions when the health plan lost money from the demonstration project, and the clinic physicians, who routinely practiced cost-efficient medical care, experienced a dangerous loss in the financial reserves of the clinic and health plan and saw a significant reduction in their personal income.

Other reports about Marshfield's program invariably faulted the AAPCC formula and adverse selection. Many observers argued that Marshfield's AAPCC was well below the national average because it was efficient, not because it was rural and had low unit costs.[62] Indeed, HCFA staffers acknowledged in 1981 that their AAPCC methodology was flawed and that their use of local data might be inappropriate when an HMO such as GMCHP enrolled a large proportion of Medicare beneficiaries.[63] Others cited HCFA's failure to account for health status in its reimbursement formula. They also criticized the agency's reliance on preenrollment usage and area per capita costs for Medicare patients because both figures can be inflated by providers who order too many services and charge high fees.[64]

One reviewer of HCFA's demonstration project noted that reliance on preenrollment utilization was inappropriate for determining GMCHP's reimbursement rate because low preenrollment usage reflected either less need for care or less access to care. Equally low usage before and after enrollment suggested a healthy population, but increased utilization after enrollment suggested that enrollees had previously had problems with access and many unmet needs.[65] Poverty and fierce pride had kept many central Wisconsin Medicare beneficiaries from seeking medical attention until they could get health care coverage at affordable rates.

New Medicare Initiatives in the 1980s

As the first round of Medicare demonstration projects neared completion, Congress passed the Tax Equity and Fiscal Responsibility Act (TEFRA) of 1982, which contained several initiatives to reduce federal expenditures for hospital care. These included new peer review organizations to monitor hospital admissions and lengths of stay; a new hospital reimbursement system; and expanded Medicare coverage for less expensive alternatives to hospitalization, such as hospice care and in-home services.[66] TEFRA also revamped the incentive structure for HMO-Medicare enrollment. The new risk-contract agreements allowed HMOs to distribute their cost savings to members as reduced copayments or added benefits or to charge additional premiums for benefits not covered by Medicare. HMOs serving Medicaid and Medicare beneficiaries no longer had to meet federal qualifications, but they were still subject to many regulatory and quality controls. HMOs could pay hospitals by using the new reimbursement system or they could negotiate more favorable rates based on a presumption of using fewer hospital services.[67] TEFRA also removed some onerous data collection and reporting requirements and offered HMOs more recruiting and marketing assistance.[68]

However, TEFRA left many barriers to HMO-Medicare contracting intact and added others. When new federal regulations took effect on 1 January 1985, they made no provision for a health status adjustment in the AAPCC formula.[69] HMOs were required to open their enrollment for at least thirty days and to accept applications on a first-come, first-served basis, but they were not allowed to reserve any savings derived from efficient operation for protection against risk exposure in the future.[70] The regulations also continued a troublesome clause that restricted Medicare and Medicaid enrollment from exceeding 50 percent of an HMO's membership, thereby preventing expansion of HMO services in low-income and medically underserved areas.

HCFA issued its second call for Medicare demonstration proposals in 1982 after TEFRA's enactment. Fifty-two plans from twenty states responded, and HCFA selected forty plans for its new National Medicare

Competition program.[71] The twenty-seven projects that ultimately accepted patients were all located in counties where medical costs and AAPCCs were high.[72] Capitations in those areas were so generous that only about one-third of the participating HMOs had to charge premiums or copayments for standard Medicare benefits. HMOs accepting only relatively healthy applicants in exceptionally high reimbursement counties showed a profit even when they offered extra services, like free prescription drugs and health club memberships.[73] The National Medicare Competition demonstration project was plagued by controversies about HCFA's capitation methodology and a major fraud in Florida, where four HMOs accounted for approximately half of the enrollment in the National Medicare Competition. When beneficiaries' complaints forced the General Accounting Office (GAO) to review Florida's projects, it uncovered many problems involving coordination of Medicare and HMO payments to physicians and hospitals. The GAO advised HCFA to correct the problems before their adverse effects on beneficiaries and providers dissuaded others from HMO-Medicare participation.[74]

In February 1985, a month after TEFRA released its regulations but while the National Medicare Competition demonstration was still underway, the Department of Health and Human Services formally initiated a full-fledged program to expand Medicare-HMO contracting. Within four months HCFA had 183 contracts, including many former demonstration projects; by the end of the year 1.5 million Medicare recipients belonged to HMOs, mostly in California, Minnesota, and Florida, all states with high reimbursement levels.[75] HCFA acknowledged that TEFRA regulations continued the AAPCC disparities and permitted HMOs to engage in favorable selection practices. Although such policies increased initial program costs, HCFA expected that the disparities would disappear as HMOs enrolled more high-risk beneficiaries and those subscribers aged. Despite the detrimental effects of adverse selection on HMO contracting and competition, HCFA staffers refused to modify their capitation formula, forcing some observers to conclude that long-term risk contracting was not sustainable on a large scale.[76]

Legislative meddling and administrative lethargy are both to blame for inequitable access to prepaid health care among the nation's elderly. Employee contributions to the Medicare system and beneficiary premiums for Part B physicians' services are uniform throughout the country. Yet the AAPCC formula favored providers who treated only healthy patients in high-paying reimbursement areas and discriminated against patients and providers in low-paying areas. While some seniors paid no premiums for HMO membership and often received many extra benefits, others paid high premiums for a very modest array of Medicare services. Still others were denied access to HMOs because they had health problems or could not afford the premiums.[77] Equal contributions by taxpayers to the Medicare program during their many years of employment did not ensure that they would have equal opportunities for comprehensive care in retirement.

For an all-too-brief period in the early 1980s, leaders of the Marshfield Clinic were able to offer affordable high-quality care to all the residents in GMCHP's service area, regardless of their age, income, or health status. GMCHP's two Medicaid programs, one in the mid-1970s and another in the early 1980s, brought comprehensive health care services to very poor families. The Marshfield Family Health Center enabled marginally poor families, and eventually individuals, to receive the health plan's benefits along with other services for monthly premiums that were priced to fit their financial circumstances. And Greater Marshfield's risk-contracting demonstration with HCFA gave Medicare beneficiaries affordable access to the health plan through their usual doctors. Regardless of their payment method, all GMCHP enrollees received the same quality of medical care. Even without adjustments for adverse selection, the Medicaid and Medicare programs could have continued if capitations had been anywhere near what other HMOs received. Instead, the clinic's vision of a health care utopia evaporated all too quickly.

Marshfield's experiences reveal a deep-seated failure of state and federal policy to promote prepaid health care and serve those who most need care. In the early 1970s promoters of federal HMO legislation were convinced that enrollment of Medicare and Medicaid beneficiaries in prepaid health care programs would reduce the government's costs and provide those citizens with better medical care. GMCHP's initial experiences with those two programs were short lived but worth studying because they show why so few HMOs enrolled public beneficiaries during the 1970s and 1980s.

GMCHP's participation in Medicaid and Medicare cost the Marshfield Clinic millions of dollars, but the clinic had hoped it would be able to help state and federal administrators devise equitable reimbursement formulas for serving all public beneficiaries regardless of their location or health status. However, changing and inconsistent public policies, state and federal agency inertia, late payments resulting from decisions in the original Medicare legislation to hand reimbursement services to the insurance industry (Blue Cross), failure to adjust formulas for serving high-risk patients, and unreasonably low compensation levels for cost-efficient providers made long-term participation impossible. HMOs elsewhere in Wisconsin and the nation enrolled a small number of public beneficiaries but only in areas where high provider costs inflated reimbursement levels or when patients with serious health problems could be denied enrollment. Despite incredible turmoil among medical and insurance providers and state and federal governments, the potential for HMOs to offer better and less costly care to Medicaid and Medicare beneficiaries remained unrealized.

Chapter 11 revisits HMO contracting with federally funded health care programs in the 1990s, showing why a continuing failure of public policy prevented HMOs from meeting their intended mission. But before we get to that, chapters 6 and 7 will examine HMO administrative and management problems and then will attempt to evaluate the quality of prepaid health care during the 1970s and 1980s.

Chapter 6

Entering a Management Revolution

> The comprehensive nature of HMO services is at once the essence of an HMO and the source of its management difficulties.
>
> Lawrence D. Brown

Few people had the requisite skills and experience to administer HMOs when the movement began to attract national attention in the 1970s. Those who did know something about prepaid health care generally agreed that successful HMOs needed to have well-defined operational goals, an administrative structure with clear lines of responsibility, a knowledgeable governing board with capable managers, and processes in place to control utilization and ensure high-quality care.[1] Few organizations came close to meeting these criteria in principle or practice. The failure of many new health plans to survive or thrive during the 1970s motivated Congress to allocate funding for HMO management training in its 1978 amendments to the HMO Act.

This chapter describes the problems that the Marshfield Clinic experienced in making the transition from a model of medical care that derived from internal standards to one controlled by external market conditions, laws and regulations, and the behavior of powerful insurers. GMCHP achieved remarkable results during its first decade of operation despite a lack of administrative expertise in prepaid care, but other young HMOs were not so fortunate.

Well-defined Organizational Goals

GMCHP had no clearly stated goals. Instead, its three partners—the Marshfield Clinic, Blue Cross Associated Hospital Services of Wisconsin, and Saint Joseph's Hospital—had widely disparate reasons for participating in the health plan. The leaders of the Marshfield Clinic initially viewed GMCHP as an experiment to test the feasibility of providing economical, high-quality, and comprehensive prepaid care to residents in its immediate service area. Blue Cross executives were eager to start the Marshfield plan because it offered opportunities to capture the prepaid health care market in central Wisconsin and to demonstrate their ability to operate a successful rural HMO.[2] Blue Cross had pressured administrators at Saint Joseph's Hospital to participate in the health plan, so their role in GMCHP's development and operation was largely passive. They simply wanted to control their own affairs and protect their institution from any losses that the plan might incur. That the clinic and Blue Cross had disparate reasons for wanting to start GMCHP seemed inconsequential in the beginning because both partners were eager for the health plan to succeed. Conflict arose only when the clinic changed its expectations for the health plan.

The Marshfield Clinic's goals began to shift shortly before GMCHP celebrated its second birthday when Dr. David Ottensmeyer was elected president and James Ensign, who had previously worked at the Blue Cross Association's national headquarters in Chicago, was hired as executive director. Because both men had strong business instincts, they urged their staff to exploit GMCHP's potential for increasing referrals by promoting its expansion into surrounding communities.[3] The health plan's physician-founders balked at the idea of using it for corporate gain, preferring to emphasize the social benefits of providing area residents with affordable care.[4] GMCHP's marketing became more proactive, but clinic doctors waited until 1980 to adopt a policy calling for aggressive expansion of the health plan in order to promote and solidify their referral base. By then GMCHP was serving patients in seven counties.[5]

For a time during the early 1970s the Marshfield Clinic and Employers Insurance, which operated the North Central Health Protection Plan (NCHPP) forty miles away in Wausau, considered joining forces. They also considered the possibility of Employers' replacing Blue Cross as GMCHP's insurance partner or developing a referral arrangement between their two plans. However, nothing came of their discussions, and the two health plans went their separate ways.[6] Employers established other health plans in Green Bay and Milwaukee in eastern Wisconsin, and in Eau Claire, Chippewa Falls, and La Crosse to the west. Meanwhile, GMCHP grew into new communities, often in conjunction with expanding clinic services.

One such expansion involved Mosinee, a small paper mill community located between Wausau and Marshfield but traditionally in the Wausau market. In 1976, after a succession of doctors had established practices in Mosinee but then moved to Wausau, village leaders asked the clinic to help them recruit a physician willing to settle permanently in their community. Marshfield agreed to assist on condition that doctors from Wausau and nearby Stevens Point also participate in the search. Within a week, however, a family practitioner visited Marshfield because he was looking for a small-town practice where he could be associated with the clinic. Soon after the clinic hired him and established a satellite service in Mosinee, the local paper mill transferred its employees' health coverage from NCHPP to GMCHP. The Wausau Medical Center realized too late that it should have made a greater effort to find a permanent doctor for Mosinee.

At a meeting in Wausau the following year, officials of the Wausau Medical Center told their counterparts at the Marshfield Clinic that the Wausau medical community had lost $1.5 million in revenue since the clinic moved into Mosinee.[7] For financial as well as political reasons, the Wausau Medical Center had to install one of its own physicians in Mosinee. The clinic refused to withdraw from Mosinee but offered to share its office space or develop a cooperative agreement whereby paper mill families enrolled in GMCHP could continue to use their Wausau physicians. Soon after that discussion Employers Insurance and Marshfield drafted a "free-flow" affiliation arrangement whereby NCHPP and GMCHP subscribers could use services from either plan.[8] Leo Suycott, the president of Blue Cross, was so convinced that the proposed arrangement, as initially drafted, would violate antitrust regulations that he withdrew his staff from the negotiations.[9] He also hired a team of attorneys to evaluate the GMCHP-NCHPP affiliation agreement; it concluded that the proposed marketing and billing arrangements, as Blue Cross understood them, raised serious antitrust issues. Before their free-flow agreement took effect, the clinic and Employers deleted all references to marketing territories.[10] That agreement was the first, and for many years the only, such arrangement in the nation.[11] Suycott was furious with the clinic for entering GMCHP into an agreement with Employers without first obtaining approval from Blue Cross and Saint Joseph's Hospital.

Just before the two health plans announced their reciprocal arrangement, Suycott chastised Lewis for joining forces with Blue Cross's major central Wisconsin competitor. After expressing his fears about antitrust violations again, Suycott warned Lewis that Employers would use the agreement to undersell its policies to healthy groups, leaving GMCHP with all the high risks. (NCHPP did attract a few small groups from the Marshfield plan by offering lower rates, but the effect on GMCHP was insignificant.) Suycott said that his efforts in Marshfield had cost Blue Cross a great deal of money but that the clinic's leaders had failed to appreciate how he had worked to increase their business and attract more than forty thousand subscribers to their health plan. If the clinic wanted to go out on its own, Suycott threatened to market a competing experience-rated prepaid health plan in GMCHP's coverage area. The conversation left Lewis with the impression that Blue Cross now viewed the Marshfield Clinic as a major threat to its business interests.[12]

In fact, GMCHP's rapid expansion had already eroded standard Blue Cross policy sales in the state's northern counties and had invaded markets that Blue Cross had targeted for its own Compcare prepaid program. And each time GMCHP expanded into a new territory, residents in surrounding communities pleaded with the Marshfield Clinic to extend much-needed medical services and health plan coverage to them as well. Lewis invariably responded that GMCHP "limited expansion to those areas covered by physicians willing to participate" in the plan.[13] Blue Cross grew progressively more intolerant of the clinic's efforts to expand GMCHP's coverage. In 1986 it dissolved their partnership. The administrators of Saint Joseph's Hospital objected to the clinic's domination of the partnership but not to the health plan's expansion, which inevitably brought more tertiary referral business to their facility.[14]

Clear Lines of Administrative Responsibility

GMCHP had no formal organization or power to act on its own. Annual contract agreements described its remarkably loose administrative structure and lines of responsibility. Blue Cross kept the books, marketed the health plan, collected premiums, maintained membership files, disbursed payments to affiliated hospitals and out-of-area providers, and distributed capitation payments for all outpatient care to the Marshfield Clinic. The clinic was responsible for medical management of the health plan and maintenance of agreements with affiliated providers. By 1980 the clinic's capitation covered all services furnished by GMCHP's affiliated physicians, optometrists, and podiatrists, as well as dentists who performed oral surgery procedures; outpatient and inpatient services provided by affiliated mental health and alcohol and drug abuse centers; skilled nursing and home care; and miscellaneous charges for ambulance services, durable medical goods, and prosthetics. Saint Joseph's Hospital was GMCHP's exclusive provider of inpatient services until the health plan expanded and affiliated with other hospitals.

The partners met in Marshfield three or four times a year to discuss problems and policy issues, review financial statements, and set premium rates for the coming year. Blue Cross representatives at these meetings included Leo Suycott, his chief financial officer, and someone from his marketing or actuarial departments. The president and comptroller of Saint Joseph's Hospital, and often the administrative director of the Sisters of the Sorrowful Mother in Milwaukee, attended on behalf of the hospital. Later, administrators from the health plan's two affiliated hospitals joined them.

Invariably, the clinic was overrepresented at these meetings. Its delegation included Lewis, the clinic's president, its executive director, and various health plan staff members. After GMCHP became involved with federally subsidized programs, the administrators of those programs at the Marshfield Medical Research and Education Foundation attended as well. All three partners rotated the chair and contributed to the agendas, but the clinic's overrepresentation at meetings troubled Suycott. He often insisted that key individuals from each organization withdraw into an executive session for more balanced discussions. In 1978 Suycott proposed that GMCHP establish a nine-member policy committee, composed of three representatives from each partner who would elect their chair annually and decide all major policy issues by a "three-quarters majority vote."[15] Lewis opposed the executive sessions, believing that his staff "should be exposed to important decisions," and he rejected the idea of a policy committee because he did not want outsiders to be dictating any aspect of the clinic's internal affairs.[16]

In another effort to achieve a more formal organization, Suycott proposed that GMCHP join Blue Cross's Compcare in seeking federal qualification. The intent of federal qualification, as described in a provision of the HMO Act of 1973, was to ensure the financial stability of health plans receiving federal funds and enhance their marketability to companies seeking to purchase group contracts for their employees. The clinic's leaders debated the advisability of federal qualification for several years and eventually decided not to apply, in part because they did not want a more formal relationship with Blue Cross. Even without qualification, GMCHP had access to federally subsidized programs through the Marshfield Medical Research and Education Foundation, and it had an extraordinarily high level of enrollment in its marketing area. Moreover, the application process and reporting regulations for federally qualified HMOs were exceedingly burdensome.[17] When the Kaiser Foundation Health Plan applied for federal qualification in 1977, for example, Joseph A. Califano, then the secretary of health, education and welfare, reported that Kaiser's application packet weighed more than six hundred pounds and was almost six feet high.[18]

Until the 1976 amendments to the HMO Act relaxed mandates for open enrollment, community rating, and specific benefits, only a few large, well-established health plans bothered to qualify.[19] The criteria for achieving federal qualification did not guarantee fiscal solvency: Six of 108 plans lost their qualified status in the late 1970s, and four went out of business. Although fewer than half of the nation's HMOs were federally qualified by 1980, those plans served more than two-thirds of the nation's enrollees in prepaid plans.[20]

GMCHP received no federal development funds and was therefore under no obligation to follow federal mandates. Nevertheless, it held open enrollment periods, used community rating to set its premiums, and offered a generous array of benefits throughout the 1970s and early 1980s. Moreover, it remained in good fiscal condition except for a brief time during and after its ill-fated experiments with Medicaid and Medicare.[21]

A Knowledgeable Governing Board and Capable Managers

During GMCHP's early years Lewis virtually managed the health plan's medical affairs out of his back pocket, in his dual role as medical director of both the clinic and GMCHP. In addition to reviewing all out-of-area referrals and responding to questions about appropriate care and coverage, Lewis worked hard to cultivate good relations with the health plan's growing number of affiliated providers.[22] Even though the clinic expected Lewis to maintain an active part-time practice in obstetrics and gynecology, his only administrative assistant was Don Nystrom, the health plan's manager. Lewis had hoped for more help when James Ensign became executive director of the clinic in 1973, fresh from the national Blue Cross office. However, Ensign was not particularly interested in the health plan and devoted little time to it. David Ottensmeyer, the clinic's president, appointed a new committee to assist Lewis with day-to-day decisions, but its members routinely deferred to Lewis's judgment and left him to manage the plan on his own.[23] "Nobody gave me a mandate to run the plan. I just did it," Lewis said.[24]

Dr. Ben Lawton, who was instrumental in founding GMCHP, was re-elected clinic president in 1975. After a flurry of administrative changes that year and the next, the doctors appointed Frederick Wenzel, formerly director of the Marshfield Medical Research and Education Foundation, to serve as executive director of the clinic and GMCHP. Unlike his predecessors, Wenzel was eager to control the health plan's management. After promoting Nystrom to business manager for the clinic, Wenzel hired David Gruel, who was working in membership services at Blue Cross in Milwaukee, to coordinate the health plan's day-to-day operation. According to Gruel, Blue Cross wanted someone familiar with its operation working in the Marshfield health plan office.[25]

Despite the administrative changes, Lewis complained to Lawton in 1977 that the health plan still had a "vague status within the Clinic framework." Now that the plan accounted for 20 percent of the clinic's business, Lewis said, "it can no longer be handled by a few people with no authorization or accountability." Lewis also objected to vesting the clinic's executive committee with the authority to set policy for the health plan. Physicians serving on that committee were fully involved with clinic issues, and few had taken the time to learn about the health plan's operation. Lewis therefore asked Lawton to appoint a five-member committee consisting of three physicians and two lay administrators who were genuinely interested and willing to participate in the health plan's policy management.[26] Lewis also asked Lawton to divide his job as medical director into two positions, one for the clinic and the other for the health plan. After submitting his resignation as the clinic's medical director, Lewis prepared what turned out to be the first of many drafts of a job description for GMCHP's medical director. As he recounted years later, "Nobody knew what my job was, including me."[27]

In retrospect, Lewis thought that his long tenure as medical director was an important factor in GMCHP's growth. It enabled him, during literally hundreds of meetings throughout the state, to nurture valuable relationships with physicians and other providers. Conversely, he thought that the clinic's lack of leadership continuity was its biggest weakness. Clinic policy required annual election of the president, and during the 1970s it limited tenure to three consecutive terms. Former presidents who had already served three terms were sometimes reelected later, but Lewis thought that such discontinuity prevented the clinic's chief spokesperson from developing ties with the wider medical community and with federal and state decision makers. In effect, he said, "The Clinic is running a $250 million business with people who are only in office for a few years." The frequent turnover also had a negative effect on Lewis and his meager staff because each new president came to office with a different agenda for the health plan.[28]

Lewis received some relief in 1978 when he won approval to hire a nurse-clinician to assist with some of his administrative tasks. He also convinced Lawton to appoint a new "policy group" consisting of five physicians; five administrators from the clinic, health plan, and research foundation; and a representative of Saint Joseph's Hospital. Lewis hoped that the new group would advise him on "problems and politics of the health plan and Clinic," but it proved ineffective and was dissolved by the next president two years later.[29]

Most HMOs struggled to find knowledgeable governing boards and capable managers in the late 1970s and early 1980s. A national survey in 1980 reported that all health plans with more than twenty thousand members were planning to make or had made changes in their governance and relationship to their medical organizations. These changes often included a stronger administrative structure with segregated medical services and an elected executive committee; appointment of a medical director to ensure physician responsibility for clinical operations; and appointment of administrators who were not physicians to oversee the management of medical groups.

When the clinic elected Dr. Nelson Moffat as president in 1980, he replaced Lawton's policy group with a GMCHP executive committee that reported to the clinic's executive committee. Moffat hoped to introduce "young blood" with fresh ideas while keeping the new committee small and efficient. He soon found it politically expedient to include several "old-timers," as well as the usual health plan and medical research foundation managers.[30] Lewis and Wenzel suggested that GMCHP develop a mission statement and an education program to help new committee members address health plan policy issues. And in conjunction with the clinic's newly adopted corporate strategy for GMCHP expansion, they proposed the hiring of an associate director, noting that the new position would require clarification of the roles of the medical and administrative directors.[31]

Lewis approved of these changes in principle, but he opposed Wenzel's attempts to give lay managers more control of the health plan. Lewis told Moffat that GMCHP's new associate director ought to be a young doctor with administrative training who would report to GMCHP's medical director rather than the clinic's executive director.[32] Lewis explained his position in a letter to a dean at the University of Wisconsin Medical School in Madison, who had developed a program in administrative medicine. "Because physicians are too busy taking care of sick people," Lewis wrote, "they have allowed many administrative functions to fall into the hands of lay administrators, who have been all too willing to take on this responsibility. We need to realize that medical administration is an important part of our profession.[33]

Suycott objected to the clinic's hiring any sort of administrator for GMCHP on its own. Instead, he repeated his demand for a separate structure with an administrator responsible to all three partners. The clinic's executive committee decided that a formal partnership agreement with Blue Cross and Saint Joseph's Hospital would be "incompatible with the organization, structure and practice" of the clinic. Then, ignoring Lewis's advice, the committee hired a lay health plan administrator who was to report to Wenzel, not Lewis. The committee also directed Lewis (or whoever served as GMCHP's medical director in the future) to report to the clinic's medical director. Job descriptions for GMCHP's medical director and a newly created assistant medical director position required doctors accepting those assignments to maintain an active practice for at least 20 percent of their time. The new job descriptions also limited the medical director's appointment to three-year terms, subject to annual review and term renewal by the clinic medical director and GMCHP's executive committee.[34]

Moffat appointed Dr. Dean Emanuel, a cardiologist at the clinic, to serve as assistant medical director in 1981, intending that Emanuel would take over when Lewis retired. Emanuel had no particular administrative training, but he was extremely interested in the health plan and eager to develop better methods for monitoring the quality of care that affiliated physicians provided to GMCHP subscribers.[35] Emanuel found that the managerial duties were too burdensome, however, and resigned in 1984, leaving Lewis and the health plan without a replacement.

The qualifications and responsibilities of HMO medical directors received considerable attention from health plan organizers and administrators in the early 1980s. Medical directors of most HMOs were responsible for maintaining physician cooperation, high-quality service, and consumer satisfaction. More specifically, they were required to negotiate with providers, help establish treatment protocols, respond to patient complaints, and approve out-of-area referrals. Physicians generally agreed that the ideal medical director was a respected clinician, "a doctor's doctor," who was well organized and able to inspire efficiency and equity in coworkers. The position also required a person with management skills; a knowledge of financial planning, budgeting, and marketing; good health; endurance; and, because of the job's demands, an understanding family.[36] "People didn't appreciate how much work was involved in the job," Lewis said. "It could be intolerable if you didn't like that sort of thing.[37]

Wenzel's new associate director who was nominally in charge of the health plan's administrative management, also had a relatively short tenure. According to Lewis, the relationship between Wenzel and GMCHP lacked clear definition, and "Wenzel got his nose under the tent more each year."[38] In 1984 Wenzel hired Robert DeVita to fill the new post of associate director in charge of the health plan. DeVita had interned with GMCHP as part of his training in the first National HMO Fellowship Program at Georgetown University in 1980–81. He was working for a Blue Cross plan in Tennessee when Wenzel brought him back to Marshfield.[39] Chapter 9 discusses DeVita's management reforms, which significantly changed many of GMCHP founding principles, for better or worse.

Ability to Control Quality and Utilization

Controlling quality of care and utilization costs were key functions for a successful HMO. Hospital services were the mostly costly aspect of medical care, but most administrators focused their efforts on physicians' behavior. Doctors, who received only 20 percent of health care dollars, were responsible for ordering nearly all services—and few had any idea how much those services cost.[40] In an early attempt to control hospital services ordered by doctors, Blue Cross of Western Pennsylvania, the Allegheny County Medical Society Foundation, and the Hospitals Council of Western Pennsylvania developed a "utilization review" process in 1959 to determine whether patients received appropriate levels of hospital care. Assisted by physician-reviewers, the Pennsylvania providers analyzed individual hospital records and summaries of utilization data after patients were discharged. That information enabled them to establish practice norms, modify the behavior of overzealous doctors, and reduce hospital costs.[41]

The HMO Act of 1973 required federally funded HMOs to use a peer review process and develop the capacity to measure quality based on health outcomes. Health plans also had to report information about the availability, accessibility, and acceptability of their services. In order to assist HMOs in assembling meaningful information, HEW contracted with the Harvard Center for Community Health and Medical Care from 1972 to 1975 to develop a format and system for collecting the required data.[42] The Marshfield Medical Research and Education Foundation was one of eight participants in the Harvard project. Marshfield had taken an early lead in collecting information about GMCHP's enrollees and their patterns of utilization because the health plan had been established as an experiment to determine the cost of providing prepaid care to a rural population. The foundation hired Greg Nycz, a biostatistician, to be its comptroller in 1972 and named him director of information systems three years later. Nycz routinely prepared reports detailing, for example, the demographics and utilization patterns of GMCHP's subscriber population.

Data Processing: A Critical Tool for Controlling Costs and Quality

Technological improvements in computers during the 1970s greatly enhanced the ability to measure internal performance and make comparisons with other plans. Some activities that I describe in this section would not have been possible without the development of increasingly more sophisticated data-processing systems. Data collected during the first fifteen months of GMCHP's operation, when the plan included only a few affiliated physicians and no outlying hospitals, showed that health plan enrollees used fewer hospital days but had many more clinic visits than did their fee-for-service counterparts.[43] Computerized data enabled several specialty departments to conduct outcome studies that increased the cost efficiency of their treatment protocols, and a newly organized cost control committee was able to reduce GMCHP's use of hospital services.[44]

One low-tech attempt by the cost control committee to shorten the length of hospital stays was a total failure. It involved placing stickers on local residents' charts to advise doctors that early discharge was appropriate because visiting nurses were available to monitor their patients at home in a much less expensive recovery setting. Lewis disliked the stickers because he believed that they gave the perception of unequal treatment based on geographic proximity to the Marshfield Clinic. Other clinic doctors simply ignored them.[45]

A few years later, when hospital utilization data showed alarming rate increases, Lewis proposed that GMCHP offer out-of-town patients who were not yet ready to return home the option of continuing their recovery under nursing supervision in a local motel. Blue Cross advised Lewis that paying for patients to stay in a local motel rather than the hospital until they were well enough to travel home might cost the health plan less for those particular patients but would free up hospital beds for other patients to use. Because doctors could then fill those empty hospital beds with other patients, using motels ultimately would increase costs to the health plan. As an alternative, Blue Cross suggested that the hospital use some of its beds to create a self-care unit for convalescing patients. Patients would be in a hospital environment and accessible to doctors, but their care would cost considerably less.[46]

GMCHP members had lower hospital utilization rates than Blue Cross fee-for-service policyholders in Wisconsin.[47] However, its rates were higher rates than those of other HMOs for several reasons: The new addition to Saint Joseph's Hospital had created a surplus of beds, allowing residents on the hospital's house staff and newly hired clinic physicians who were unfamiliar with the clinic's policies of limiting admissions and inpatient care, to keep patients hospitalized too long.[48] GMCHP's affiliated doctors made liberal use of their outlying hospitals with no concern for costs.[49] Perhaps most significant was that GMCHP's direct-pay subscribers, who accounted for one-third of its membership, used 60 percent more hospital days per person on average than its group enrollees.[50] A consultant who reviewed Marshfield's utilization records in the mid-1970s said that the health plan could not compare itself with other HMOs because others had "little experience with direct-pay patients.[51]

By 1980 GMCHP utilization review nurses were using data-processing services to monitor daily activity and issue weekly reports about the frequency of admissions and duration of stays at Saint Joseph's Hospital and affiliated hospitals. To expedite discharges from Saint Joseph's Hospital a nurse coordinator helped doctors transfer patients to less expensive accommodations whenever appropriate. Those options included nursing homes, round-the-clock home nursing care, visiting nurses, outpatient rehabilitation services from Saint Joseph's Hospital, and a home care center for newborns with congenital defects.

Saint Joseph's Hospital also introduced three-day and same-day surgery protocols. Under the three-day protocol patients had their surgical procedures—such as coronary arteriograms; oral surgery; uterine dilation and curettage; and breast, liver, and kidney biopsies—on the day of admission and were discharged two days later if they had no complications. The same-day surgery protocol enabled patients to have procedures performed on the day that they were admitted and to be discharged if their physical condition posed no significant anesthetic risk and they lived within thirty miles of Marshfield.[52] (By the 1990s doctors in many parts of the county were performing most of these procedures on an outpatient basis.) Same-day surgeries performed during the program's first five months, long before it had reached its full potential, saved the health plan $37,000.[53] All these cost-saving measures enabled the hospital to successfully cope with Medicare's new reimbursement system a few years later.[54]

Data processing also helped administrators monitor outpatient visits, which HMOs encouraged in order to reduce hospital admissions. HMO subscribers averaged 3.8 visits a year, compared with 3.2 visits for patients in all systems of care, but individual patients, physicians, and health plans showed enormous variation.[55] Administrators at Kaiser Permanente reported that high outpatient users, whom they called the "worried well," usually lacked a medical diagnosis appropriate for the frequency of their office visits. These patients attached special meaning to their symptoms, changed doctors regularly, and subjected themselves to many diagnostic tests and medications but rarely followed their doctor's advice. To control unnecessary visits Kaiser Permanente first assessed a small fee for each visit but then in the early 1980s assigned all new patients to a primary care team that assessed and monitored each patient's progress.[56]

Marshfield researchers reviewed the charts of 116 GMCHP enrollees, each of whom had twenty-five or more documented visits during one year, and found that the number of visits and care generally were appropriate for their condition. Six exceptions were four depressed patients with psychosomatic complaints who never received a referral for psychiatric evaluation or antidepressant drugs and two patients with chronic back pain who obtained manipulation from "outside providers" rather than "more common physical therapy measures.[57]

Data processing was essential for profiling utilization patterns of clinic and affiliated physicians so that GMCHP could identify those who ordered too many tests, treatments, or hospital admissions. The availability of this information often provided sufficient motivation for doctors to change their practice patterns. In 1979 GMCHP asked its insurance committee to conduct peer reviews of affiliated physicians, in addition to its other duties of credentialing new affiliates and setting maximum reimbursement limits. At each meeting the physicians reviewed a sampling of patient chart profiles that were coded to disguise the patient's and doctor's names. When concerns arose about patient care, Lewis reviewed the charts and asked the physician to explain what appeared to be inappropriate or questionable practices. Insurance committee members reviewed his reports at their next meeting, when they might issue a warning, refuse payment for specified services, or could disaffiliate the provider from the health plan. GMCHP rarely took punitive action against a doctor. Instead, Marshfield Clinic physicians who served on the committee used the chart review process and nonconfrontational private discussions to advise affiliated providers about standard diagnostic and treatment protocols.[58]

GMCHP and Wausau's North Central Health Protection Plan formed a joint utilization review committee shortly after the two health plans signed their reciprocal agreement. The review committee was independent of either plan's internal peer review system. Usually, two to four doctors and one or two administrators from each plan met about four times a year for dinner at an area supper club. The meetings were cordial and often congenial, although the participants sometimes worried that the "other plan" had ulterior motives or was overcharging them for services. In addition to discussing problems with their affiliation agreement or problems common to both operations, the doctors reviewed profiles of randomly selected charts in order to identify duplicated services, aberrant charges, inappropriate referrals, and questionable treatments. The reviewers took questions back to their health plan's doctors for clarification and reported the results of their investigations and remedial action at their next meeting.

After NCHPP reorganized as a cooperative in 1980, the Marshfield Clinic's leaders feared that the Wausau group would dissolve their affiliation agreement because the cooperative's new president saw no advantage to it and thought that the clinic's fees were too high.[59] However, their affiliation continued, and the two plans finally signed a new agreement 1983.[60] A year later NCHPP discontinued reimbursements to three of GMCHP's affiliated clinics because their doctors persistently overused hospital services and referred patients to providers not associated with either health plan.[61] NCHPP also notified the Marshfield Clinic that it anticipated a fiscal year loss of $450,000 in its physicians' reimbursement fund and would therefore assess the clinic and its Mosinee satellite approximately $76,000 to offset their share of the year-end deficit.[62] Although the actual losses were somewhat less than anticipated, Marshfield avoided further assessments by accepting a capitation in lieu of fees for treating NCHPP subscribers.[63]

Chapter 10 covers the antitrust implications of Marshfield's continuing affiliation with Wausau, but it is important to note the joint review committee's significant accomplishments here. James Coleman, who worked for NCHPP before moving over to GMCHP in 1985, believed that the committee's meetings provided a highly constructive forum for peer review for both plans.[64] Indeed, research by Paul Ellwood's InterStudy confirmed that physician involvement in discussions and decisions about costs was invariably more effective than subjecting doctors to financial risk when they overused or giving them bonuses when they performed in a cost-conscious manner.[65]

The joint review committee changed physicians' practice behaviors and improved patient care in both health plans and throughout central Wisconsin's fee-for-service system. Elsewhere, competition from HMOs was forcing fee-for-service practitioners to improve their performance.[66] But in the counties covered by GMCHP and NCHPP cooperation between the two HMOs promoted better, less expensive care for all residents.

The administrative problems that GMCHP encountered during its first ten years were typical for HMOs that developed in the 1970s, before and after federal funding became available. During the first decade of the HMO movement new health plans rarely had well-defined organizational goals because each sponsor had its own motivations and needs. Almost none of the plans had administrators or governing boards equipped to deal with the very different and complicated requirements of prepaid care. The HMOs also lacked the tools that they needed to measure quality, keep track of utilization, or convince physicians to adopt cost-conscious treatment practices. Few new plans attracted sufficient enrollment to show a profit. Plans that organized later faced equally difficult challenges, but they at least had the benefit of their predecessors' experiences and administrators trained in HMO management.

Chapter 7

Assessing HMO Quality and Consumer Satisfaction in the 1980s

HMOs have not proved to be solutions to health care problems of many poor, sick, old, unemployed, rural or central-city underserved.

Lawrence D. Brown

After private and public health insurance programs became widely available in the 1950s and 1960s, most physicians grew accustomed to ordering tests and treatments without regard for cost. Although an occasional cynic accused the medical profession of promoting unnecessary services in order to make more money, most Americans accepted whatever their doctors advised, equating more care with better care.[1] Indeed, physicians who tried to economize invited malpractice litigation.

Hardly anyone thought about the quality of medical care until the early 1970s when Congress began to consider federal funding for HMO development. Critics of such legislation claimed that HMOs might jeopardize their patients' welfare by restricting medical care in order to save money. Despite a growing body of evidence showing that prepaid, cost-effective care did not harm patients, the critics' warnings alarmed many legislators, regulators, and consumers.[2] Quite suddenly, quality of care became an important public issue and a major preoccupation for many researchers. Few people knew how to define or measure the quality of medical care in the 1970s and early 1980s, but that did not deter researchers and consumers from trying to evaluate HMOs with the tools at hand. As health plan administrators and consumers began to appreciate the significance of these evaluations and realize that physicians' motives, judgment, and performance were open to question, the sacrosanct bastions of the medical profession's sovereignty slowly eroded.

Definitions and Measurements of Quality

In 1966 Avedis Donabedian, a researcher at the University of Michigan School of Public Health, devised what most observers believe was the first conceptual model for evaluating everyday care. According to Donabedian, medical care depended on the interaction of three elements: structure, process, and outcome.[3] Researchers used these criteria, for example, to evaluate how prenatal care administered in a variety of clinical settings affected the health of mothers and their newborns.[4] Donabedian's research and writings created the theoretical underpinnings for many health care system assessments that followed.

The federal Office of HMOs reviewed the two previous decades of research in 1979, using Donabedian's structure, process, and outcome measurements to compare fee-for-service and prepaid health care. The agency identified nineteen major studies, twenty-five reports, and sixty-nine quality variables. HMOs fared very well compared to fee-for-service care: nineteen reports ranked the general quality of HMO care as superior, and six others found that the two delivery systems were comparable; none found overall care offered by HMOs to be inferior.[5]

Researchers at the Rand Corporation concluded in the late 1970s, however, that structural and procedural variables, considered alone or together, were not valid measurements of quality because improvements in these variables did not always promote better health outcomes.[6] Rand began to develop more precise criteria for measuring treatments and outcomes, but until the think tank published its results in the mid-1980s, many researchers continued to evaluate HMOs by using earlier variables, such as access to appropriate, affordable, and timely medical care and consumer and provider satisfaction.[7] Although researchers usually examined HMO accessibility in terms of availability of services to members, health plans could also be evaluated from a social perspective, that is, how accessible they were to potential subscribers.

The Social Perspective of HMO Accessibility

Most HMOs failed the social test of accessibility in the 1970s because they marketed policies only to employee groups.[8] Very few health plans offered individual policies to Americans who had to buy their own insurance because they were out of work, self-employed, or held low-paying jobs that offered no benefits.[9] The HMO Act of 1973 required federally funded HMOs to provide one 30-day open enrollment period each year for nongroup subscribers, but waivers allowed health plans to ignore that mandate if it jeopardized their economic viability. As a result the number of direct-pay enrollees was minuscule.[10] The North Communities Health Plan (North Care) of Evanston, Illinois, was one of a very few federally financed health plans that briefly offered an unrestricted (no screening for health status) open enrollment period. When more than twelve hundred direct-pay subscribers joined North Care in 1975, their unusually high hospital costs increased the premiums for all nine thousand policyholders by 20 percent. Thereafter, North Care denied admission to applicants with significant health problems.[11]

Amendments to the HMO Act did not improve the situation for direct-pay consumers. In 1976 Congress allowed health plans to defer open enrollment until they had been in business for five years or reached a membership of fifty thousand (whichever came first) and had operated without a deficit for one full year. And in 1980 provisions added to the HMO Act enabled the Department of Health and Human Services (HHS) to grant open enrollment waivers whenever the agency determined that such a practice would cause undue financial burden.

HMOs were beyond the means of many people who had to purchase their own coverage, even though prepaid plans were often less costly than traditional insurance policies requiring copayments, deductibles, and other out-of-pocket expenses. In 1980, when the median annual income for U.S. families was approximately $4,700, the average annual family premium among fifteen HMOs surveyed by the American Medical Association was $1,222, far beyond the means of many family budgets.[12] In addition, as I noted in chapter 5, HMOs were virtually inaccessible to most Medicare and Medicaid beneficiaries in the 1980s because the federal government and most states had not yet developed adequate mechanisms for prepaid contracting.[13]

Several studies in the 1980s examined why some people, when given a choice, joined HMOs, whereas others preferred to stay in the fee-for-service system. Some researchers reported strong correlations between specific subscriber characteristics and health benefit choices,[14] but most found that decisions about HMO enrollment were difficult to predict because the process involved many interrelated variables: out-of-pocket costs, personal choice of physicians and hospitals, anticipated health care needs, geographic accessibility, breadth of benefits, convenience of services, and advice from family and friends.[15]

Central Wisconsin residents were an exception to national HMO enrollment patterns largely because the Greater Marshfield Community Health Plan had an exceedingly liberal enrollment policy and offered subscribers care by all physicians and hospitals in its coverage area. Moreover, GMCHP was the only HMO in Wisconsin and one of few in the nation where group and direct-pay enrollees paid the same monthly premium, based on an area-wide community rate.[16]

GMCHP's liberal enrollment policy became a significant issue when Marshfield and Wausau's North Central Health Protection Plan (NCHPP) signed an affiliation agreement in 1978, allowing their members to use the services of either plan. Unlike Marshfield, NCHPP had marketed exclusively to employers during its first seven years. Shortly after NCHPP announced the new affiliation agreement, one of its administrators informed Lewis that several Wausau residents wanted to enroll in the Marshfield plan so that they could obtain coverage for care that they received in Wausau. Presumably fearing that Marshfield would market to Wausau individuals, the administrator asked Lewis to delay his next open enrollment period until NCHPP started one of its own. Lewis said that GMCHP would enroll new subscribers shortly but did not intend to market beyond its present coverage area.[17] Although Lewis hoped the new agreement would enhance the clinic's tertiary referral base, he had no desire to capture NCHPP's potential subscribers, healthy or otherwise.[18]

Marshfield's obsession with open and direct-pay enrollment demonstrated how HMOs could make themselves broadly accessible. In 1980 GMCHP's membership in all or portions of seven central Wisconsin counties represented 46 percent of the residents sixty-four or younger.[19] Just two years earlier seven prepaid health plans in the Minnesota Twin Cities—a hotbed of prepaid activity and home base of the HMO promoter Paul Ellwood—were serving only 10 percent of that area's population.[20]

Subscriber Accessibility to Medical Services

HMO subscribers who lacked the means to evaluate the technical features of their health plans often judged a plan by the accessibility of its services: the distance to medical facilities, availability of round-the-clock care, how long they waited for an appointment or to see a doctor when they had an appointment, how readily they were referred to a specialist, and how well they communicated with their physician.

Distance to health care facilities was an issue of particular concern for inner city and rural residents. The Office of HMOs required federally qualified health plans to define their enrollment area by a radius of thirty minutes' travel time from primary health care services. Those theoretical constraints were irrelevant as late as 1980 because more than half the nation's population still lived in metropolitan or rural areas that had no HMOs.[21] GMCHP was not bound by this federal mandate, but its policy of affiliating with local providers placed primary care reasonably close to most enrollees. In 1979 GMCHP's forty-five thousand subscribers living beyond commuting distance to Marshfield had access to thirty-three solo practitioners and five small clinics scattered throughout a three-thousand-square-mile area.

Appointment scheduling was a major reason why HMO subscribers were dissatisfied and often left their health plans. Kaiser Permanente blamed "the worried well," members who abused their unlimited access to physicians, for long delays in getting appointments.[22] After Kaiser instituted small copayment fees and hired paramedics to reduce unnecessary outpatient visits in the early 1970s, new patients' accessibility to physicians increased twenty-fold and appointment waiting times decreased from six to eight weeks to one or two days.[23]

The medical directors' division of the Group Health Association of America (GHAA) devoted its entire 1979 conference to subscribers' accessibility to care. The delegates learned that prepaid and fee-for-service provider groups of similar size had an equal number of appointment scheduling problems. Large medical groups had more difficulties than small groups and spent significantly more resources measuring waiting times and patient perceptions of waiting times. HMOs surveyed for an AMA study that year usually reserved time for same-day urgent care, but waits for routine appointments averaged seven to ten days and waits for complete physical examinations were four to twelve weeks.[24]

In the late 1970s the Marshfield Medical Research Foundation interviewed patients treated by the Marshfield Clinic and GMCHP-affiliated
physicians, all of whom offered both fee-for-service and prepaid care. Patients using affiliated physicians in solo and small group practices had significantly shorter waiting times for appointments but longer office waits
than the Marshfield Clinic patients did. Fee-for-service and prepaid patients were equally satisfied with their care, but the patients using solo and
small group practitioners expressed more satisfaction with access and the
social and emotional dimensions of their care than patients using the
clinic's large multispecialty facility. The foundation attributed the clinic's
low patient-satisfaction score to its bureaucratic structure and the inability of 42 percent of clinic patient respondents to name the physician who
coordinated their care.[25] The inability of patients to identify a particular
doctor was common but usually involved individuals who lacked a regular
source of health care.[26] The clinic subsequently implemented a series of
reforms that decreased the waiting time for appointments and established
each patient with a personal physician.[27]

Most HMOs required new enrollees to select a pediatrician, internist,
or family practitioner as their primary care physician. These doctors, sometimes called "gatekeepers," were supposed to coordinate diagnostic tests,
treatments, and referrals to specialists in order to prevent unnecessary services. HMOs usually required referrals before they would cover services
that their subscribers obtained from specialists and unaffiliated providers.
GMCHP did not require referrals for its enrollees to visit any Marshfield
Clinic or affiliated physician. In fact, for several years after GMCHP began,
Lewis allowed enrollees to seek treatment from reputable physicians who
were not associated with the health plan if they did not duplicate previous
diagnostic work. Lewis believed that his flexible referral policy, which cost
the clinic about 5 percent of its capitation, created goodwill among subscribers and enhanced the health plan's marketability.[28]

Availability of Comprehensive Benefits

HMOs typically covered a full array of health care services. The range
of benefits, and methods by which health plans decided what specific
treatments to cover, were both measures of HMO quality in the 1970s.
During GMCHP's first fifteen years administrators were asked to consider
coverage for 111 new, experimental, or questionable medical procedures,

ranging from acupuncture and artificial insemination to liver transplants and weight reduction programs.[29] In making its decisions, GMCHP relied on the clinic's specialty department protocols and the coverage standards advocated by Blue Cross and the Group Health Association of America.

In addition to standard benefits, some HMOs provided coverage for prescription drugs, oral surgery and other dental care, eyeglasses, contact lenses, and medical appliances. The 1973 HMO Act required federally funded HMOs to provide preventive dental care for children, but the U.S. Department of Health, Education and Welfare (HEW) ignored that mandate because it was ambiguous and would have been difficult for most HMOs to implement.[30] HMOs offering a prescription drug benefit frequently charged enrollees a few dollars for each prescription and limited the total annual value of their benefit.[31] To save money these plans also encouraged physicians to prescribe generic rather than brand name drugs and to use only those medications on an approved list, or formulary. By 1978 thirty-two states allowed, and five states required, pharmacies to sell generic drugs.[32]

Historically, treatment for affective disorders and substance abuse has been among the most contentious health benefits. Insurance companies and HMOs had many reasons for wanting to limit coverage for these conditions.[33] There was no consensus on the causes or classification of many mental disorders. Psychiatric illness was often difficult to diagnose. Many who might have benefited from treatment did not seek, or actively rejected, help. Treatment methods varied considerably in cost, and few objective evaluations of their therapeutic value were available. In addition, some health care insurers and providers held substance abusers responsible for their condition and found them difficult, sometimes impossible, to treat.[34]

The federal government had few requirements for insurance coverage of mental health services until the 1980s. Among states, fewer than half required insurance carriers or HMOs to provide treatment for psychiatric disorders or substance abuse. HEW regulations weakened the modest requirements for mental health care in the HMO Act of 1973 by exempting psychiatric treatment for chronic alcoholism, even though federally funded HMOs were expected to treat medical problems associated with that disease.[35] Eighty-seven percent of HMOs responding to a 1978 survey provided outpatient and hospital mental health benefits as part of their basic plan or as supplemental coverage, while the remaining 13 percent

offered only outpatient care or nothing at all. Health plans with both ambulatory and inpatient services varied in the amount of care that they offered but averaged about twenty ambulatory visits and forty-five hospital
days per year. Almost none of the HMOs required copayments for hospital care, but one-third collected fees for outpatient services. Prepaid group
practice plans generally offered more benefits and reported greater mental health care utilization than IPAs and other types of HMOs.[36]

Mental health problems are widespread and often cause physical ailments. According to a psychiatrist formerly with the Alcohol, Drug Abuse
and Mental Health Administration at the U.S. Department of Health and
Human Services (HHS, successor to HEW), in the 1980s almost 25 percent of the U.S. population had specifically diagnosable mental disorders
and 15 percent had stresses that taxed their ability to cope. Approximately
10 percent of adult Americans sought counseling each year.[37] A Marshfield Medical Research Foundation study of patients with untreated affective disorders found that males had more digestive system disorders
and females had more genitourinary problems than mentally healthy patients in the same age groups. Many observers believed that comprehensive mental health benefits were cost effective because they significantly
reduced the use of medical services while adding only about $10 per year
to the average HMO premium.[38] GMCHP's mental health benefits were
very generous by HMO standards in the 1970s, but the clinic's psychiatric
department frequently sought to have unlimited benefits for its patients,
analogous to GMCHP's benefits for medical problems. The health plan
never expanded coverage beyond its initial levels, but Lewis usually ac-
commodated patients in rare instances when they needed more than their
allotted number of mental health visits or hospital days.

Treatment for alcoholism is expensive because it often involves extended inpatient care. However, the reasons for treating alcoholics are
compelling. Compared to nonabusers, alcoholics suffer from more psy-
chosocial and chronic physical problems, experience more accidents and
violence, and use many more medical services.[39] Rand Corporation studies published in the 1980s reported that alcoholics and their families used
medical services one-and-a-half to two times more frequently than nonabusers and their families. Family use of medical services declined by as
much as 75 percent when an alcoholic family member received treatment.[40] GMCHP's policy with regard to the treatment of alcoholism was
also very generous.[41] Before Saint Joseph's Hospital developed an inpatient treatment facility for alcohol and other drug abuse, Lewis referred

patients who might benefit from inpatient therapy to treatment centers in other communities. He estimated that such referrals accounted for nearly one-third of GMCHP's out-of-area referral costs, about $300,000 annually in the early 1980s.[42]

GMCHP initially covered smoking cessation and weight reduction programs provided by clinic psychologists who used hypnosis for behavior modification, until the department abandoned both programs in the early 1980s because of their relatively high costs and low success rates. About that time a clinic endocrinologist who was working with obese diabetic patients started a weight reduction program involving a prepared dietary formula for initial weight loss, nutrition education by dietitians, and exercise training by a nurse-clinician who was an exercise specialist. GMCHP eventually agreed to cover program costs for enrollees who were at least fifty pounds overweight and received a referral from their physician. The health plan revised its coverage of the weight-loss program in 1986; thereafter, patients paid for the program but received full reimbursement when they completed it.[43]

HMOs generally offered better coverage for health promotion services than did traditional insurance plans.[44] Some HMO promoters believed that such services were appropriate benefits, but others were quite skeptical. For example, Dr. Ernest Saward, medical director for the Kaiser Foundation Hospital in Portland, Oregon, called health maintenance a "political euphemism."[45] Although HMO medical directors generally favored Pap smears, mammograms, and immunizations, they sometimes questioned the cost benefits of too-frequent screening.[46] Health plans frequently published newsletters urging subscribers to obtain appropriate immunizations, quit smoking, eat a balanced diet, exercise, practice moderation, recognize early warning signs of disease, wear seat belts, and take responsibility for their personal health and safety.[47] The administrators of these plans hoped that these health promotion efforts would change subscribers' lifestyles and reduce utilization costs, but the health economist Odin Anderson was pessimistic. "Hedonistic habits are difficult to change," he said, "for many people believe they make life worthwhile."[48]

Consumer Satisfaction

Whatever subscribers thought about attempts to change their lifestyle, their general level of satisfaction remained the most important measure of HMO evaluation in the 1970s. Favorable perceptions undeniably helped

HMOs attract and retain enrollees.[49] Several surveys during the 1970s and early 1980s found that consumers were generally happy with whatever type of insurance they held until they got sick and had to use their policies. Consumers were also more likely to judge doctors by their bedside manner than their technical expertise.[50]

Few consumers had an opportunity to choose their own policies because employers purchased most of the nation's private health insurance, and their selection criteria seldom gave priority to quality of care. Ninety-seven percent of employers responding to one large survey in 1975 said they considered cost when selecting policies, whereas only 29 percent considered quality as well as cost. Union contracts and the availability of other options further compromised consumers' choice.[51]

Many observers considered membership termination a significant indication of consumer displeasure. But when 14 percent of GMCHP's members left one year, independent researchers found that one-third were involuntarily terminated because they were no longer covered by their parents' policies or that they had turned sixty-five and GMCHP had not yet made arrangements to serve Medicare beneficiaries. Another third left the health plan because they moved from the area or got a job with an employer who did not offer GMCHP membership. And the remaining third left because they could no longer afford the premiums or were dissatisfied with some aspect of the health plan's coverage. No patients left because they were unhappy with their care.[52]

Nationally, the average annual rate of HMO terminations in the late 1970s was about 10 percent. When the Kaiser Family Foundation commissioned the pollster Lou Harris to survey some of the twelve million Americans enrolled in HMOs, Harris reported that 89 percent of HMO members were satisfied with their care and expected to renew their membership. "Looking at the data," Harris said, "I must tell you we are looking at a success story."[53] That assessment may have been true for HMO sponsors and their members, but it certainly did not apply to the approximately twenty-six million Americans who lacked any form of health care coverage in the late 1970s.[54]

Cracks in the Bastions of Professional Supremacy

The AMA opposed passage of the HMO Act in 1973 and of its 1976 amendments, which removed some impractical features of that act. Many health care advocates challenged the medical profession to end its chronic, conditioned defiance of reforms and take the lead in promoting better health care for all Americans. For example, Richard H. Egdahl, director of the Health Policy Institute in Boston, warned members of the American Surgical Association at their 1977 annual meeting:

The basic question is whether private practice medicine as it currently exists can long survive without the development of strong management organizations with both financial and other incentives built into practice patterns so physicians regularly assess the economic as well as quality impact of their services. The medical profession will increasingly be held to standards which will require demonstrations of efficacy in terms of patient outcomes for diagnostic and treatment procedures. It seems clear that if the profession itself does not provide some answers to the cost control problem the government will. The only alternative for organized medicine is to seize the initiative and provide a cost-effective alternative to a government-run national health care service.[55]

The year 1978 was disastrous for the AMA's conservative leaders, who favored traditional fee-for-service practice. A survey of physicians by the AMA's *Medical World News* reported growing acceptance of prepaid health care among younger doctors.[56] The association had to disavow a highly critical report on HMOs that it had commissioned after federal employees exposed the author's egregiously wrong data and assumptions. Finally, the Federal Trade Commission launched a suit against the AMA, alleging that it had conducted a fifty-year campaign to impede development of "non-fee-for-service contract practices," violating section 5 of the Federal Trade Commission Act.[57]

At the AMA's annual convention in June 1978 its House of Delegates approved the "concept of a neutral public policy and fair market competition among all systems of health care delivery." Further, delegates urged their board of trustees to "seek an objective assessment of HMOs, including IPAs and other group arrangements, with respect to their impact on access, quality and cost of health care."[58] The HMO assessment published two years later by the AMA's Council on Medical Services was well documented and highly supportive of prepaid care in general and prepaid group practices in particular.[59]

Despite the council's favorable report, some doctors feared that HMO restrictions on what they prescribed for their patients would expose them to allegations of malpractice. Malpractice law was more troublesome for innovative and cost-conscious providers than for traditional practitioners during the 1970s and early 1980s. Practice patterns varied greatly throughout the nation, and the profession had no generally accepted standards of performance. Furthermore, the legal standard of "customary medical practice," derived from a fee-for-service system that paid little attention to costs, did not address cost-effective treatment protocols. Indeed, juries often penalized physicians who failed to go beyond accepted standards or simply got poor results. Jurors' attitudes were also biased by the perception that HMOs stinted on care in order to make more money. In the early 1980s the courts still offered no consistent legal position on who was ultimately responsible when HMO patients sought recourse for an unsatisfactory outcome.[60]

Some legal scholars suggested that certain HMO characteristics had the potential to increase the incidence of malpractice claims. For example, subscribers who believed an HMO's promises of comprehensive and preventive care might sue if they got sick. Additionally, patients might be more willing to take legal action against a large impersonal organization than an individual doctor in private practice. But other characteristics seemed to explain why prepaid health plans had historically experienced relatively few malpractice claims. These features included member ownership or participation in the governance of health care cooperatives; the availability of peer review programs for monitoring quality; and consumer access to grievance procedures.[61]

In evaluating physician satisfaction with HMOs critics often wondered whether prepaid group practices attracted doctors with certain personality traits and beliefs or whether such practices shaped physicians' attitudes and patterns of care. Doctors in prepaid group practices of all sizes tended to share many of the same characteristics. Compared with physicians in traditional settings, these doctors were younger and included more women, who may have been attracted by opportunities for flexible scheduling. They were more likely to be generalists than specialists. Although they usually earned less money than did physicians in fee-for-service practice, they had comparatively better fringe benefits, educational opportunities, and retirement plans. Their lower incomes reflected their shorter workweek and greater leisure time. On average prepaid group practice physicians in the late 1970s performed relatively fewer procedures, spent less time in hospitals, and relied more heavily on paraprofessional and administrative assistants. They had more contact with health care professionals and were more likely to seek advice from other doctors than were their peers in solo practice.[62] For doctors who participated in IPAs, the greatest advantage of prepaid care was a reduction in bookkeeping and collection costs; the greatest disadvantage was the potential for financial risk if their health plans lost money. Physicians in both prepaid group practice and IPAs reported problems with lay administrators who tried to control their medical decisions.[63]

The pollster Lou Harris reported in 1984 that participation and acceptance of HMOs had grown among physicians during the preceding four years. Although many doctors who remained in traditional practices viewed their HMO counterparts as inferior and less well qualified to give quality care, Harris found that HMO physicians were as likely to be board certified and experienced as other doctors in their community. Harris found that HMO practitioners were less content with their income but more satisfied with their professional peer support and leisure time than traditional fee-for-service doctors. Highly specialized physicians were least satisfied with prepaid care, and primary care physicians were the most unhappy with their inability to control their work pace. A Blue Cross and Blue Shield poll that same year found that doctors who had joined HMOs believed that they could cut costs and maintain quality, whereas those who avoided participation in such plans thought that cost cutting resulted in poor-quality health care.[64]

Variables used to evaluate HMO services in the 1970s and early 1980s provided compelling evidence that prepaid health care was equal to or, in many instances better than, care in traditional settings. HMOs tended to have benefits that were more comprehensive, and their care, especially in group practice plans, was apt to be better coordinated and more cost effective than in the traditional fee-for-service system. Indeed, several studies suggested that patients who were exposed to fewer tests and less aggressive treatment, and spent less time in hospitals, recovered faster than patients who received more services.[65] Although HMOs covered fewer than 7 percent of Americans by the end of the 1980s and had yet to prove their social value, they had challenged traditional notions about good medical care. The revolution's challenge to physician autonomy was clearly underway.

Chapter 8

Idealism Confronts Realities

Believe me, some of us involved in this from the beginning have deep regrets about the way things have been happening in the last few years.

Dr. Russell Lewis, 1982

The full impact of the U.S. health care revolution hit central Wisconsin during an economic recession in the early 1980s when Marshfield's medical utopia collapsed. GMCHP found 1982 to be a watershed year for many reasons. Its state and federal reimbursement formulas for prepaid Medicaid and Medicare services proved grossly inadequate and threatened the health plan's operating reserves. The federal Bureau of Community Health Sevices (BCHS) discontinued subsidies for inpatient care, leaving Marshfield's Family Health Center enrollees without hospital coverage. In addition, employers' demands for less expensive premiums forced GMCHP to abandon community rating, open enrollment, and uniform subscriber benefits.

Some long-time clinic physicians and administrators believed that the clinic lost its heart and sold its soul to the health care market when GMCHP compromised the cherished principles that had set it apart from all other plans. Younger voices argued that change was necessary if the health plan was to survive in an increasingly competitive environment. The need for HMOs to compromise their principles is a recurring theme in the struggle of health plans to stay alive.[1] In fact, GMCHP did not survive. Competition to control prepaid markets in northern Wisconsin set the Marshfield Clinic and Blue Cross on a collision course that led to a dissolution of GMCHP's partnership in 1986 and formation of Security Health Plan, an organization solely owned and operated by the Marshfield Clinic.

Greater Marshfield's experiences during the 1980s recession are note-worthy because they demonstrate how the loss of a community-wide risk pool and federal subsidies to care for the poor quickly eroded its ability to provide affordable, comprehensive services to those who most needed care.

Hard financial times and increasing competition forced GMCHP to monitor the services and charges of its affiliated providers more closely. My return to problems with affiliates in this chapter underscores the fail-ure of medical licensing and examining boards to protect the public from unqualified and unscrupulous physicians and the extremes to which clinic doctors were willing to go in their efforts to help other doctors improve their care of patients.

Goodbye to Founding Principles

Employer spending on health benefits in the United States nearly doubled, from $49 billion in 1980 to $93 billion (11 percent of the nation's payroll) in 1984.[2] Faced with corporate losses and international competi-tion, some companies reduced their workforces, eliminated fringe bene-fits, or both. Others required workers to pay more of their insurance costs or select less costly options.[3] Many large firms bypassed insurance carriers entirely, developing self-funded plans and negotiating directly with pro-viders for services at discounted rates. The number of employees enrolled in company-operated plans doubled, from 21 percent in 1981 to 42 per-cent in 1985.

Self-insured plans were more expensive than purchased policies, even when they offered fewer benefits and required workers to pay higher de-ductibles and copayments.[4] Nevertheless, such plans held many advan-tages for interstate companies. The Employment Retirement and Income Security Act of 1974 (ERISA) exempted them from burdensome state in-surance laws. They did not have to pay state taxes on premiums, contribute to state insurance programs for high-risk policyholders, provide state-mandated services, or maintain state-specified financial reserves. Budget-ing was relatively straightforward because their aggregate claims varied little from year to year, and they could keep their money until they needed it to pay claims. Their high deductibles and copayments discouraged usage, and data-processing systems could track usage and the costs that individual employees incurred.[5] Firms operated their health plans entirely in house or purchased claims processing, utilization review, and other "third-party" administrative services from HMOs or insurance carriers.[6]

Most companies that held contracts with GMCHP were too small to self-insure. Instead, they switched to traditional insurers that were able to sell them lower-cost, experience-rated policies. In fact, some central Wisconsin agents reduced policy costs significantly when companies agreed to keep workers with serious health problems enrolled in GMCHP. (Workers elsewhere often preferred traditional insurance policies that allowed free choice of physicians, but most central Wisconsin workers wanted to remain in GMCHP because it included all the doctors in their area and provided comprehensive coverage.) Such predatory insurance practices left GMCHP's community risk pool with a progressively sicker population. In order to cut the projected rate increases needed to cover a riskier pool in 1981, the clinic accepted a capitation that was well below its anticipated costs and pledged to cut hospital use by twenty-five days for each one thousand enrollees during the coming year. Failing that, the clinic said it would reimburse the health plan as much as $500,000 for excess days of hospital care.

The clinic's leaders refused to accept rate reduction proposals from Blue Cross that year. Lewis reminded E. Everett Edwards Jr., the Wisconsin Blues' new president, "We got into this venture with Blue Cross because insurance companies had failed to meet their obligations to a large segment of our population. Traditionally, they have excluded people with health risks whenever possible. For those reasons, we insisted on four basic principles, which you have probably heard *ad nauseam:* community rating, open enrollment, no identification of enrolled patients, and no co-payments or deductibles."[7]

The clinic's refusal to modify those principles caused GMCHP's premiums to rise 23 percent for the 1981–82 fiscal year. As a result group enrollment fell 4 percent and direct-pay enrollment dropped 12 percent during the first six months.[8] The heads of many families in the direct-pay program lacked work-related health benefits and were too sick or poor to buy traditional insurance. Charity care was available from the clinic and other area providers, but people who did not have insurance deferred treatment until they were seriously ill.

During rate negotiations for the next fiscal year Blue Cross actuaries warned that premiums would increase as much as 22 percent unless

GMCHP changed some of its policies.[9] Backed against a wall, the clinic's leaders agreed to reduce open enrollment from two 30-day periods each year to two weeks in 1982 so that fewer people would be able to join the direct-pay program. And, after much impassioned debate, clinic leaders also agreed to abandon community rating and first-dollar coverage in its direct-pay program.[10] Thereafter, all direct-pay subscribers were assessed deductibles and copayments: the first $150 in charges for doctor visits, the first $150 in charges for hospital care, and $25 for each emergency room visit. To avoid out-of-pocket costs and increased premiums, many farm families transferred from the direct-pay program into GMCHP group policies offered by their dairy cooperatives. The movement of farmers, with their large families and significant health problems, into cooperative contracts significantly increased the risk in the group subscriber pool.[11]

Clinic officials also allowed the health plan to introduce "Health-share," a less expensive group benefit package with deductibles and co-payments, designed, like those in the direct-pay program, to discourage usage.[12] The partners hoped that Healthshare would attract small firms, but only a few purchased that option, perhaps because union negotiators found that the cost-sharing component was unacceptable.[13]

One irate labor leader wondered why GMCHP attributed premium increases to overuse by subscribers, when, he said, the clinic and Saint Joseph's Hospital had failed to control their operating expenses.[14] That accusation had some clinic physicians nodding in agreement—they had abandoned their uniform salary plan in 1980 because they were unable to attract certain types of specialists who were in great demand and commanded high incomes. The doctors had chosen uniform salaries in 1954 because they considered their services of equal value to patients, but the plan's failure to acknowledge earning-power differences among specialists twenty-five years later deprived the clinic of talent it needed.[15] A new salary scale that reflected market norms enabled the clinic to recruit specialists and in some instances raised the fees and incomes of physicians already on the staff.[16] Some long-time clinic doctors thought that their health plan could have avoided high premiums and out-of-pocket charges if their younger peers had not been so eager to increase their salaries. However, the costs of GMCHP's medical services were remarkably similar to those of other HMOs.[17]

The loss of farm families and other subscribers too poor to afford the new nongroup premiums caused direct-pay enrollment to decline from fourteen thousand in 1982 to less than six thousand in 1983. Nearly everyone who responded to a survey after leaving the direct-pay program attributed her or his defection to higher premium costs, the imposition of out-of-pocket payments, or both. That only 60 percent of the respondents had purchased new insurance suggests that they were having problems finding affordable coverage elsewhere.[18] An unemployed social worker whose family was in the direct-pay program wrote to Lewis that her family had subscribed to the health plan for four years, hanging on and borrowing money from other family members when necessary to pay their premiums. But she did not know how they could possibly manage another rate increase.[19]

Older individuals not yet eligible for Medicare tried to remain in the direct-pay program as long as possible, despite its rising costs, because their health problems denied them access to other types of coverage. As relatively young subscribers left the program for less expensive policies, the proportion of direct-pay subscribers aged fifty-five to sixty-four quickly increased, from 13 percent to 33 percent.[20] GMCHP tried to slow the exodus of young people by charging relatively low rates to healthy individuals and families and higher rates to older folks with significant medical needs. After underwriting began, the new rates for older enrollees with health problems were still not high enough to cover their medical costs.[21]

All these changes and defections of medically needy subscribers deeply distressed the doctors and staff members who had started the plan. Lewis told a friend, "I think we made a sad mistake, but our new leadership did not have enough guts to stick with what had always worked in the past. They caved into a continual clamor to involve the patient in the cost of care."[22] Dr. Gerald Porter, a pediatrician at the Marshfield Clinic, and Dr. Richard Sautter, director of the Marshfield Medical Research and Education Foundation, advised the clinic to acknowledge that its experiment had been a failure and publish the results.[23] Dr. Ben Lawton, who had worked closely with Lewis in developing GMCHP, found the changes so disgusting that he thereafter referred to the health plan as "that slick insurance company."[24] Greg Nycz had argued against the changes as much as anyone but was perhaps more realistic than some. "The dream had lasted for almost ten years," he said, "but employers couldn't afford our premiums anymore."[25]

Nycz was much less sanguine when his Family Health Center enrollees lost their inpatient benefits in 1982. At the time Marshfield's Family Health Center was one of nearly eight hundred federally funded health
centers in the nation but one of only a few dozen providing comprehensive prepaid services, including hospital care, for a monthly income-
adjusted premium. When appropriations for the Bureau of Community
Health Services stagnated during the Reagan administration, funding was
insufficient to keep up with inflation and growing needs. The bureau
therefore discontinued inpatient subsidies so that it could provide outpatient services to more people. Bureau staffers reasoned that intervention
early in the course of illness would reduce the need for hospitalization.
When health center clients required hospital care, they could turn to institutions that were obliged to provide charity care under the Hill-Burton
Hospital Construction Act.[26]

Most of Marshfield's Family Health Center enrollees in 1982 had incomes well below the federal poverty level.[27] Unemployment rates in their
area were substantially higher than in the state or nation, and nearly one-
third lived in areas designated as medically underserved by federal standards. Sizable reductions in federal dairy price supports and high interest
rates threatened the solvency of many family farms. Because of cutbacks
in Wisconsin's Medicaid program and on-going reductions in federal support, the Family Health Center had more than two thousand eligible individuals on its waiting list.[28]

Marshfield's center never received enough money to serve all the
people eligible for enrollment. Because families with the greatest needs
were most likely to join the program, the Family Health Center's patients
were much sicker and required more services than GMCHP's other subscribers. The clinic's leaders considered the program successful despite
funding shortfalls because it afforded poor families comprehensive health
care without the stigma of charity and paid providers who might otherwise
have given away their services. The Family Health Center had to terminate its contract with Greater Marshfield when it could no longer offer
hospital care. Instead, the center signed separate agreements with the
Marshfield Clinic for outpatient services and with Blue Cross for emergency care and administrative services.[29] While similar in some respects
to the former arrangement with GMCHP, the new contracts contained
no provisions for hospital care or subsidies from the health plan through

community rating. Henceforth, the center's operating funds came entirely from BCHS grants, enrollee income-adjusted premiums, and Marshfield Clinic contributions.[30]

Nycz said the clinic never refused his requests for program assistance, but he had less success with Saint Joseph's Hospital, where the Sisters of the Sorrowful Mother Ministry Corporation used profits from its Marsh-field hospital to finance programs elsewhere. After the Family Health Center lost its inpatient benefits, Nycz said, "the hospital only collected about fifteen percent of its usual charges from FHC patients who were hospitalized. I tried to convince them to provide care for twenty percent of costs, about five percent more than they usually collected. Some of the hospital's administrators were supportive, but [hospital president David] Jaye was afraid FHC patients would overuse hospital services."[31]

Jaye later agreed with that assessment and said he resented the manner in which Nycz pressed for his cooperation.[32] The hospital never reduced its charges to the Family Health Center for inpatient care but eventually gave the program a 5 percent discount for the more limited emergency room and hospital outpatient services still covered by the Family Health Center. Although Saint Joseph's Hospital provided some charity care to indigent patients, Porter, the pediatrician who was a Catholic and vocal advocate for the poor, thought the hospital could be "pretty tough" on patients who failed to pay their bills.[33]

Even as GMCHP struggled with rapidly rising premium costs, the hospital refused to give its health plan a significant discount or accept the risk of capitation, probably because it had no competition in the immediate area.[34] Jaye recalled that he "always had 524 beds and 524 patients" in his hospital until 1983, when Medicare introduced its new prospective payment system.[35] Rather than paying hospitals for the care that patients actually received, Medicare's new system based payments on the estimated inpatient treatment costs for each of approximately five hundred diagnostic-related groups of illnesses (DRGs). Hospitals could make money by treating Medicare patients expeditiously but incurred losses when treatment costs exceeded the maximum reimbursement for each illness. Hospital administrators therefore urged physicians to assign diagnoses with high reimbursement levels to Medicare beneficiaries. This strategy of "DRG creep" dramatically increased the proportion of older patients hospitalized with apparently serious conditions.

The introduction of the prospective payment system created a sudden demand for Medicare's extended care facility benefit.[36] Congress had enacted this largely ignored benefit seventeen years earlier to reduce the length of hospital stays by moving patients into less intensive and costly settings. To reduce their expenses and reap higher profits from DRG reimbursements, hospitals encouraged doctors to discharge patients to extended care facilities as soon as possible. As their acute care patient volume dropped because of early discharges, hospitals converted empty units into extended care facilities that qualified to receive additional Medicare reimbursements.

Prospective payment encouraged efficient care and short hospital stays but offered no incentives for doctors to reduce hospital admissions.[37] To address that need Congress created a network of peer review organizations that had the authority to apply sanctions and deny payments when doctors ordered inappropriate hospital care for Medicare patients.[38] (GMCHP's experience with the Wisconsin Peer Review Organization, which I describe later in this chapter, suggests that these agencies rarely used their vested authority.)

Largely as a result of the new prospective payment system, hospital occupancy across the nation dropped from a long-time average of 75 percent to 67 percent in 1984.[39] When Saint Joseph's Hospital experienced an unexpectedly low occupancy rate in 1983, Jaye asked GMCHP to cover his losses. His request triggered a vehement discussion among the partners regarding the hospital's role in the health plan.[40] Jaye subsequently agreed to give GMCHP a significant discount and accept the risk of capitation. However, the Wisconsin Hospital Rate Review Committee, which was jointly operated by Blue Cross, the Wisconsin Hospital Association, and Wisconsin Health and Human Services, refused to approve the agreement because it gave "undue advantage to the health plan."[41] Because members of hospital review boards in other states represented the same interests, they tended to favor discounts for Blue Cross indemnity plans but not for HMOs.[42] When GMCHP decided to capitate the hospital without a discount, its reimbursement proved so generous that the hospital needed no increase for inflation the following year.[43]

GMCHP's group premium rates compared favorably with those of other HMOs in Wisconsin despite its problems with the hospital, financial losses from publicly subsidized and direct-pay programs, and a relatively unhealthy enrollee population. Monthly family premiums for group contracts around the state ranged from $140 to more than $200. All the other fifteen plans provided prescription drug benefits, experience-rated their groups, and assessed copayments for certain benefits. GMCHP's community-rated family group benefit package required no copayments and cost about $176 per month or $180.50 if employers added a drug benefit.[44]

GMCHP's administrators continually sought ways to cut costs so they could attract more group contracts, but their efforts had little effect on clinic physicians who believed that they practiced cost-efficient care and felt no need to alter their behavior for the health plan.[45] Lewis, who was more concerned about losing direct-pay subscribers than enrolling new groups, issued a wake-up call to the clinic doctors in January 1984. Unless they wanted to participate in a health plan that refused to care for people who were sick, old, or poor, he told them, they would have to change their ways.[46]

Getting Serious about Cost Containment

In the 1980s researchers began to identify problems associated with providing too much care, but talk of reducing medical services continued to raise concerns about quality. Because well-qualified physicians showed wide variations in treatment patterns and disagreed about the right amount of care, administrators directed most cost-saving strategies toward reducing expensive, easily identifiable hospital services.[47] While the Marshfield Clinic doctors had become quite adept at testing and treating patients during a single visit, the GMCHP's affiliated physicians still relied quite heavily on hospital services.

Sparked by losses from Medicaid and Medicare, GMCHP had taken uncharacteristically aggressive steps to reduce admissions and lengths of stay at Saint Joseph's Hospital. In 1984 the clinic opened its Ambulatory Surgery Center to reduce surgical and hospital costs further and capture profits from procedures. Clinic surgeons preferred the center to the same-day surgery facility at Saint Joseph's Hospital because it gave them more control over scheduling, anesthesia, and case management.[48] A comparison of ambulatory surgery charges at the hospital and clinic the following year found that five of six procedures frequently performed in both settings were less expensive at the clinic, sometimes by as much as half.[49] (When the Marshfield's nationally accredited Ambulatory Surgery Center celebrated its twentieth anniversary in 2004, it and surgery centers at three other clinic locations were performing more than 20,000 proce-dures each year.[50]) As a result of these and other belt-tightening measures at Saint Joseph's and the affiliated hospitals, GMCHP's inpatient utiliza-tion rates were less than 50 percent of the national average by 1985.[51]

GMCHP also tried during the postrecession period to reduce out-of-area referrals, which were another large drain on its resources. Lewis was initially lenient about such referrals because he wanted to keep doctors and patients happy. As the number of affiliates and the cost of referrals in-creased, he urged doctors to refer their GMCHP patients to Marshfield whenever possible and otherwise to the Mayo Clinic and university med-ical centers in Wisconsin and Minnesota, where he had arranged dis-counts for services unavailable in Marshfield.[52] Many affiliates ignored Lewis's request that they obtain approval before referring health plan sub-scribers to out-of-area providers, probably because he usually approved such cases retroactively and rarely withheld payment. Unapproved out-of-area charges continued to escalate until 1986 but then suddenly dropped by 12 percent when Lewis announced that he would withhold the monthly reimbursement of any affiliate who repeatedly violated the rules.[53]

The opening of a drug and alcohol treatment unit at Saint Joseph's Hos-pital in 1984 had little effect on GMCHP's total benefit costs. Lewis con-tinued to refer patients to facilities out of the area when he thought these patients would benefit from anonymity or a different treatment setting. He also gave retroactive approval to "patients who simply turned themselves in at other centers because they were ready to start treatment."[54] His benevolent attitude recognized the far-reaching social costs of addiction and that patients respond to treatment best when they are receptive.

Attempts to Reform Affiliates

The Marshfield plan was ambivalent about how aggressively to pursue utilization and cost-containment with its affiliated physicians because the health plan relied upon them to provide primary care in outlying commu-nities and the clinic depended upon their goodwill for referrals. But the quality of care that some affiliates provided sometimes posed a real dan-ger to patients and reflected negatively on the clinic and its health plan. Clinic physicians informally monitored the performance of their cowork-ers when providing coverage for their patients, but Lewis believed that

GMCHP's affiliated doctors were at a disadvantage because they practiced "in a vacuum," with little peer oversight and few opportunities for
continuing education.[55]

To make matters worse the affiliates were an expensive drain on the
clinic's capitation; their charges were so unexpectedly high some years
that the clinic recovered less than 80 percent of its own costs.[56] One physician advised Lewis that some of his fellow affiliates were charging for
more services than they provided and urged him to examine their practice
patterns. Lewis replied that profiling of clinic physicians' services had
saved money and that he hoped to do the same with the affiliates in the
near future.[57]

Shortly after that exchange of letters, auditors reported that services
performed by the health plans' affiliates cost the Marshfield Clinic $5 mil-
lion to $7 million a year. Although clinic physicians provided ample docu-
mentation of patient care with appointment logs, routing sheets, patient
files, and an annual audit to confirm accounts, GMCHP's affiliates offered
no evidence for their activities other than their bills. The auditors therefore urged the clinic to protect its assets by developing confirmation procedures for the affiliates.[58]

GMCHP administrators initially focused on one group of affiliated
doctors that appeared to provide the greatest number of inappropriate
services, even though all were board certified in their specialties and the
credentialing committee had approved them. Lewis asked the Wisconsin
Peer Review Organization (WIPRO) for help because he wanted to ensure
that the physicians would have a fair, disinterested evaluation. WIPRO
agreed to perform a review and directed Lewis to submit nearly five dozen
randomly selected hospital records of patients seen by doctors in the
group during a two-month period.[59] The four independent physicians who
examined those records for WIPRO identified many problems with patient care: poor quality and high utilization rates; relatively few appropriate admissions to their local hospital; physical findings that did not support
the degree of severity reported by examining physicians; inappropriate
tests for presenting symptoms; overuse of chest x-rays; inappropriate diagnoses; poor documentation; and inappropriate treatments by physicians
who seemed unaware of adverse side-effects. Further, the WIPRO reviewers concluded that the doctors should make greater attempts to manage care on an outpatient basis.[60]

WIPRO's report caused considerable anguish among the clinic and health plan leaders. They felt an obligation to improve the quality of care that those doctors were providing to their patients, but the clinic doctors were also reluctant to continue their affiliation with physicians who were causing obvious harm to GMCHP subscribers. A couple of clinic physicians volunteered to help the affiliates and the administrator of their hospital set up a quality assurance program and then ask WIPRO to reevaluate the group's progress. GMCHP's partners agreed to terminate the affiliation of the group and its hospital if those steps failed to improve care.[61]

When Lewis, Jaye of Saint Joseph's Hospital, and a Blue Cross representative first met with the group to discuss their report, the affiliates were greatly upset with WIPRO and insisted that its reviewers explain their evaluations on a case-by-case basis. The director of the affiliated hospital, who had hired an attorney to represent his facility and the doctors, refused to meet with WIPRO staff or allow them further access to his records.[62]

On the second visit by GMCHP representatives, the affiliates said that their situation had improved but offered no evidence of change. They also claimed that WIPRO had libeled them and questioned the credibility of its physician-reviewers. Lewis told the group that GMCHP intended to ask for another review of its hospital records, together with those from another small affiliated clinic and—to be completely fair—the Marshfield Clinic and Saint Joseph's Hospital. "This is a serious matter," he warned in a follow-up letter. "We have an obligation to participants in our plan to reach a conclusion as rapidly as possible."[63] The affiliates agreed to meet with WIPRO reviewers in Madison but refused to participate in a second audit. Lewis countered that another review "was necessary to determine if changes have been made."[64]

After reading WIPRO's report, Dr. Sidney Johnson, the Marshfield Clinic's medical director, urged Lewis to end the affiliation of the errant group. But Lewis hoped to improve the group's performance and therefore pressed for the second, more comprehensive audit involving the three hospitals. WIPRO was extremely reluctant to pursue the matter because its reviewers "had never been so verbally abused by a group of physicians or a hospital administrator." In fact, its regional director said that the group was so "extremely rude" that many staffers and reviewers vowed to leave the agency before submitting to another such experience.[65] When WIPRO finally did agree to another audit, the hospital director involved in the first review assured Lewis that "90 percent of the problems had been resolved and there were no real quality problems."[66]

Lewis waited more than a year for WIPRO to conduct the second audit. Meanwhile, GMCHP utilization nurses documented numerous cases of questionable care and inappropriate billing by the two affiliated groups slated for review.[67] The original group showed exceptionally high rates of caesarean sections and induced deliveries, and the serious mismanagement of three cancer patients.[68] Caesarean section is an appropriate surgical procedure for shortening labor when there is evidence of impending danger to the mother or child, but its risks can be justified only under such conditions. This group also had four particularly egregious billing errors, with physicians and assistants charging for surgeries in which they had no role.[69]

Frustrated by WIPRO's inaction, Lewis asked a clinic physician whether the Wisconsin Medical Examining Board, on which he served, would investigate the case of a cancer patient who had received "highly inappropriate care" or whether Lewis ought to ask the State Medical Society or Wisconsin Medical Licensing Board for help. Given the past performance of his board, the clinic physician advised Lewis, disciplinary action by the medical society or licensing board would occur only when care "fell below the minimum standard, not the standard of excellent or average care." Furthermore, Lewis's adviser said there was "little chance of getting satisfaction from the Medical Examining Board in a timely manner."[70]

Eighteen months after issuing its first report but before beginning its second audit, WIPRO asked the Marshfield Clinic to "indemnify it against all liability or loss, and against all claims or actions based upon or arising out of damage or injury caused or sustained by Marshfield HMO or its personnel in the performance of services under this Agreement." Reed Hall, the clinic's legal counsel, thought that WIPRO was trying to abdicate its responsibility, but the partners decided to proceed under the agency's conditions.[71] Six months later the WIPRO reviewers, who refused to be identified, reported that ten of twenty-five cases that they sampled at one affiliated hospital and six of twenty-five at the other had been inappropriately managed. In addition, many of the forty-nine records that they had gathered from Saint Joseph's Hospital–Marshfield Clinic charts were incomplete, although only "a few cases" showed evidence of inappropriate care.[72]

Upon examining the cases selected from Marshfield, the clinic doctors discovered that whoever collected the records from Saint Joseph's Hospital missed significant information contained in the clinic's portion of each patient's chart. The doctors also noted that WIPRO's comments about the few cases of inappropriate care in Marshfield were minor compared with its criticisms about care at the two other sites.[73] Johnson urged Lewis to bring the two affiliated groups before GMCHP's insurance (formerly credentials) committee for further evaluation and possible expulsion from the health plan.[74]

When presented with its WIPRO reports, the original group of affiliated doctors took issue with the conclusions and said that information leaked to physicians and the public had damaged their reputation. Furthermore, they felt that the insurance committee, which represented the standards of their peers, should have conducted their reviews. Lewis replied that GMCHP had chosen WIPRO in order to spare them embarrassment and protect their confidentiality.[75]

Most of GMCHP's relationships with affiliates were more rewarding than those that I have described here. Indeed, some practitioners provided exemplary care and were very cooperative. The clinic ultimately decided to keep the affiliates with aberrant practice behaviors in its health plan so that it could monitor and improve the quality of care that those providers gave to all their patients, not just those enrolled in the health plan. That decision, like so many others made by Marshfield doctors during the early 1980s recession, involved unpleasant compromises between doing what might be best in a medical utopia and what was beneficial for the most people under existing conditions. Monitoring affiliated providers was costly and time consuming, but abandoning patients to doctors who lacked adequate professional oversight was not an acceptable alternative for the clinic doctors. Their commitment to quality patient care is a model, especially for the changing construct of medical practice, which suggests that all physicians take responsibility for upholding professional standards when regulatory agencies fail to do their job. It contrasts sharply with the attitude of HMOs that routinely dismiss affiliated physicians who practice substandard care.

Health Care Competition Increases

In 1981, just as the recession was starting, President Reagan's newly reorganized Department of Health and Human Services (HHS, formerly HEW) allowed funding authorization for HMO development grants and loans to expire and instructed the Office of HMOs to promote private investment.[76] Federal support had given prepaid health care a legitimacy that it previously lacked, but the government's $270 million investment in HMOs since 1970 had yielded only a few hundred marginally viable health plans.[77] Although that investment failed, the recession ignited an explosive growth of prepaid plans, especially privately funded IPAs and preferred provider organizations (PPOs).[78] PPOs are similar to IPAs in that they both provide care to enrollees through a network of independent physicians and hospitals, but they also allow subscribers to use the services of non-network providers for an additional charge. Many doctors favored IPAs and PPOs because they could remain in private practice and collect fee-for-service reimbursements. Investors liked these types of organizations because they used existing facilities and were relatively inexpensive to develop. Consumers found them more flexible than staff model HMOs.[79] On the down side, IPAs and PPOs had many of the same problems controlling utilization that GMCHP had with its affiliates and seldom were fully integrated delivery systems. Staff and group practice HMOs sometimes required large start-up investments, but they afforded the best long-term potential for cost control and quality assurance because their patient records and information data bases were centralized.

Effects of Competition on HMOs and Insurance Companies

Public offerings for various types of for-profit HMOs began to attract considerable interest on Wall Street in the early 1980s. Before that, just a few large multistate HMOs operated by the nonprofit Kaiser Permanente and Blue Cross plans insured about three-quarters of the nation's prepaid subscribers. Private investment quickly weighted the balance in favor of for-profit HMOs. More than a dozen for-profit insurance carriers developed health plan networks in several states or within a single state. In addition, some smaller nonprofit HMOs joined to form for-profit corporations that increased their operational efficiency and opened new markets.[80]

Ninety nonprofit and three hundred for-profit HMOs organized during the last half of the 1980s. Commercial insurance carriers were responsible for most of the for-profit growth.[81] HMO market share nearly tripled, from 4 percent in the early 1980s to 11.5 percent in 1987 because of a growing employer demand for less expensive medical care and an increasing familiarity with prepaid care among consumers and investors.[82] Perhaps following GMCHP's example, some relatively small health plans expanded into rural markets by establishing primary care satellites or affiliating with primary care providers in outlying communities.[83] Despite some progress, physician recruitment problems and lack of hospitals continued to retard HMO development in most rural areas.[84] As in central Wisconsin, competition forced HMOs to improve their operations. The term *managed care* entered the American lexicon as newly trained lay administrators applied business management tools to prepaid health care.[85] Purchasers' demands for discounts motivated doctors and hospitals to be more cost efficient.[86] Computerized information systems became essential for evaluating utilization patterns and monitoring financial outlays.[87] Health plans offered a variety of "products" featuring different benefit levels, premiums, and cost-sharing features to fit their customers' needs. By the mid-1980s more than half of the nation's HMOs had diversified and were offering services such as third-party administration.[88]

In the wake of growing commercialism and competition, HHS allowed federally qualified health plans to abandon all semblance of community rating (such as for similar industries within their coverage area) and underwrite each group contract separately.[89] Those very few HMOs offering direct-pay enrollment to individuals and families not covered by employee benefits dropped such policies or substantially raised those premiums to reflect high utilization costs. Many insurance carriers also phased out individual and family policies that were more expensive to market and administer than group contracts.[90] TransAmerica, Allstate, and New England Mutual withdrew from the health care market entirely.[91] Other carriers tolerated low profits from their health policies if their sales volume was sufficiently high or they needed a health care product to compete successfully in the fringe benefit market.[92]

All health insurance companies lost policyholders during the economic recession, but Blue Cross and Blue Shield plans fared much worse than most commercial carriers did. In addition to losing 889 million policyholders between 1981 and 1982, competition from self-insured firms and new HMOs eroded the Blues' ability to obtain favorable discounts from providers.[93] When their public service obligations to serve the sick outweighed the advantages of their tax-exempt status, many Blues reorganized into for-profit corporations. Others established for-profit subsidiaries through which they could market a wider variety of services.[94] Distinctions between HMOs and other insurers blurred as insurance carriers adopted managed care strategies and HMOs increased copayment requirements.[95] By the late 1980s costs for various types of health care coverage were comparable.

Effects of Competition on Hospitals

The locus of health care shifted from hospitals to outpatient settings in the 1980s.[96] By the end of the decade Americans were nine times more likely to see a doctor in an office than in a hospital.[97] Governments, employers, HMOs, and insurers all encouraged doctors to limit hospital admissions and discharge patients as quickly as possible. Many services formerly performed in hospitals—such as emergency care and minor surgical procedures—were moved into less expensive, often freestanding, outpatient clinics.[98] Nearly one-fifth of all surgeries in the United States were performed on an outpatient basis by 1985, and some observers thought that amount could easily triple.[99]

Hospitals adopted various strategies to cope with revenue losses. They discouraged physicians from admitting "unprofitable" patients who were Medicaid or Medicare beneficiaries, uninsured, or seriously ill with a number of complicated health problems.[100] They discharged Medicare patients from acute-care beds as soon as possible in order to maximize savings from prospective payments. And they transformed empty beds into skilled nursing and self-care units so that the hospitals could capture additional revenue from newly discharged patients. Hospitals with nonprofit status also established for-profit subsidiaries for activities such as drug and alcohol treatment, home nursing and therapy services, and hospital equipment rentals.[101]

Large urban hospitals generally fared well under Medicare's prospective payment system, but some small inner city hospitals and many rural hospitals had to close because they lacked sufficient reserves to absorb the costs of even a few Medicare patients requiring extraordinary amounts of care.[102] Several for-profit hospital chains faltered badly during the mid-1980s and had to reorganize. Others formed networks or linked their services to vertically structured organizations offering a cafeteria of health care services, including skilled and intermediate nursing care, extended care, congregate housing, and assisted living. Institutions belonging to multihospital systems increased from 10 percent in 1970 to 44 percent in 1987.

Although the proportion of for-profit hospitals remained at about 13.5

percent throughout the 1970s and 1980s, many observers worried that the growth and diversification of hospital corporations would have an adverse effect on quality of care.[103] The National Academy of Sciences' Institute of Medicine studied this issue at length in the mid-1980s. A report largely influenced by health care providers on the committee found no appreciable difference in quality between for-profit and nonprofit hospitals, although nonprofits played "a valuable role" in medical education, research, and tertiary care. The report recommended that federal and state governments redistribute the burden of charity care that was falling to particular hospitals.[104] Many of the committee's academic members thought that the data used to make quality comparisons were inadequate. They warned that a substantial increase in for-profit care would reduce medicine's service orientation.[105] One advocate of competition thought that commercial and nonprofit hospitals gave equal amounts of charity care, although some in each category were clearly more generous than others.[106]

Effects of Competition on Physicians

Physicians and other "learned professions" were thought to be exempt from federal antitrust laws until 1975 when the Supreme Court ruled otherwise in *Goldfarb v. Virginia State Bar.*[107] However, few legal scholars in the 1980s understood the full effect of antitrust laws on the medical profession.[108] Although doctors still controlled the delivery of most care, employers, governments, and insurers clearly determined what health care benefits their workers, beneficiaries, and policyholders were entitled to receive.[109]

Managed care organizations created a great demand for primary care physicians, who were supposed to coordinate patient care and restrict unnecessary referrals to specialists. In general, medical schools responded to market forces reluctantly. They refused to teach cost-efficient care and continued to produce an unduly high proportion of specialists. As a result many specialists had to advertise, an activity that the profession had previously prohibited, in order to create patient demand for their services.[110]

Many doctors feared for-profit health care because they thought that it was impossible to serve the interests of patients and investors simultaneously.[111] Observers outside the profession argued that doctors in the traditional fee-for-service system had always faced a moral dilemma because their income depended upon the number of services that they provided.

Some saw as much inherent conflict between prepayment and underutilization as between fee-for-service and overutilization. The economist Uwe Reinhardt described the medical profession "a role model" for for-profit enterprise in the health care industry. Although taxpayers largely financed the training of physicians, he noted that most doctors felt no obligation to provide community service or treat patients for inadequate compensation. The profession claimed to hold a central role in protecting patients' interests, but physicians were not the only ones capable of such trust. Reinhardt said that for-profit managers could be equally committed to the welfare of the patients that they served.[112]

Older physicians with leadership positions in organized medicine strongly opposed the new marketplace trends. Dr. John L. Cory Jr., the incoming AMA president, told an interviewer in 1986, "The AMA has always been in favor of cost-effective medicine, but there is a limit to how far you can shave costs without endangering quality. The AMA is saying to third party payers, 'Enough is enough.'"[113] By then his association spoke for only 40 percent of the nation's practicing physicians, and growing numbers of members and nonmembers were joining the managed care movement.[114]

Effects of Competition on Consumers

Lewis told employers at a 1984 business forum in Milwaukee that "managed care systems wanting to make money and remain competitive are not interested in people who are poor, sick or old because they cost too much money to serve. But one measure of quality service is accessibility to all groups."[115] His words probably fell on deaf ears. Corporate efforts to control health benefit costs during the recession of the early 1980s challenged the social perception of health care as a right. Millions of workers and their families lost health coverage when employers laid them off or discontinued their benefits or when insurance carriers dropped their policies or priced them out of the market.[116]

Workers had to pay more money for fewer benefits after the recession.[117] The proportion of health plans charging deductibles and copayments doubled, from 30 percent in 1982 to 63 percent in 1984. More than two-thirds of the self-operated company plans required workers to pay a deductible of at least $100.[118] Employers justified such out-of-pocket charges as a way to reduce utilization and "make people who used the system pay for it," rather than spreading risk among many in order to support those few needing care at any given time.[119] According to the Rand Corporation, it is impossible to predict when any individual might be among that 1 percent of the population who consumes a catastrophic 28 percent of health care costs each year.[120]

Most employers who purchased care from HMOs were satisfied with the overall performance of their health plan, but labor unions were displeased with the way that companies forced workers pay a share of their benefit costs.[121] Several studies in the early 1980s confirmed that cost sharing reduced utilization. The Congressional Budget Office reported that families that had to pay 25 percent of their bill up to a specified maximum amount spent 19 percent less on services than those with full coverage. Copayments also motivated patients to seek out less expensive and sometimes less effective services.[122] The Rand Corporation found that the amount that patients paid for ambulatory visits was inversely proportional to the number of visits that they made each year. When cost sharing was applied equally across all income levels, low-income groups showed the greatest reduction in utilization. The effect of copayments was unclear, however, because Rand researchers did not yet fully understand the relationship between utilization and quality of care.[123]

Economic strategies used by employers and health plans to save money clearly had a serious effect on equity. As the 1980s ended, thirty-five million Americans—14 percent of the nation's population—were uninsured, most often because they were unemployed, lacked on-the-job benefits, or were too sick to purchase affordable coverage; many of the uninsured were children living in poverty.[124]

Should Governments Ensure Equity?

Several observers argued that governments ought to play a more active role in meeting the needs of Americans who lacked insurance. In 1979 the legal scholar Clark Havighurst, a long-time proponent of open markets, observed, with his colleagues James Blumstein and Randall Bovbjerg that "rare cases where consumers were unable to pay for uncovered but necessary treatment could be easily handled by the health care system's remaining capacity for extending free care." By 1986 Havighurst was willing to concede a "more formal role" for government intervention because competition had reduced the ability of providers to offer charity care.[125] According to an Institute of Medicine report released that year, "The importance of health care for all people, but particularly for those with few resources, is too essential to a nation's well-being and to people's welfare to be left wholly to the marketplace."[126]

The health economist Alain Enthoven and others identified several conditions for an equitable but competitive market, which they referred to as "managed competition." A standard benefit package would allow consumers to evaluate differences among plans and assess the value of add-ons. Community rating and pricing systems would remove incentives for adverse selection and level the playing field for all insurers. An annual enrollment period with adequate information for comparison-shopping would enable dissatisfied consumers to change insurers. Health plans could vary their services beyond the standard package but would require some mechanism, such as certification, to ensure their quality and fiscal stability. And, because public policymakers cannot rely on private institutions to provide charity care, Enthoven said governments would need to supply subsidies to ensure equitable, universal coverage.[127]

Marshfield's experiences during the 1980s showed that HMOs cannot reach their full potential when insurers are allowed to engage in predatory practices and when government subsidies for disadvantaged populations are inadequate. Many needy people lost their insurance coverage or ability to secure charity care. Workers had to pay more for insurance choices over which they often had no control. Lay administrators far removed from their consumers acquired authority to make treatment decisions about patients they did not know. Competition among health care providers during America's health care revolution left a trail of victims, and in central Wisconsin led to GMCHP's untimely demise.

Chapter 9

Competing Values
Doom a Partnership

Marshfield was unique. We showed it could happen and be successful in a rural area, but the experiment didn't justify all the problems we had. We finally had to raise the rates, change the structure and keep out the lame and blind when they were on stretchers.

Blue Cross president Leo Suycott, 1995

Some major players in the partnership that developed and operated the Greater Marshfield Community Health Plan were wary of the alliance from the start. Lewis served as GMCHP's medical director throughout its lifetime and developed strong personal ties with his Blue Cross partners; while the Blues' record-keeping problems sometimes bothered him, he promoted their participation in the plan to its end. Health plan employees in Marshfield, who had to deal with their Milwaukee counterparts on a day-to-day basis, were much less tolerant and often hostile to the arrangement. Yet GMCHP lasted fifteen years and was remarkably successful by any number of standards, especially as a rural HMO. Perhaps it was too successful for its own good.

Changing Corporate Goals

Leo Suycott, who headed the Blue Cross arm of GMCHP's partnership for most of its years, believed that its dissolution began on opening day. "The doctors, especially Ben [Lawton] and Russ [Lewis], were unwavering in their support of us," he said, "but the staff people were suspicious about outsiders' taking advantage of the clinic." Suycott thought that Frederick (Fritz) Wenzel appreciated Blue Cross efforts while he was director of the Marshfield Medical Research and Education Foundation. But after Wenzel became the clinic's executive director, Suycott said, "The staff began to think they could do everything themselves. I used to say, 'They'll only be satisfied when they have a clinic in Milwaukee.' I could see their desire to expand. Maybe that drove them all along. It was unfortunate but inevitable when you bring together two big companies."[1]

The clinic's desire to expand its services and health plan, if not into Milwaukee at least into more of northern Wisconsin, eventually collided head-on with Blue Cross ambitions to control the state's prepaid market with its own Compcare health plan. The conflict had to do with an uneasy tension between doctors and payers. The doctors wanted to provide better medical care to more people regardless of the cost, and to do that they believed that they had to extend their services to reach new populations and expand their referral base to support the growing number of specialists required to provide state-of-the-art care: They had to be big to be good. The Wisconsin Blues simply wanted to increase their share of central Wisconsin's market for financial gain, and they began to show their true colors when they shed their nonprofit mantle.

The road to commercialization of Blue Cross and Blue Shield began in 1978 when the two national organizations began a four-year merger process that culminated in the formation of the Blue Cross Blue Shield Association (BCBSA). Walter J. McNerney, who had presided over Blue Cross for many years, was a highly regarded health insurance leader and social reformer. When the Blues lost $889 million during the 1980 and 1981 recession, he had a falling out with his board and resigned. The newly organized association board then turned the reins over to Bernard R. Tresnowski, a market-oriented business executive who presided over a radical transformation in the Blues' values.[2] Under Tresnowski BCBSA developed networks of new managed care plans and introduced several highly commercial product lines. Many state and regional Blues retained their nonprofit subsidiaries but reincorporated as mutual insurers, sometimes consuming weaker plans in order to enlarge their markets.[3]

In Milwaukee the Blue Cross Associated Hospital Service merged with Blue Shield Surgical Care in 1980. Reorganization two years later created the United Wisconsin Group, a for-profit holding company and the parent organization for Blue Cross Blue Shield United of Wisconsin

(BCBSU) and other subsidiary corporations. BCBSU named former Blue Cross president Leo Suycott its president and chief executive officer. E. Everett Edwards Jr. became vice president and chief operating officer, and Thomas Hefty, formerly with the Wisconsin Office of the Commissioner of Insurance, assumed the duties of vice president for legal and corporate affairs. When BCBSU started its Compcare plan in western Wisconsin in 1982, Suycott told a local reporter, "Expansion of the program into Eau Claire is a major step in the firm's goal to develop a statewide network."[4]

The Marshfield Clinic made health care accessibility for medically underserved residents in north-central Wisconsin its number one corporate goal in 1983. That goal implied expansion of GMCHP because residents in outlying areas often needed affordable or subsidized health care coverage. Blue Cross strenuously objected to the clinic's making unilateral expansion decisions and providing services to other HMOs. At a 1979 partnership meeting Leo Suycott asked Lewis to tell GMCHP's affiliated providers that it was inappropriate for them to contract with multiple HMOs, and he asked the Marshfield Clinic to sign an exclusive contract with GMCHP in order to "prevent further proliferation of HMOs in GMCHP's service area." Suycott also suggested that his GMCHP partners target areas for growth so that Blue Cross could avoid them as it expanded its own prepaid network.[5] Instead of responding to his requests, the clinic officially adopted a policy the following year for using GMCHP to strengthen its referral base. BCBSU's Edwards told clinic leaders that they ought to keep their corporate strategy separate from that of the health plan and urged the partners to adopt joint guidelines for GMCHP's expansion.[6]

Other Sources of Conflict

Conflicting corporate goals was just one of the problems confronting the partners in the 1980s. Marketing practices were another. Blue Cross initially went along with the clinic's efforts to enroll sick people in GMCHP. Such practices were unsound from an insurance perspective but tolerable while the health plan had a sufficient number of healthy subscribers in its community risk pool to keep rates low. But after Greater Marshfield lost several company contracts and its rates climbed in the early 1980s, a former Blue Cross staffer said, "the Blues were in a terrific position to sell its

[Blue Cross and Blue Shield] indemnity policies to employers." In fact, their salespeople were supposed to market the policies of GMCHP and the Blues to the same groups. Blue Cross tried to minimize this conflict of interest in discussions with its Marshfield partners, but according to the former staffer, Blue Cross sales goals "were expressed differently in Milwaukee."[7]

BCBSU's data processing was also an enormous problem for clinic administrators. Fritz Wenzel, the executive director, calculated that reconciliation of Blue Cross data with the clinic's system cost the two institutions an estimated $2.8 million in fiscal year 1982–83.[8] After the Blues signed a contract with Ross Perot's Electronic Data Systems (EDS) in June 1985, conversion problems made the situation even worse. Within the next five months a clinic staffer who audited GMCHP's programs for processing discrepancies found more than five thousand membership, billing, and payment errors.[9]

Lewis hoped that BCBSU would resolve its computer problems so that the partnership could survive the mounting discontent among the clinic's administrators about Blue Cross data-processing failures and discrepancies. He worked behind the scenes, sending copies of clinic-generated discrepancy reports to a Blue Cross administrator because, he said, "you have to know what the problems are in order to fix them." Nearly a year after EDS won the BCBSU contract, Lewis told his Blues' contact that "one set of unreconciled problems involves some $45 million, but the encouraging word was that things seem to be improving."[10] This situation did not improve for some time, however. At the end of 1986 the Wisconsin Office of the Commissioner of Insurance was still receiving twice as many complaints from Blue Cross subscribers than it did before EDS installed its system.[11]

Many of those close to GMCHP's operations during the mid-1980s blamed much of the partnership strife on personnel changes at Blue Cross and the Marshfield Clinic. The Milwaukee people with whom Lewis and Lawton had dealt during the early years were gone, and new administrators in both camps viewed their counterparts as competitors rather than collaborators. Although the original relationship between the clinic and Blue Cross had been built on faith and trust, Lewis eventually decided to involve at least three people whenever he had conversations with Blue Cross staffers so as "to keep everyone honest."[12]

The operational inefficiencies in Milwaukee frustrated the clinic's new

health plan managers, many of whom came from Blue Cross and other insurers, because they were the ones who had to deal directly with subscriber
and provider complaints. James Coleman, who arrived from Employers of
Wausau in 1985, was also "alarmed by the clinic's lack of interest in the bottom line." He said, "Numbers of subscribers were not the criteria for success, because the health plan had to show a profit."[13] The bottom line was
receiving more attention from new administrators in Milwaukee too. Dealing with Marshfield staffers who wanted to run the plan and doctors who
clung to outmoded insurance principles was not worth the trouble, particularly when GMCHP represented only 1 percent of the Blues' business.[14]

Lewis was sometimes ambivalent about dissolution. He wanted to retain a relationship with Blue Cross but was unwilling to let it control the
clinic's future.[15] In his search for answers Lewis frequently conferred with
members of the HMO Clinic Club, an organization that he had helped to
form in 1983 while attending a Group Health Association of America meeting in Dallas. He and the medical directors of the Carle Clinic in Urbana,
Illinois, and the Scott & White Clinic in Temple, Texas, decided it would
be helpful for multispecialty clinics with health plans such as theirs to
have a forum for discussing mutual concerns.[16] The club soon expanded
to include the Geisinger Clinic of Danbury, Pennsylvania; St. Louis Park–
Nicolet Clinic in Minneapolis; Dean Clinic in Madison, Wisconsin; Virginia
Mason Clinic in Seattle; and Ochsner Clinic in New Orleans. The medical
director and chief administrator of each health plan met in separate sessions
at a host clinic twice a year to share information and discuss solutions to
problems that were often peculiar to their types of organizations.[17]

Despite encouragement from other club members who owned and
operated their own health plans, Lewis worried about Marshfield's ability
to run a plan and assume the attendant risks.[18] In addition to diluting
GMCHP's risk, the partnership with Blue Cross gave GMCHP a national
identity. Blue Cross also controlled half the state's insurance and covered
many of the clinic's fee-for-service patients.[19] Some doctors feared that
dissolution would have a serious financial effect on the clinic and that Blue
Cross would be a formidable competitor. "If we wound the Blue Cross
ego," Dr. Richard Sautter warned, "they [its administrators] will find a way
to make us pay."[20]

Blue Cross prepared a long-range planning report for GMCHP in
1985 that identified several issues that the partners needed to resolve.
These included the health plan's governing structure, competition from

other HMOs, and marketing conflicts between GMCHP and Compcare. Blue Cross also proposed that the three partners form a new corporate entity that would give each partner three seats on a nine-member board that would hire an executive director responsible for oversight of existing markets and territorial expansion. Alternatively, the Blues said that they and the clinic could form a separate corporate entity without Saint Joseph's Hospital to "serve as a vehicle for statewide expansion of GMCHP." In areas where local providers or employers did not accept GMCHP, Compcare would seek to initiate its own contracts and agreements. But where Compcare and GMCHP were in direct competition, Blue Cross said that it would "assure that providers could participate in both plans."[21]

Ownership and control issues concerned all three partners. The Blues and Saint Joseph's Hospital wanted a partner-owned corporation.[22] The clinic wanted to own and manage the plan, assisted by an advisory policy board representing the Blues, hospital, and clinic.[23] Lewis recalled that Blue Cross argued that "a policymaking board with veto powers was at the heart of a true partnership," but the doctors refused to give their two partners the power of a veto or majority rule in decisions affecting their clinic.[24]

When negotiations with Blue Cross deadlocked in February 1986, the clinic's executive committee voted unanimously to terminate the GMCHP partnership. However, before the board of directors (all the clinic doctors) could meet to affirm that vote, Lewis sent them a memo outlining his own arguments against termination. In an accompanying memo Sidney Johnson, president of the clinic, said that the executive committee had reviewed Lewis's arguments before its vote and he hoped that the rest of the clinic's physicians would agree with the executive committee's decision to terminate the partnership and establish a health plan that would be owned and operated by the clinic. Perhaps in deference to Lewis, the board of directors tabled the issue pending further negotiations.[25]

One young and very angry doctor called the board's decision "a death knell for Marshfield Clinic as a growing, vibrant organization." He said, "What we saw was a coalition of old men who rallied together to deal a death blow to prospects for future growth. We who are younger must rally support for our elected Executive Committee and very competent administrators against the reaction of overly risk-averse physicians who will retire in a few short years."[26] After drafting one letter that he signed "old man Lewis, M.D.," Lewis responded with another version in which he wrote, "Clinic management is frustrated by their dealings with the Blue Cross organization, and they're willing to lay their jobs on the line to separate. As physician owners of the Clinic, we may lose more than a few management jobs if we fail. If Blue Cross refuses to give us full management authority, we may have to break, but we should try to continue our alliance if possible."[27]

The clinic's vote to table the negotiations produced mixed reactions. David Jaye, president of Saint Joseph's Hospital, wanted the hospital to serve on a policy board if the partners restructured GMCHP, and he supported clinic management of the plan. A member of Jaye's hospital board wondered why the clinic would want Blue Cross to handle GMCHP's marketing when the insurer was selling competing products. "'If I'm the salesman,'" he said, "'I can't serve two masters.'"[28] Everett Edwards from Blue Cross was happy to hear that the clinic had not terminated the partnership. He thanked Lewis and Lawton for their efforts, saying that he attributed the board's decision to the respect in which they were held within the clinic organization. Lewis replied that he was pleased with the results but wanted to meet with Edwards privately to discuss some lingering concerns.[29]

Johnson and Wenzel immediately set out to convince the board of directors to reconsider and vote for dissolution of the partnership. They scheduled two special meetings of the board in March 1986 and distributed to the directors large packets of material reviewing past negotiations and analyzing the clinic's options. Wenzel gave several reasons why he thought it was time for the partnership to dissolve. Blue Cross and the clinic no longer shared the common objectives necessary for a successful joint venture. The clinic was in a strong financial position, and its staff had developed considerable insurance expertise. BCBSU had significant problems with staffing and data processing, and the company was losing money as well as the esteem of Wisconsin providers and customers. Conversely, the clinic and GMCHP had "significant brand name loyalty," and provider acceptance was at an all-time high.[30]

Negotiations languished for several months until Thomas Hefty replaced Edwards as BCBSU's president and CEO in the fall of 1986. At that point Thomas Gazzana, a Blue Cross vice president in charge of health management operations, presented the partners with a final offer and asked them to respond within a week. He said that Blue Cross had lost money for the past five years and was unable to meet reserve requirements for the Office of the Commissioner of Insurance. Therefore, his company was reducing management staff and salaries and seeking financial relief from its vendors and partners. Because Hefty expected GMCHP to lose $500,000 during 1987, Blue Cross would have to reduce the health plan's advertising expenses and clinic's capitation and would require Saint Joseph's Hospital to accept a risk contract. Gazzana said that Edwards might have done anything to keep the GMCHP contract, but Hefty had his limits.[31]

Farewell to Founding Partners

When significant differences remained at week's end, Gazzana suggested that the partners spend their next meeting exploring outstanding issues. If the partners decided to dissolve the plan, they would all benefit from a carefully planned process, he said.[32] But before their next meeting Hefty sent a letter requesting termination of the partnership, and Gazzana told the partners that BCBSU wanted "a quick out" with as little negative publicity as possible.[33] The clinic administrators were prepared for such an outcome. They had applied several months earlier to the state insurance commissioner for permission to operate GMCHP and some of its subsidiary plans if negotiations failed. In September 1986 the state insurance commissioner granted the Marshfield Clinic a certificate of authority to establish and operate Security Health Plan of Wisconsin, Inc., in eighteen counties.[34] The clinic had to assign a new name to its health plan because Blue Cross refused to allow continued use of GMCHP.

The dissolution agreement called for BCBSU to continue as a partner and share one-third of all gains or losses until the end of 1986, when the clinic's new Security Health Plan (SHP) would assume GMCHP's contracts. The Blues also received approximately $1.8 million, the net value of the plan on 30 September 1986.[35]

Greg Nycz was incensed to find that another provision in the agreement allowed Blue Cross to keep half of FHC's year-end reserves, money that the Bureau of Community Health Services had designated for low-income patients. He argued that the Blue Cross–FHC contract was with the Marshfield Medical Research and Education Foundation, not with GMCHP or the clinic.[36] BCBSU refused to discuss the matter, and the foundation eventually wrote off the loss.[37]

Officials at Saint Joseph's Hospital and its Ministry Corporation were also upset. Hospital administrators had agreed to terminate the partnership because clinic personnel had led them to believe that the hospital would be included in the new corporation established by the clinic. The expectation was apparently mutual until several clinic administrators decided that the clinic ought to have sole ownership and responsibility. Lewis wanted the doctors to have full control of the new plan, but he had hoped that SHP would cooperate with the hospital because it needed to keep the hospital's three thousand employees, its largest subscriber group, and cultivate the hospital's expertise.[38] David Jaye and Sister Lois Bush of the Ministry Corporation called upon the doctors to involve their hospital in the new health plan's governance, but their appeals were ignored.[39]

Recalling the partnership some years later, Jaye said he was disappointed when it dissolved. "We'd been together for fifteen years, and it was a pretty smooth operation. We had a good relationship with [Ben] Lawton, [Russell] Lewis, and [William] Maurer but an adversarial relationship with others. Lewis was under a lot of pressure from the clinic, but Lawton's charisma would have prevented the split if he'd still been alive."[40] (In fact, Lawton was very ill and died after the dissolution.)

Nycz thought that GMCHP had been a positive experience because it had stimulated demand for service and improved patient care. However, he said that its greatest strategic value was in "motivating Clinic leadership to address the problems of rising health care costs. What was done with respect to hospital utilization had immense value to this community."[41]

Joseph Voyer, vice president for fiscal affairs at Blue Cross before he retired in the early 1980s, was heavily involved with GMCHP's development and early operation. He, Lewis, and Lawton shared close ties and mutual respect. "The clinic expansion treaded on Blue Cross and Blue Shield markets," he said. "We figured if they ever left us, we'd have a big doughnut hole where Marshfield is because we didn't have anything there. You help an organization get started, but then they want to be on their own. When new administrators took over in Marshfield and Milwaukee, they lost the personal contacts and forgot what we went through. That happens when you get too big."[42] According to Leo Suycott, clinic administrators "built Blue Cross into a big bad bear. Jealousy and pride got in their way."[43]

Security on Its Own

The Security Health Plan (SHP) set off on its own with more than seventy-three thousand former GMCHP subscribers and a confusing array of thirty different benefits packages.[44] The clinic gained much-needed actuarial expertise and some inside information when it hired Robert Mimier in October 1986, just as the partnership was dissolving. Mimier started at Blue Cross in the late 1960s and had helped calculate GMCHP's rates before it began operations in 1971. He lost his job during the company's downsizing, after he had worked on GMCHP's rates for the 1986–87 fiscal year. "The partners were still running the health plan," he said, "but Blue Cross had already identified which groups had healthy workers. If the partnership failed, they intended to 'pick off' those groups, leaving the high-risk ones with Marshfield." The dissolution agreement prevented Blue Cross from entering SHP's market until January 1988, but after that, Mimier said, "SHP's community rating system made it a sitting target for Blue Cross. In order to prevent the Blues from 'cherry picking,' we dropped community rating in the new fiscal year and experience-rated all groups with more than one hundred employees."[45]

Before the split in 1986 Robert DeVita, the administrator of the clinic's health plan, had urged the GMCHP partners to tighten medical underwriting and raise premiums for certain groups. "We do not need to be as competitive as we are," he said, "because our enrollees cannot get comprehensive health insurance elsewhere without a pre-existing condition waiting period."[46] SHP adopted his proposals in 1987, but it also had to increase rates by an average of 16 percent.[47] Later improvement in the clinic's information systems eventually enabled SHP's sales force to develop products tailored to meet individual employers' specific coverage needs.[48] Blue Cross picked off a few healthy groups when it was able to market in SHP's territory, but three other groups with a combined total of twenty-four hundred members dropped SHP because underwriting for the high-risk nature of their work significantly increased their premiums.[49]

Dr. William Maurer, who became SHP's medical director when Lewis retired in 1987, attributed the higher rates to increasing utilization, coverage of expensive procedures such as organ transplants that were no longer experimental, and the comprehensive nature of SHP's coverage. Special rates for farmers and farm families, he said, had to reflect the high-risk nature of farming and its frequent and costly claims.[50]

SHP raised its rates again in 1988 for high-risk direct-pay enrollees and farmers who enrolled through their dairy cooperative. In order to cover the medical cost of farm families with serious health problems, the health plan increased their premiums 25 percent and introduced age-related underwriting and copayments.[51] At midyear half of SHP's financial losses were the direct result some very sick enrollees in the direct-pay pro-gram, which by then accounted for only 5 percent of SHP's subscriber population. SHP administrators calculated that they would need to in-crease the direct-pay premium by 70 percent to cover those losses, but their governing board voted to raise the premium just 50 percent. Even so, direct-pay enrollment declined precipitously the following year.[52]

Nycz feared that continuing losses would force SHP to drop its direct-pay program. His analysis of usage by participants in that program showed some had "very manageable health care expenditures," but seventy-eight patients had incurred an average cost of more than $22,000, or a collective cost of more than $1.76 million, during 1987. Although the health care needs of most people varied from year to year, Nycz predicted that many of these individuals would continue to incur high costs. To avoid "probable collection problems" when these enrollees lost their insurance coverage, he proposed that Saint Joseph's Hospital and the clinic provide a substan-tial discount to the direct-pay program in order to ensure its continuation.[53]

Nycz also recommended that SHP refer subscribers with extensive medical needs to the Wisconsin Health Insurance Risk-Sharing Plan. The state legislature created that program in 1979 to provide coverage for state residents younger than sixty-five who were unable to obtain private health insurance because of serious health problems. The program's funding came from general purpose revenues, subscriber premiums, assessments of insurance companies and HMOs doing business in Wisconsin (though not multistate plans operated by employers), and discounts from hospitals and medical professionals who participated in the program. Lawmakers originally limited the cost of policies to no more than 130 percent of the amount paid for standard health care coverage in Wisconsin's private mar-ket, but the program's high deductibles and copayments placed it beyond the financial means of many people. The legislature increased the pre-mium cap to 150 percent of standard rates in 1983 but simultaneously cre-ated a premium subsidy system for low-income households. It raised the cap on unsubsidized premiums still further in subsequent years.[54]

Risk-sharing plans in Wisconsin and elsewhere were supposed to solve the problems created by insurance carriers that were unwilling to cover people in poor health, but these plans offered no incentives for insurers to enroll people who had serious health problems.[55] Although SHP served more high-risk patients than were enrolled in the Wisconsin Health In-surance Risk-Sharing Plan, the state required Marshfield to contribute to the state risk-sharing plan.[56] In the late 1980s SHP finally diverted its high-risk applicants to the state plan and began to market its direct-pay program only to relatively healthy individuals. Within twelve years the program had nine thousand nongroup enrollees, but only one hundred were individuals who had belonged to the program before the new enrollment policy took effect.[57]

Maurer and DeVita instituted many other new cost-containment measures as well. SHP identified all subscribers' medical charts in order to remind doctors to observe health plan protocols for nonemergency hospital admissions and out-of-area referrals. "Any plan that doesn't identify their members is operating in the dark ages," Maurer said. "If you're a provider, you better know who the payer is."[58] SHP established new protocols for ancillary services, preoperative laboratory tests, unusual drug therapies, and organ transplants. It required precertification for many hospital procedures and moved others to outpatient care. It encouraged enrollees unable to get immediate appointments with their own doctors to use the clinic's newly opened urgent care center rather than the hospital's emergency department, where services were much more expensive. It placed greater emphasis on home care, nursing home care, and hospice services.

With the help of more sophisticated information systems, SHP was able to track and provide detailed reports of clinic and affiliated physicians' utilization patterns.[59] The Security Health Plan also adopted new, tougher standards for its affiliated providers and devoted increased attention to credentialing them and assessing the quality of the care that they provided. New reimbursement arrangements required most affiliates to give the health plan a 15 percent discount but paid them promptly twice a month.[60] However, some things never seemed to change. Despite Maurer's efforts to restrict out-of-area referrals to services unavailable from the clinic or other health plan providers, the cost of such referrals rose from more than $289,000 in 1988 to nearly $535,000 in 1990.[61]

Changing Times, Changing Mission

Rising medical costs, intense competition among health insurers, and new profit-oriented administrators demolished any altruism that the Marshfield health plan had left after the reorganization. SHP's new mission bore little resemblance to the vision held by GMCHP's founders, who had especially wanted their plan to serve the poor and sick. Ronald F. Pfannerstil, the clinic's director of fiscal affairs, had followed the plan since it was four years old and had witnessed many changes in its mission. From his vantage point the plan had become an integral part of the clinic's operation, a way to finance its patients' health care. "We don't go out of our medical care service area to secure SHP business," he said. Although the health plan had lost its social conscience, he noted that "clinic support of the Family Health Center and its provisions for charity care are very generous."[62]

David Gruel, a longtime Marshfield health plan administrator, described SHP's mission as a "buffer between physicians and the rest of the world." He said, "Many organizations want to manage care, but no one is willing to let physicians make decisions about what care to give. The physicians in this organization have total control over the quality of their services."[63] Robert Mimier in actuarial services concurred, saying, "Fewer doctors have ownership and control of HMOs today, but the doctors here make decisions about where we're going."[64]

The doctors' governance of their health plan nevertheless frustrated SHP's medical director, Maurer. Like Lewis before him, Maurer believed that the clinic's executive committee, which also served as SHP's governing board, was far too busy with other matters to devote sufficient attention to the health plan. Furthermore, he said, "what's good for the clinic is not always good for the health plan. The clinic ought to set expectations and cost parameters, but it should let the plan hire its own personnel and manage its own affairs. Publicly, we say our mission is to develop the best outcome quality care for a good price. When we're designed to move money into the clinic, we're at odds with our mission."[65]

During debate about continuation of the direct-pay program in 1988, Gerald Porter reminded the clinic president that GMCHP had started as an experiment to see whether it was possible to serve whole populations. He added:

We have proven that was not realistic. But we also started the plan because some of us were convinced that people who lived "within the shadows of the medical complex" were not receiving minimum or adequate medical care. We help migrants, serve on Ship *Hope* and so forth, but we need to do missionary work right here. Since we dropped community rating three years ago, more and more people refuse care or won't come in because they have no coverage. Since we recently received 501(c) (3) status, the hospital and we must act like charity organizations,

and serve the uninsured and near poor who need help. Security Health Plan—
whose security—the Clinic's?[66]

Porter's letter referred to the Marshfield Clinic's receiving tax-exempt
501(c) (3) status from the Internal Revenue Service in 1987. The clinic
had been granted nonprofit 501(c) (4) status seven years earlier and
earned tax-exempt status largely because of its growing commitment to
charity care, research, and education.[67] The Security Health Plan obtained nonprofit 501(c) (4) status soon after it was organized. But when it
sought tax-exempt status the following year, a legal adviser told Reed Hall
that SHP was "probably not eligible for tax exemption" because "it did not
have a history of community rating and open enrollment for the entire
community to meet the charitable test." As Hall noted in the margin of a
memo he sent to Lewis, "We have seen the enemy and it is us."[68]

Changes in the health plan that he had helped create saddened and
angered Lewis. In 1990 he wrote to the clinic's president,

When I left the health plan, I thought the medical director position was castrated
by the administration, which is now calling the shots. Although it makes good
sense for the health plan to show a profit, the Executive Committee's insistence
that it show a 5 percent profit is 180 degrees from the original philosophy of the
plan—to take care of people who were not getting care because they couldn't
afford to come in. Now, increasing numbers of people are dropping out of the
health plan because they can't afford its cost.[69]

Security Health Plan still had nearly sixty thousand enrollees in 1990
despite its membership losses after dissolution of GMCHP. It remained
one of the largest rural health plans in the United States, second only to
the Geisinger Health Plan in Pennsylvania, which had eight-eight thousand subscribers. The average size of nonmetropolitan HMOs in the nation that year was only about 15,700.[70]

The clinic, Blue Cross, and Saint Joseph's Hospital had set out in 1971
to prove that they could build an HMO in rural Wisconsin, and they succeeded. Their health plan grew and survived until changing corporate
goals drove two of the partners to compete in the clinic's growing sphere
of influence. SHP maintained financial stability in a progressively more
competitive environment because its administrators adopted strategies
common to other managed care organizations. In effect, it kept premiums
affordable for corporate customers by introducing underwriting and co-

payments to the direct-pay program. Before enacting these policy revisions, GMCHP's community rating system had subsidized the direct-pay subscribers, enabling them to purchase coverage for the same cost as group policies. No amount of charity from the clinic or subsidized care from the Family Health Center could plug the hole created when competition forced the health plan to abandon direct-pay subscribers who were too poor or sick to purchase coverage elsewhere.

Perhaps the clinic physicians had been too idealistic when they started their health plan in the 1970s, but they willingly sacrificed clinic profits and their incomes to do what they felt was right. Competition in the ensuing health care revolution stripped them of their vision, leaving hundreds of battlefields, in central Wisconsin and elsewhere, littered with Americans who no longer had access to health care coverage.

A few years after GMCHP's dissolution Thomas Hefty, president and CEO of BCBSU, was back in Marshfield, trying to contract for medical services with the clinic so that he could market his Compcare Health Plan in northern Wisconsin. Marshfield's unwillingness to accept Hefty's terms prompted hims to warn that refusal to do business with his company would be an antitrust violation.[71]

Chapter 10

The Perils of Antitrust in the Health Care Marketplace

We live in the age of technology and specialization in medical services. Physicians practice in groups, in alliances, in networks, utilizing expensive equipment and support. Only as part of a large and sophisticated medical enterprise such as the Marshfield Clinic can they practice modern medicine in rural Wisconsin.

Judge Richard Posner, U.S. Court of Appeals for the Seventh Circuit

The U.S. health care revolution created more adversarial relationships between health care providers and insurers, especially the Blues. Before the HMO movement began in the early 1970s, physicians and hospitals had cozy arrangements with Blue Shield and Blue Cross boards, allowing the boards and doctors to set generous reimbursement rates not only for themselves but also for the entire health care industry. Furthermore, the Blues' nonprofit status and their dominance in the field enabled them to obtain larger discounts than competing insurers by using a "most favored nation" clause in contracts with physicians and hospitals. The rules of engagement changed when providers and insurers became competitors, but the adversaries did not yet understand all the rules. As a result some Blues plans continued to flex their muscles as they had in days of yore.

Thomas Hefty, CEO and president of Blue Cross Blue Shield United (BCBSU), visited Marshfield shortly after he resolved his data-processing problems in 1990 to propose a new partnership in which his company would resume its administration of Marshfield's health plan. When the clinic declined, preferring to manage its own plan, Hefty asked for discounts on medical services for Compcare, his company's prepaid health plan. His terms required Marshfield to assume full financial risk for cost overruns and grant his company "most favored nation" status. Because Hefty would not disclose information essential for determining a capitation rate, the doctors refused to discount their services to Compcare.

Hefty, who had a background in antitrust enforcement, periodically reminded clinic leaders during their negotiations that they controlled a substantial share of central Wisconsin's health care market. Thus their refusal to deal with his company would force him to take legal action.[1] When Hefty rejected an offer from the clinic that would have limited its risk to 5 percent of its fee-for-service charges, the doctors consulted legal advisers in Washington, D.C., about their options and decided to hold their ground. Faced with another refusal to meet their demands, the Blues threatened a "firestorm of litigation." In February 1994 they filed an antitrust lawsuit in federal court.[2] So began a five-year battle through largely uncharted legal territory.

Antitrust Confusion

A scene at the 1993 National Forum on Hospital and Health Affairs in Durham, North Carolina, illustrates just how confusing the antitrust issue was for health care providers. Dean Harris, who was from the School of Law at the University of North Carolina at Chapel Hill and an expert on such issues, tried to clarify the situation. Harris told his audience:

Antitrust laws are designed to protect the competitive market in order to insure that consumers will be able to obtain goods and services of the highest quality at the lowest possible price. . . . For years many people in the health care field were absolutely convinced that antitrust laws did not apply to the field because, as we all know, health care is so different from other industries. It is not like hotdogs and steel and mufflers.

But the United States Supreme Court has made it absolutely clear time and time again that antitrust laws do apply to the health care industry in the same way, not withstanding the unique characteristics of the health care marketplace. . . . It doesn't matter that the laws of supply and demand don't really work the same ways as they would in a competitive market. And it doesn't even matter if what you are doing is designed to contain health care costs. . . . That's not a defense. The antitrust law is applied the same way to health care as it is to other parts of the economy, and so cases in other areas give us guidance.

Asked by a conference participant for some "rules of thumb," Harris replied, "There are no hard and fast rules. And I recommend not getting hung up on the numbers game . . . because the rules for that game were written by the Department of Justice for other industries that are very different from health care."[3]

The Sherman Antitrust Act of 1890, as interpreted by subsequent court rulings and antitrust enforcement agencies, holds certain commercial activities—such as price fixing, boycotts, or refusals to deal—to be illegal "per se," that is, inherently illegal. Other activities are illegal because they suppress or destroy competition under a "rule of reason."[4] Organized medicine had several encounters with antitrust law in the 1940s and 1950s when the courts halted practices by the American Medical Association and its local chapters that prevented physicians from participating in prepaid health care plans.[5] But medical practitioners were largely immune from charges of monopoly until 1975, when the U.S. Supreme Court ruled in *Goldfarb v. Virginia State Bar* that antitrust law applied to the "learned professions."[6]

Before *Goldfarb* health care was considered one of the least competitive markets in the U.S. economy. The tenth edition of *Merriam-Webster's Collegiate Dictionary*, defined a *market* as an economic area of activity in which buyers and sellers of a commodity come together and the forces of supply and demand affect prices. However, economists, antitrust officials, lawyers, and judges often have conflicting definitions for *buyers, sellers,* and *commodity* when considering a specific case. Physicians thought that they were protected from commercial pressures and conflicts of interest by the professional standards that they had developed during the nineteenth century. These standards were based on the doctors' belief that patients were not ordinary consumers and that doctors had an ethical responsibility to regulate their own behavior. Organized medicine maintained professional quality by controlling the training and licensing of new practitioners and enforced ethical standards by prohibiting such activities as fee splitting and advertising. Doctors believed that these measures protected their patients' welfare, but skeptical observers regarded these rules as monopolistic behaviors motivated by self-interest.[7]

After *Goldfarb* the Federal Trade Commission (FTC) and courts challenged many of the profession's self-regulatory activities as illegal restraints on competition. For example, in 1982 the Supreme Court upheld a 1975 FTC ruling that ended the American Medical Association's ban on physician advertising. Additional rulings and investigations in the late 1970s and early 1980s reached into other areas of physician domination. The FTC prohibited agreements on fee schedules. It reduced the profession's influence on Blue Shield and hospital boards. And it challenged physicians' control of hospital practice privileges and state licensing boards for allied health professions.[8]

The Health Maintenance Organization Act of 1973 appeared to encourage anticompetitive economic strategies by allowing physicians to practice in closed panels and set maximum reimbursement levels for their services.[9] However, a 1977 FTC report on the economic benefits of HMOs suggested that cost-saving strategies used by prepaid health plans promoted competition. The report noted that the presence of prepaid health plans in nine study areas had stimulated development of new HMOs by physicians' groups, Blue Cross plans, and other entities and that a "significant" HMO presence usually lowered health care costs of both HMO subscribers and fee-for-service patients.[10] But in another 1982 ruling, in *Arizona v. Maricopa County Medical Society,* the Supreme Court found that physicians had engaged in illegal price fixing when they established maximum fee schedules for their health plan.[11]

After the decision in *Maricopa,* the courts and enforcement agencies regarded physician-operated networks with fee schedules as antitrust violations per se unless participating doctors were in a common business venture with pooled capital and shared risk of loss.[12] The McCarran-Ferguson Act of 1976 raised new questions for HMOs because it exempted certain practices within the "business of insurance" from antitrust laws.[13] The courts were then left to decide whether an HMO's financial arrangements constituted illegal price fixing or were covered by the "business of insurance" exemption as contracting for preferential prices.

Health insurers and for-profit sponsors started many managed care plans during the 1980s, but physicians largely avoided such business ventures, fearing expensive lawsuits. Potential investors hoped that the Clinton administration's health care reforms would deliver antitrust relief in the early 1990s. When those reform efforts failed, litigation involving HMOs accelerated.[14] The Department of Justice and FTC acknowledged confusion surrounding antitrust regulation of health care in 1994 when the two agencies published joint statements describing "safety zones," where they would not challenge certain types of activities. These guidelines addressed several concerns but left many others unresolved until

1996, when the outcome of the Blue Cross lawsuit against the Marshfield Clinic raised new antitrust issues for insurers, physicians, and HMOs.[15]

Blue Cross v. Marshfield Clinic

BCBSU's lawsuit, filed in U.S. District Court in Madison on 16 February 1994, charged that exclusive contracts between the Marshfield Clinic and its four hundred employee-physicians and nine hundred affiliated physicians prevented Compcare from forming physician panels in Security Heath Plan's market. Furthermore, the suit alleged, control of the market enabled the clinic to set high prices and overcharge Blue Cross indemnity plans. BCBSU therefore sought "millions of dollars in damages" and a court order forcing the clinic to divest itself of its seventy-thousand-member health plan and twenty-one satellite facilities.[16] For undisclosed reasons Blue Cross named Saint Joseph's Hospital as a co-conspirator but not a defendant.

The lawsuit was unusual in many respects. Insurers rarely sue clinics to gain access to their doctors; typically, doctors sue insurers for being excluded from managed care panels. The lawsuit challenged the right of health care providers to refuse to participate in a managed care contract that they considered financially unacceptable.[17] More broadly, the suit questioned the conditions under which a multispecialty clinic could legally provide integrated services in a predominantly rural area. Sellers of services are not obligated to deal with a buyer unless the buyer needs the sellers' services in order to compete successfully in the market. For that reason some legal observers thought BCBSU could force the clinic to sell services to its Compcare HMO (at discounted prices, no less) if it could prove that the clinic and its physicians' services were "essential facilities" that the Blues needed in order to compete successfully in the central Wisconsin market.[18]

The Marshfield Clinic responded with two motions in July and September 1994, asking the federal court to dismiss the lawsuit on the ground that the charges were unwarranted. The clinic did not control doctors in ten northern Wisconsin counties because all the physicians affiliated with SHP were free to participate in other health plans. SHP had not prevented physicians in other cities, or large referral centers in Madison, Milwaukee, and Minneapolis, from competing successfully for patients in its marketing area. Contrary to the Blue Cross allegations, the clinic held contracts with a number of HMOs, including one operated by Blue Cross in western Wisconsin. The clinic had offered Compcare capitation terms more favorable than those enjoyed by its own health plan. And, last, the clinic said that its charges were in line with those of other highly advanced tertiary referral clinics in the Midwest and were routinely accepted as "usual and customary" by other Wisconsin insurers.[19] U.S. District Judge John Shabaz denied the clinic's motions and scheduled a jury trial during the last half of December, with a brief recess for Christmas.[20] Marshfield's negotiators met with Blue Cross in November to discuss a possible out-of-court settlement but reached no agreement.

While waiting for the trial to begin, the clinic tried to counteract unfavorable publicity from the lawsuit with an ambitious public relations campaign. For example, it arranged to link a meeting of Donna Shalala, secretary of health and human services, and the National Press Club via a video conference connection to several of the clinic's regional centers, where clinic staff, local officials, and news reporters could see it. Shalala used the occasion to announce that Marshfield's newly expanded medical research center was to be named for Melvin Laid, the former member of Congress and defense secretary. She also praised the Marshfield Clinic for "reinvesting in rural health care to address the needs of our rural residents." Clinic administrators in Marshfield then reviewed the clinic's seventy-eight-year history, noting that they had invested $100 million to create a network of 430 doctors at twenty-five clinic locations in economically and medically disadvantaged areas of the state. Irritated by such activity, Hefty said, "Marshfield has sought publicity in an attempt to make this [lawsuit] into a national debate, which it's not. We don't think it's appropriate to try the case in the media."[21] He soon had his day in court.

After a nine-day trial and jury deliberations lasting only four hours and fifteen minutes, the jury affirmed all the BCBSU charges against the clinic on 30 December 1994. During a separate hearing on damages a few days later, the jury awarded the Blues $16.1 million, somewhat more than the $15.5 million that they had requested. Those damages were tripled under federal antitrust law to more than $48 million, and BCBSU's legal fees were added to the clinic's penalty. Reactions from the litigants were predictable. Hefty told a reporter, "The jury understood our concerns about encouraging competition in the marketplace. This is a major step toward low health care costs for people throughout north and north central Wisconsin."[22] While announcing that the clinic would appeal, Richard Leer, president of the Marshfield Clinic, said, "We are confident the relevant facts presented during the trial will result in a reversal."[23]

Authors of a book that went to press before the lawsuit reached an appeals court said the jury and damage verdicts rendered in Shabaz's courtroom showed that "federal courts are awakening to the monopolization of contracts with providers by managed care organizations. When a single insurer controls a market by sweeping up all providers," they warned, "quality may suffer."[24] A Blue Cross representative from Milwaukee said, "This is not a case about who controls health care in Wisconsin. It is a case that asks who obeys the law." However, an article published in the *Milwaukee Journal* disagreed, saying the case raised "questions about the future of health professionals banding together to run health plans that threaten the profits of insurance companies."[25] The general counsel for the American Medical Association thought that the Marshfield Clinic was being punished because it was successful. "If Blue Cross wanted to make the investment," he said, "there would be no way to keep them out of any market they wanted to go into."[26] Another observer called the Marshfield case "a chilling example of the problems providers face as they try to develop more competitive and innovative health service plans. Rural areas with sparse populations can easily become dominated by a provider." He noted that at least seventeen states had approved or intended to approve laws allowing partially integrated systems and/or doctor networks to apply for exemptions from state and federal antitrust rules if they submitted to state supervision.[27]

Reed Hall, the clinic's corporation counsel, said that the damage award had surprised the jury, two members of which had written to Shabaz after the trial to say that they had not received enough information about laws governing the case to make intelligent decisions and had not realized that their award would be tripled.[28] Hall was critical of the tight schedule on which the trial had been conducted, with sessions lasting until late at night during the holiday season. "I didn't envy the jury having to hear this case," he said. "The arguments involved detailed and complex antitrust theories, including market and pricing issues." Hall thought that BCBSU's lead attorney, James R. Troupis of Michael, Best & Friedrich in Madison, succeeded with the jury by rephrasing extremely complex legal issues into simple questions requiring yes or no answers. [29]

After the clinic filed its appeal, Shabaz upheld the jury's verdict on 16 March 1995 but reduced the damages from $48.5 million to $17 million. He called the jury's award "monstrously excessive," even though jurors were unaware that their damages would be tripled. Shabaz denied BCBSU's request for an order that Marshfield divest itself of two large satellite clinics in northern Wisconsin (which the clinic had established at the request of local providers), but he voided the Marshfield Clinic's agreements with three independent clinics in central Wisconsin and its "free-flow" arrangement with Wausau's North Central Health Protection Plan. Shabaz also froze any plans by the clinic to administer, supervise, or acquire any new facilities or health plans during the next three years. He ordered the clinic to stop collaborating with Saint Joseph's Hospital with regard to allocation of products or services or the setting of fees. He voided a noncompete clause for salaried physicians who left the clinic's employ, as well as agreements forcing affiliated physicians to refer patients other than SHP subscribers to Marshfield. (The clinic had no such agreements with its affiliated physicians.) And he ordered the clinic physicians to provide coverage when independent physicians in their area wanted to take a night off. Sharing coverage is usually a reciprocal activity; clinic physicians would not cover or share calls with some independent doctors because of malpractice and liability concerns. While refusing to "micromanage the health care economy in north central Wisconsin," the judge directed the clinic to "negotiate favorable terms" with BCBSU for providing medical services to its clients. Last, he told the clinic to meet with its employees and send letters to all physicians, hospitals, and employers in north and central Wisconsin explaining his orders.[30]

Three months after Shabaz issued those rulings, the Marshfield Clinic bought full-page ads in dozens of northern Wisconsin newspapers to thank "literally thousands of individuals" who had written letters, telephoned, and given their personal assurances of support. BCBSU countered with full-page ads in the area's five major newspapers that explained what the judge and jury "really said" about the clinic. A Blue Cross spokesperson said that his company's $25,000 ad campaign was meant to counter the clinic's claims that it did not deliberately monopolize health care. "We believe the steady diet of misinformation presented by the clinic cannot go unchallenged," he added.[31] The Marshfield Clinic filed a motion asking Shabaz to stop BCBSU's ads, claiming that the insurer had taken quotations from clinic documents out of context and violated pretrial agreements not to use certain internal information "outside of the public trial." The judge refused to penalize Blue Cross for the ads because evidence presented for trial had become a matter of public record. Shabaz also refused to delay enforcement of the clinic's penalties while the case was on appeal.[32]

One month later the U.S. Court of Appeals for the Seventh Circuit, sitting in Chicago, ruled that none of the lower court's orders was enforceable while it considered the case. In arguments before that court the Marshfield Clinic's lead trial lawyer emphasized six major points. BCBSU had failed to establish markets or market power in the case. Compcare had failed to prove its claim that the Marshfield Clinic was an "essential facility." Blue Cross lacked standing to recover for alleged overcharges. Compcare had failed to prove that it had suffered damages in the amount claimed. And the federal district court had granted improper injunctive remedies.[33]

Marshfield's appeal was supported by two friend-of-the-court (amicus) briefs. One, submitted jointly by the State Medical Society of Wisconsin, American Medical Association, and Medical Group Management Association, advanced four arguments. The district court's order would stifle development of physician networks and limit access to health care in rural areas. The establishment of satellite clinics by multispecialty physician group practices is an effective method for delivering quality health care in rural and other areas and should be encouraged. Vertical integration of physicians into the health care financing market fosters competition. Finally, the brief maintained that condemnation of Marshfield's noncompete covenants for doctors who left the clinic's employ meant that medical groups would be unable to protect their substantial investment in recruiting and training new physician-employees.

In a separate amicus brief the American Group Practice Association (AGPA) argued five points in support of Marshfield. The growth of multispecialty physician group practices fosters competition. The "essential facilities" doctrine rarely, if ever, applies to group practices. The lower court had failed to distinguish a group practice's role as a purchaser from its role as a provider. Mere evidence that a group practice charged above-average prices does not reflect monopoly power. Finally, the AGPA brief argued that "product market" definitions vary from one locality to another.

The Health Insurance Association of America (HIAA) and the Blue

Cross and Blue Shield Association (BCBSA) submitted briefs on behalf of Blue Cross. HIAA argued that a health insurer suffers direct antitrust injury when a health care provider engages in monopolistic activities to secure market power. Exercising that power by refusing to enter into direct contracts for services at competitive prices forces the insurer to pay inflated amounts for its policyholders' health care. The appellate court rejected BCBSA's brief without giving a reason.

While three appellate judges read through dozens of boxes of evidence and testimony, attorneys for the clinic, BCBSU, an independent law firm, and the FTC appeared together on a panel for a seminar at the annual convention of the State Bar of Wisconsin in 1995. Charles E. Burroughs, chair of the bar's Health Law Section, said at the time, "The Marshfield case is to my knowledge one of the few antitrust lawsuits in the health care industry that has been decided by a jury verdict. . . . Most cases to date have been decided at the motion stage. Because of the depth and breadth of the many issues litigated, it is likely the lessons taught by this case will significantly impact how lawyers advise their clients in the future."[34]

Just before BCBSU and Marshfield were due to present oral arguments to the Court of Appeals, Blue Cross invited clinic leaders to a meeting in Milwaukee. Hefty offered to settle for $15 million, rather than the $17 million judgment plus the rapidly accumulating legal fees and interest owed his company. Marshfield countered with a $1 million offer that Hefty rejected.[35] On 18 September 1995 the three-judge panel substantially reversed the Shabaz jury's verdict. Writing on behalf of the panel, Chief Judge Richard Posner said:

If an entire county has only twelve physicians, one can hardly expect or want them to set up in competition with each other. We live in the age of technology and specialization in medical services. Physicians practice in groups, in alliances, in networks, utilizing expensive equipment and support. Twelve physicians competing in a county would be competing to provide horse-and-buggy medicine. Only as part of a large and sophisticated medical enterprise such as the Marshfield Clinic can they practice modern medicine in rural Wisconsin.[36]

Posner, a highly regarded economist and antitrust scholar, determined that the clinic was not an "essential facility" because it did not control even 50 percent of any properly defined market. He said that nothing in antitrust law prevented a firm from refusing to do business with a buyer that considered it the "best." The clinic was under no obligation to provide cross-coverage for other doctors because it "maintains a reputation for high quality by being selective about the physicians to whom it entrusts its customers."[37] Disregarding what Posner called "various furbelows and arabesques" in the Blue Cross claims, he found that the clinic had not colluded with its affiliated physicians to raise prices above competitive levels. There was evidence, "though a little scanty," that the clinic had colluded with competitors, in particular Wausau's North Central Health Protection Plan (NCHPP), to divide markets.[38] Posner therefore invalidated all judgments against Marshfield except one involving the free-flow agreement with NCHPP. On this one issue he ordered a new trial to determine whether BCBSU had suffered any damage because of that agreement. "The burden will be on Blue Cross to show how much less it would have paid the Clinic had the Clinic refrained from that illegal practice," he said.[39]

Posner also criticized the unusual speed with which the jury brought in a verdict just short of $20 million, to which the trial judge added "sweeping injunctions." Posner warned judges and lawyers in his jurisdiction "not to imitate" the way this case went to the jury. "The verdict form contained eighteen questions. If the jury wanted to find for the plaintiff on every contested point, all it had to do (and all it did do)," he said, "was to write 'yes' eighteen times. A verdict so configured . . . does not invite the jurors to use their heads."[40]

Physicians were almost universally pleased and relieved by the reversal. Reed Hall found the appeals court ruling "very comforting" and said that he "didn't expect the retrial to award Blue Cross any substantial sum at all."[41] James Troupis, the lead attorney for Blue Cross, put a positive spin on the appeals court verdict. He said that an order sending one issue back to the district court confirmed that the clinic had violated antitrust laws to the detriment of health care consumers. "This means we have won. Marshfield Clinic has been found to violate the United States antitrust laws. This is not an issue on whether we suffered damages; the question is how much damages did we suffer?"[42]

Shortly after Blue Cross asked Posner to reconsider the case, its lawyers wrote that it "was virtually impossible to reconcile [Posner's] decision with existing antitrust guidelines" promulgated by the Justice Department and FTC. "The centerpiece of the court's market analyses appears to be the belief that PPOs [preferred provider organizations] and HMOs are easily substituted for each other," an interpretation that Blue Cross rejected. Further, the lawyers argued, "the court's holding that Marshfield does not have a monopoly in physician services was based on its failure to consider the Clinic's relationship with and control over many physicians whom it does not employ." The Blue Cross lawyers also criticized Posner for believing that "most favored nation" clauses could foster competition when the Justice Department and FTC viewed them as anticompetitive.[43]

At least in the Marshfield case the clinic's lawyers agreed with Posner's description of "most favored nation" clauses, which they described as competition-fostering devices that payers use "to try to bargain for low prices by getting the seller to treat them as favorably as any of their other customers, . . . the sort of conduct antitrust laws seek to encourage." In their defense of Posner's findings, the clinic's lawyers wrote, "The results of that case seemed to be consistent with the government's standard. Once the court defined the product market as all health insurance, Marshfield Clinic and Security [Health Plan] did not have a dominant share of any relevant insurance market as shown by the fact that Security accounted for only 6 percent of the income of the 900 physicians who provided services to Security under nonexclusive contracts."[44]

Posner's decision did not satisfy the Justice Department and FTC, which promptly filed a brief supporting BCBSU's request for a rehearing of the case by the original three-judge panel or the entire circuit of the Court of Appeals. The agencies noted in their brief that they had jointly filed more than twenty antitrust suits against health care providers in the previous eighteen months and were conducting at least another eighty investigations. They asked Posner to clarify two issues involving a separate HMO market and the legality of "most favored nation" clauses between HMOs and their providers.[45] A Blue Cross press release quoted Troupis as saying that he took the antitrust agencies' involvement in the case to be a sign of vindication for the Blues. "That the Federal Government has entered the case—and they can only do that when it is a matter of concern to all consumers—is highly significant," he said.[46] According to a press release from the Marshfield Clinic, its trial counsel said that the government agencies did "not support Blue Cross's motion to reinstate the verdict." Instead, the agencies' motion for clarification was "entirely inconsequential to the dispute between these parties." Reed Hall added that the Justice Department and FTC were solely concerned about how Posner's decision would affect enforcement throughout the country.[47]

On 13 October 1995 Posner denied BCBSU's request to reconsider the case and agreed to delay the district court's retrial to determine whether the Blues had suffered any damage as a result of Marshfield's free-flow agreement with Wausau while the Blues appealed his decision to the U.S. Supreme Court. By way of clarification Posner said that his interpretation of HMO markets and the "most favored nation" clause applied to Marshfield but not generally to all cases involving health care providers, HMOs, and antitrust laws.[48]

BCBSU's petition to the Supreme Court on 11 January 1996 emphasized the precedent-setting importance of the case for the health care industry. More immediately, the Blues argued that the case directly affected the health care system for 500,000 residents of northern and north-central Wisconsin.[49] Wisconsin attorney general James Doyle, acting on behalf of Wisconsin and twenty-five other states, supported the Blue Cross petition. Doyle argued that the appeals court decision was contrary to previous rulings by the Supreme Court. "If it stands," he said, "HMOs would be encouraged to consolidate and state antitrust lawyers would be powerless to stop them."[50] The clinic's brief opposing the petition argued that Blue Cross had not produced sufficient evidence to support a jury finding of a separate health care market for HMOs, nor had the insurer shown that contracts between Security Health Plan and its affiliated physicians restrained trade unreasonably.[51] On 18 March 1996 the U.S. Supreme Court let the appeals court decision stand without comment.[52] Richard Leer, president of the Marshfield Clinic, said, "This is an important decision for the future of health care. Providers can continue to develop integrated health delivery systems in rural areas." He called it "a victory for the residents of central and northern Wisconsin and for rural America."[53]

In light of the Supreme Court's refusal to take up the case, the FTC announced that it would undergo a substantial review of its enforcement policies. Limits on physician network size were a major source of controversy between organized medicine and antitrust enforcers. Insurers forming managed care networks were able to contract with as many physicians in an area as they wanted. But the government had limited the size of physician-organized networks because doctors technically are "sellers" of medical services and antitrust doctrine is designed to protect "buyers." However much the government disagreed, the size of Marshfield's network meant little to the appellate court because Security Health Plan's nine hundred affiliated doctors derived so little of their income from the plan.[54]

Posner remanded the case to U.S. District Judge Barbara Crabb in Madison for a retrial to determine whether the free-flow agreement had damaged the Blues. Daryl Bell, a Milwaukee lawyer not involved in the suit, called the retrial a "footnote" in the case. Otherwise, Bell said, "Marshfield Clinic's victory means rural health care delivery systems are viable even if they're large, and even if they have a high percentage of the number of doctors in the area." And, he added, "The ruling may inhibit Blue Cross in negotiating financial arrangements with HMOs, hospitals and other providers. But the possibility of antitrust litigation has aided Blue Cross in such negotiations."[55]

Before the second trial the Marshfield Clinic calculated its legal costs at $4.5 million, approximately $3.5 million for trial lawyers' fees and another $1 million for expert witnesses and other litigation-related expenses.[56] Warren Greenberg, a professor of health economics at George Washington University in Washington, D.C., had been retained by Blue Cross and served as an expert witness at the initial trial. Writing shortly after the U.S. Supreme Court refused to hear the case, Greenberg estimated that Blue Cross had spent about $3 million on the lawsuit but stood to gain at least $17.1 million in damages if it was successful. He said, "With a benefit-cost ratio of seventeen to three, Blue Cross needed less than a 20 percent chance of winning in order to bring this suit. Blue Cross of course had to take into consideration risks such as the potential evidence would not be as convincing as it believed." Greenberg maintained that BCBSU's efforts to lower medical costs and provide alternative health care plans in the clinic's area of influence were done "for the public good" and worth the risk.[57]

After several months of motions to determine the scope of the retrial, Crabb removed Compcare from the case on 10 September 1996 because the appeals court had already thrown out its claims of injury. Crabb told Blue Cross that it would have to prove that it suffered damages as a result of an inappropriate allocation of markets between the Marshfield Clinic and its competitors; however, if damage was proved, the award did not have to be restricted to the $594,883 judgment from the first trial. She voided Marshfield's agreements with competing plans or groups but allowed its legitimate joint ventures to continue.[58] A lawyer for BCBSU said that Blue Cross planned to prove that Marshfield's division of markets had caused "$4 million to $6 million in damages, which would be tripled under antitrust law." But Crabb rejected BCBSU's damages claim on 1 April 1997, saying:

It appears from the expert reports that plaintiff has filed in preparation for the new trial on damages that it views as a magnanimous invitation the small window of opportunity left it by the Court of Appeals and by the 10 September 1996 order. Far from taking the $594,883 as a starting point from which it would attempt to show how much of that amount was attributable to the anticompetitive action that the Court of Appeals has found to be a true antitrust violation, plaintiff computes its damages from scratch, with a new definition of market and two whole new constructs of damages, each amounting to more than $7 million.

It is difficult not to view plaintiff's expert reports with a jaundiced eye, given the huge discrepancy between the current damage calculations and those offered at the first trial. Plaintiff's experts have calculated damages resulting from market division seven times higher than the damages caused by market division together with monopoly, price fixing and other illegal acts at the first trial.[59]

Crabb also criticized the Blues for attributing all their losses to Marshfield's illegal conduct. She dismissed the case the following week, noting that Blue Cross "has no evidence it can introduce at trial that would enable the jury to make an informed decision about the amount of damages, if any, that it suffered from the antitrust violation at issue." Further, she said that "the plaintiff had nineteen months in which to consider the implications of the Court of Appeals' decision and to have its experts prepare to respond to them. That it put all its eggs into one basket is not the fault of defendants or any of the courts that have dealt with this case."[60] On appeal from Blue Cross, Crabb reaffirmed her decision to close the case. And because the Blues were unable to prove any damages, she removed her previous injunction limiting Marshfield's agreements.[61]

When BCBSU appealed Crabb's decision to the seventh circuit, Posner called the damage reports submitted by Blue Cross's economic experts worthless and affirmed Crabb's ruling absolving the clinic and SHP of damages. Because the clinic had been found guilty of dividing markets with the North Central Health Protection Plan in Wausau, however, he advised Crabb to restore her injunctions against Marshfield and order that the clinic pay BCBSU's legal costs for this particular issue.[62] After the U.S. Supreme Court refused to hear the Blues' appeal on 11 January 1999, Crabb voided agreements between the clinic and other providers that allocated customers, territories, or service markets. But she said that nothing in her order should be construed as prohibiting the Marshfield Clinic from retaining or entering new agreements that would be lawful under antitrust law as legitimate business ventures.

In fact, the Marshfield Clinic had engaged in several new business ventures during the lawsuit. In 1995 it acquired the Family Health Clinic of Merrill, a century-old practice in north-central Wisconsin with eleven physicians and a support staff of fifty-five employees.[63] The following year the clinic joined several health care providers in forming Aegishealth, a partnership providing "a comprehensive range of locally-accessible, high-quality and cost-competitive health service products" in several western Wisconsin communities. Planning for that joint venture began in 1994 and developed in response to research outlining the needs and demands of these communities. At its inception the Aegishealth network included 4,250 hospital, clinic, and medical office employees throughout western and central Wisconsin.[64]

SHP began marketing its policies in Wausau shortly after Shabaz's initial ruling in 1995. The following year the Marshfield Clinic signed an agreement to acquire Wausau Medical Center, pending FTC approval. At that time the center was a seventy-three-physician multispecialty group with 450 employees at five locations in two counties.[65] The Wisconsin attorney general, the Federal Trade Commission, and Judge Crabb signed off on the merger in mid-1997, and Wausau Medical Center officially joined the clinic's system on 1 October 1997.[66]

Six days later the clinic announced an agreement with the Group Health Cooperative of Eau Claire in western Wisconsin, whereby the medical practices, physicians, and staff at four Group Health locations were incorporated into the clinic's health care system, effective 1 January 1998.[67] Eighteen months later the Marshfield Clinic–Eau Claire Center opened a new $14.5 million, ninety thousand–square-foot primary and secondary health care facility for approximately seventy providers. The center also houses the Marshfield Clinic's western Wisconsin administrative offices.[68]

Piggyback Lawsuits

The clinic's leaders hailed their various acquisitions as efforts to provide Wisconsin residents with better access to high-quality, cost-efficient care, but some patients were not impressed. Shortly after Crabb received the Blue Cross–Marshfield Clinic case in 1996, a Marshfield couple filed a class action suit against the clinic and Security Health Plan.[69] That suit was quickly followed by a second, which named the North Central Health Protection Plan and Rhinelander Medical Center, as well as the clinic and SHP, as defendants.[70] Both suits claimed that the defendants had conspired to eliminate competition and raise prices among the region's health care providers. The plaintiffs asked Crabb to consolidate their cases with the Blue Cross case then before her court. She rejected their request on the ground that the issues were substantially different. Moreover, she said it would be inappropriate to delay the Blue Cross case for up to eighteen months "while the class actions unfolded."[71]

A third class action was filed a short while later on behalf of some Medicaid patients and the Wisconsin Department of Health and Family Services, which administers the state's Medicaid program. This lawsuit named the same defendants and accused them of charging "excessive, noncompetitive and unreasonable" prices.[72] Reed Hall called the case "very unusual," noting that "we're forced by the state to accept a very reduced fee schedule, which we have done for many, many years. Now the state has, in effect, accused the Clinic of overcharging."[73]

Crabb consolidated the three class action lawsuits and ruled that the case would cover anyone who had purchased health care from the defendants in eight north-central Wisconsin counties after 24 July 1992 (approximately 200,000 patients).[74] Rhinelander Medical Center subsequently settled with the plaintiffs for $57,000, and NCHPP agreed to pay them $650,000. Crabb denied a clinic motion to dismiss the case. Although the plaintiff's expert evidence of "supra competitive prices" was not compelling, she said it was sufficient to go to trial. Crabb told the plaintiffs that they could win their case by establishing several independent illegal market allocation agreements and proving that those agreements caused them to suffer.[75] The Marshfield Clinic denied any wrongdoing but offered a $4 million settlement, which the judge accepted before the case went to trial. Part of the settlement went to pay the plaintiffs' legal fees and other expenses; $1,000 went to each of the six plaintiffs named in the suits; and approximately $2.5 million was distributed to charities offering health care to low-income residents in north-central Wisconsin. Other features of the settlement approved by Crabb barred the clinic from engaging in anticompetitive practices or discriminating against nonclinic physicians. For a two-year period the clinic also agreed to limit its fee increases for medical services to approximately 5 percent each year and to maintain its current level of uncompensated charity care, which averaged $4.8 million annually.[76]

With most of their disputes settled after five years of litigation, the clinic and Blue Cross signed a preferred provider agreement in January 1999, giving BCBSU's 500,000 indemnity policyholders and Compcare's 200,000 managed care patients throughout Wisconsin access to clinic physicians. In announcing the new contract, William Hocking, president of the Marshfield Clinic, told a reporter that he had begun talks with Hefty the previous year in an effort "to put our legal issues behind us and better serve patients throughout the state." Hocking said that they had reached agreement because BCBSU had dropped its demands for a "most favored nation" clause.[77]

The clinic's claims on a $10 million insurance policy that it had purchased from Aetna and Travelers for antitrust coverage in 1992 provided an ironic ending to the case brought by the Blues. The clinic's costs in the Blue Cross and related lawsuits exceeded its policy limits, but the insurers refused to cover even the legal expenses up to those limits. A clinic lawsuit claiming breach of contract was eventually transferred to U.S. District Court, bringing the case back to Judge John Shabaz. After extensive negotiations the parties reached a settlement in which Aetna and Travelers agreed to pay all but $350,000 of the $10 million policy. Shabaz accepted the agreement and canceled a trial that he had scheduled for November 1999.[78]

Reactions to the Antitrust Lawsuit and New Enforcement Guidelines

Reactions to the outcome of the Blue Cross–Marshfield lawsuit varied widely in the legal community. Mark L. Glassman, writing in the *American University Law Review* after the Supreme Court let the appellate decision stand, said, "The ability to define the relevant product market and determine market power within that market is crucial to virtually all antitrust actions in the health care field." Because the Supreme Court refused to review the appellate decision, Glassman and others predicted that questions of how to define an HMO's market and how to assess market power were likely to be the subject of considerable antitrust litigation in the future.[79]

William M. Sage, a physician, attorney, and professor of health law at

Columbia University, criticized Posner's decision for its sweeping generalizations about health care and lack of empirical foundation. He said that the decisiveness and breadth of that ruling surprised the health care bar because it contradicted recent policy statements by the Justice Department and FTC, which share responsibility for antitrust oversight. The agencies' guidelines lack the force of law, Sage said, but Posner's decision carried considerable weight elsewhere because of his reputation "as a brilliant and respected legal scholar. . . . Empirical research in health care antitrust litigation is desperately needed to generate a clear vocabulary, to formulate a standard analytical approach, to frame the key issues, and to support or refute common assertions about managed care markets." Without such research, Sage concluded, "the application of antitrust law to managed care will be fitful at best."[80]

Clark Havighurst, a long-time promoter of health care competition, was an influential antitrust scholar at Duke University School of Law. His amicus brief in the 1975 *Goldfarb* case had urged the Supreme Court to view learned professions as purveyors of ordinary commerce. Testifying before the House Judiciary Committee in 1996, he criticized the FTC and Justice Department for restraining competition in the medical marketplace: "The irony is that the [two agencies] have yet to recognize their own success in bringing real competition in American health care, or to entrust decisions to the marketplace they have so ably fostered."[81]

New antitrust guidelines published by both agencies a short while later recognized that clinical integration could provide the same efficiencies as risk sharing and that methods of risk sharing other than capitation and withholding provider reimbursements could encourage competition and reductions in health care costs.[82] The agencies therefore agreed to review proposals for physician-operated networks on a case-by-case basis, rather than using rigid formulas, as they had in the past.[83]

Warren Greenberg, BCBSU's expert economic witness, was highly critical of Posner for overturning most elements of the lower court's jury verdict but acknowledged "how complex many of the concepts in the industrial organization of health care can be." Greenberg noted that the joint guidelines of the Justice Department and FTC, first issued in 1996, based the legality of physician networks on "rule of reason" criteria rather than defining them as price-fixing networks that are illegal per se. The "rule of reason" in these new guidelines, Greenberg explained, required antitrust authorities to take into account "significant efficiencies that benefit consumers" as well as the structure of the physician services market in a defined geographic area. "New empirical work is needed," he said, "to help calculate the benefits and costs of vertical integration as well as the variety of physician networks."[84] In effect, Greenburg acknowledged that providing quality health care services to widely dispersed, disadvantaged rural populations requires a degree of provider cooperation that might be considered anticompetitive in other circumstances.

Robert Kuttner, a health policy analyst and frequent contributor to the *New England Journal of Medicine,* observed that antitrust policy had come nearly full circle in two decades when the FTC and Justice Department liberalized their joint antitrust guidelines on health care in 1997: "Before the 1975 *Goldfarb* case, physicians were insulated from commercial pressures and conflicts of interest by professional norms that had evolved over nearly a century, buttressed by legally sanctioned self-regulation. But when the courts and antitrust agencies started to apply market principles to medicine, self-regulation came to be perceived as the enemy of healthy competition." Antitrust enforcement overturned the sovereignty of physicians in the name of consumer choice, but consumer choice suffered in the competitive system that ensued. According to Kuttner, "There is no other industry in which the consumer's purported agent supposedly maximizes the consumer's satisfaction by withholding products the consumer desires."[85]

Consumers in a competitive market usually discipline producers by making free and informed choices based on price and quality. But because of third-party insurance, the specialized nature of medical expertise, and such factors as risk selection, medicine is no ordinary market. "Now having demolished professional self-regulation as a means of consumer protection," Kuttner concluded, "the antitrust authorities have decided that physicians can have a virtuous, pro-consumer role in the marketplace after all. Doctors, at last, have a somewhat level playing field on which to pursue the practice of medicine as ordinary commerce. But doubts remain about whether medicine is, or ought to be, ordinary commerce."[86]

Posner's evaluation of health care markets in northern Wisconsin and his rulings in *Blue Cross v. Marshfield Clinic* raised many new questions about antitrust guidelines, but his vindication of the Marshfield Clinic clearly resolved several issues pertaining to rural health care delivery. Sara Rosenbaum, a professor of health care sciences at the George Washington University Medical Center, was generally supportive of Posner's decision.

Writing in *Law and the American Health Care System*, she said, "Division of markets, where proven, constitutes a per se violation of antitrust law because of its pernicious effects on competition. But consider the effects of applying this principle in a sparsely populated rural area ... where distances are great, physician practice is difficult and where there are relatively few 'insured lives' to support health care financing arrangements operating on a financial risk basis." Given the "confusing jumble of managed care products today," she wondered how HMOs fit into the health care financing market. "Regardless of that issue, the theme that continuously simmers below the surface of Judge Posner's decision in the Marshfield case is the Clinic's dominance of the geographic region in which it is located." Rosenbaum said:

The Marshfield Clinic is much more intriguing than Judge Posner's ruling is able to express. . . . In fact, the Marshfield Clinic is quite legendary, both as a model of rural health care delivery and for its impact on health care access in a large, remote rural area of the state in which more than 402,000 persons are completely uninsured and 627,000 residents can be classified as medically underserved because of poverty, lack of health insurance, or both. . . .

The Marshfield Clinic has made two important contributions to the northern region of the state. First, as Judge Posner notes, the Clinic enjoys a national reputation for the quality of its medical care. This is a particular feat given the isolation in which the area's physicians live and work. . . . Marshfield has built a sort of health care "ecosystem" for residents who otherwise would have been left with virtually no accessible care. Second, the Marshfield Clinic has undertaken these efforts not only for the region's more affluent and insured populations but for individuals who are too poor to purchase health insurance on an unsubsidized basis.

The Marshfield Clinic story is illustrative of the important policy concerns that arise when principles of competition are superimposed on a health care system in a nation that has not yet chosen to level the playing field for all consumers through a national health insurance system. With competition would come risk selection, risk segmentation and price reductions for "good risks." As a result, the small promise of universal access found in this area of Wisconsin would inevitably collapse.[87]

Some Final Reflections

The Blues challenged the Marshfield Clinic's health care system in central Wisconsin because they were willing to risk a few million dollars in legal costs to maintain their status as the state's preeminent insurer, certainly not because they had a better product, provided superior service, or wanted to assist populations in great need of care. Marshfield emerged from this skirmish scathed but emboldened by its vindication. Although the particulars of this conflict do not have broad application, the legal rulings certainly protect other rural health care providers that are attempting to serve patients in areas where returns on investment are sometimes notably low. In the course of the U.S. health care revolution, the central Wisconsin battle was one of a few instances in which the desire to provide better service bested a craving for more money, power, and influence.

Chapter 11

HMOs and Public Programs in the 1990s and Early 2000s

> Until we insist that all Americans—including the retired—contribute to the costs of their health care as far as they are able; until we acknowledge that additional benefits for those with insurance are less vital than providing basic care for the uninsured, the political finagling over health care in Washington is likely to do more harm than good.
>
> David S. Broder, 1999

HMO involvement with federally subsidized public health care programs during the 1970s and 1980s was a dismal failure. By the late 1980s HMOs were serving only about 11 percent of the nation's Medicaid population because of the problems of dealing with a constantly changing beneficiary population and lack of state-level support for prepaid contracting.[1] Senior citizens receiving care from HMOs and other managed care organizations under prepaid capitated (risk) contracts accounted for only 3.3 percent of the Medicare beneficiary population in 1990.[2] Health plans with Medicare contracts were invariably located in high reimbursement areas. Because these plans usually excluded applicants with serious health problems, their reimbursements (based on the average cost of caring for all beneficiaries in their area) were relatively high and service costs low. Instead of helping Medicare save money, these plans creamed the system.

The federal Bureau of Community Health Services (BCHS) was still subsidizing health care for low-income families and individuals in medically underserved areas but had not funded inpatient services—a necessary component of comprehensive prepaid care—since in the early 1980s. Marshfield's Family Health Center weathered a storm of funding cuts from the BCHS and was able to continue its program without a hospital care component because it obtained income from various public and private insurance programs and generous support from the Marshfield Clinic.

GMCHP's adventures with prepaid Medicaid, and a Medicare risk-contracting demonstration in the late 1970s and early 1980s, were financially disastrous for the health plan. Afterward, the clinic reverted to serving Medicaid beneficiaries on a fee-for-service basis. It also developed the Senior Security Health Plan, a program for Medicare beneficiaries financed by monthly premiums from subscribers and by Medicare's fee-for-service reimbursements, which were much more generous than Medicare's risk-contracting capitation payments.

The federal and state governments introduced several new initiatives in the 1990s to encourage more HMO involvement in Medicaid, Medicare, community health centers, and other programs designed to serve disadvantaged populations. Because it had been burned so often in the past, the Marshfield Clinic adopted a rather atypical wait-and-see approach to some of the new opportunities but enthusiastically grabbed at others. I described Marshfield's experience with Medicaid and Medicare in chapter 5 in order to illustrate why HMOs were so reluctant to enter contracts with those two programs. In this chapter I first describe how new initiatives in the 1990s were received at the state and national level and then compare those responses with Marshfield's. Before that, however, I want to review a few initiatives that failed to survive the early 1990s.

Failed Reforms in the Early 1990s

President Bill Clinton's administration proposed several health care reforms in the early 1990s that would have extended health care services to all Americans by changing funding mechanisms and requiring government compensation to insurers that incurred extra costs when accepting high-risk patients. The failure of his proposals to gain approval marked the fifth time in sixty years that Congress had refused to accept a presidential call for universal health care.[3] Instead, Congress and state legislatures enacted a series of piecemeal initiatives to reduce public costs by increasing the enrollment of public beneficiaries in HMOs.

Washington observers blamed the demise of Clinton's ambitious Health Security Bill on political miscalculations by the White House, tactical blunders on Capitol Hill, relentless attacks by special interest groups, and uncertainty among voters.[4] Extensive media ad campaigns by special interest groups demonstrated some of the most sophisticated persuasion techniques that money could buy. Highly controversial television ads by the Health Insurance Association of America featured "Harry and Louise," an ordinary couple who feared that Clinton's program would ration their health care, force them to change doctors, and create "mandatory government health alliances . . . run by tens of thousands of new bureaucrats."[5] The Health Care Leadership Council, representing major pharmaceutical companies, insurance carriers, and hospitals, launched a $225,000 ad campaign on radio stations in nine states, hoping to convince members of targeted congressional committees to oppose White House proposals for insurance price controls and health care spending limits.

The American Medical Association spent at least as much on print advertisements that were aimed at opinion leaders in the capital and other metropolitan areas and warned, "What You Don't Know Can Hurt You." The Patient Access to Specialty Care Coalition, representing eighty physician and patient organizations, lobbied to ensure that Clinton's emphasis on managed care would not restrict patients' access to medical specialists or specialists' access to patients. In addition, trade groups such as the National Federation of Independent Business, National Restaurant Association, and National Association of Wholesale Distributors encouraged their members to oppose any bill before Congress that would require employers to finance health care coverage for workers.[6]

In the midst of debate about Clinton's proposals, the veteran health policy and public opinion analyst Robert J. Blendon noted that most Americans thought that adequate health care for all citizens was an exceedingly important national goal. But he said that public support weakened when proposals for universal care introduced new financing mechanisms or limited certain types of services.[7] A Kaiser Family Foundation survey reported similar findings at the end of the decade. Sixty percent of respondents acknowledged that a growing number of Americans lacked health insurance, but just as many people erroneously believed that the uninsured came from families in which no one worked. Nearly half, moreover, were unwilling to add five or more dollars to their premiums or taxes in order to help provide coverage for the uninsured.[8]

When Robert Blendon and John M. Benson, managing directors of the Harvard Opinion Research Program at the Harvard School of Public Health, reviewed more than one hundred public opinion surveys conducted between 1950 and 2000, they found many conflicting views about the nation's health policy. The surveys showed much dissatisfaction with the health care system, private health insurance, and managed care companies, and general support for a national health plan. However, most Americans were satisfied with their current medical arrangements, did not trust the federal government to do what was right, and did not favor a single-payer type of national health plan. Confidence in the leaders of medicine declined during that period, but most Americans continued to trust the honesty and ethical standards of individual physicians.[9]

Few Americans realized that federal tax subsidies to employers, and tax-supported health insurance for the poor and elderly, paid for most of most of the nation's health care bills. According to the World Health Organization, in 2000 the United States spent about $2,500 on health care for each citizen, more than any other country in the world. Although medical costs in the United States were at least 50 percent more per person than in Switzerland, Germany, and France, and twice as much as in all other industrialized countries, American health care standards ranked a lowly thirty-seventh among the world's nations.[10] Of the ten most technologically advanced countries, the United States had the highest infant mortality rate, lowest life expectancy, and proportionally largest uninsured population.[11] Some observers contend that sufficient data are not available to make international comparisons.[12] However, comparisons clearly point to reasons for the vast discrepancies in national health status rankings. While other industrialized countries have national health systems that provide care to all citizens, 44.3 million Americans, including 11.1 million children younger than eighteen, had no health insurance in 1998 and 45 million more lacked adequate coverage, according to estimates by the U.S. Census Bureau.[13] The United States may offer some of the best medical services in the world, but its disadvantaged people clearly lack access to timely and adequate care.

Managed Care for Low-Income Americans

Millions of poor and elderly Americans benefited from Medicare and Medicaid in 2000, but many were worse off than their counterparts forty

years earlier, before those programs began. The nation's uninsured population had increased rapidly in the early 1980s because rising health care
costs forced employers to drop health benefits and competition among insurers reduced the availability of affordable coverage for patients with serious health problems. Despite a strong economy in the late 1990s, more
than half of the uninsured lived in families headed by full-time workers
who lacked on-the-job benefits and could not afford private policies. Traditional safety nets for uninsured patients deteriorated or entirely disap-
peared during this period as financial pressures from competition reduced
opportunities for doctors and hospitals to provide charity care.[14]

Congress originally intended for Medicaid to serve low-income mothers and children. However, the program has been assigned many new obligations and now influences many sectors of the nation's health care system. While poor and near-poor parents and their dependent children
represented nearly 75 percent of the program's beneficiaries in 1998, they
accounted for only 25 percent of total expenditures; two-thirds of the program's costs went for individuals with disabilities and elderly patients receiving long-term care.[15] In 1998 Medicaid paid for one-third of all births,
one-quarter of the health care for children younger than five, and nearly
half of all nursing home care. It also covered more than 45 percent of patients in public hospitals and a third of patients served by federally funded
community health centers.[16] A U.S. Supreme Court ruling in 1999 found
that states have an obligation to provide services to disabled Medicaid
beneficiaries in the least restrictive and most cost-effective setting. As a
result of that ruling Medicaid now spends more on the nonelderly disabled,
including the mentally retarded and mentally ill, than on any other group.[17]
Some observers worry that delegating the care of these vulnerable populations to HMOs that receive inadequate capitations and try to cut corners
will have serious consequences for patient welfare.[18]

Federal financing of state Medicaid plans is open ended, limited only
by the size of a state's program. Participating states receive a percentage
of their federally approved expenditures, ranging from 50 percent to more
than 80 percent, based on a federal formula linked to state revenue.[19] Tremendous disparities exist in the program because each state determines
its own eligibility requirements, enrollment and copayment policies, benefits, and provider reimbursement rates.[20] According to a national review
published in 2003, capitation for Medicaid services increased by an aver-

age of 18 percent between 1998 and 2001, considerably more than the rate increases for Medicare's managed care programs.[21] Because the U.S. population is aging, federal and state agencies expect Medicaid's 1999 spending levels for home care and nursing home care will more than quadruple by 2030.[22]

A growing conviction among policymakers that managed care could control Medicaid expenditures led to several federal and state initiatives in the 1980s and 1990s to promote HMO enrollment. Most states had at least a few contracts with HMOs, but problems from the 1980s continued unabated. Coverage and services varied widely. The managed care environment was still inhospitable for Medicaid providers.[23] Reimbursement formulas were low and failed to adjust for financial loss from adverse selection.[24] And changing eligibility status and rapid membership turnover resulted in high administrative costs.[25] Nevertheless, more than half (58 percent) of all Medicaid beneficiaries were enrolled in managed care programs by 1998.[26]

Relatively few Medicaid beneficiaries living in rural areas had access to HMOs because provider reimbursements were even lower there than in cities. The Balanced Budget Act of 1997 allowed states to choose from among several contracting arrangements that were designed to encourage rural beneficiaries to enroll in HMOs.[27] Despite such incentives, physicians were unwilling to work in sparsely settled areas where professional facilities were inadequate and poor patients ineligible for public insurance depended on doctors for charity care.[28]

HMO enrollment offered few advantages for Medicaid beneficiaries. Studies comparing cost, care, and treatment outcomes of Medicaid patients in managed care and fee-for-service delivery systems found that managed care was less expensive than fee-for-service care, but services were often substandard in both systems and outcome measures were ambiguous.[29] Some Medicaid HMOs appeared to engage in selective race and age enrollment practices that excluded black children, who died at twice the rate of white children, and infants and preschool children, who typically had greater medical needs than did older children.[30]

HMOs gained favor with state Medicaid administrators during the 1990s largely because contracts with providers willing to assume risk helped reduce program costs. As I will show later in this chapter and in chapter 12, the relative tranquility in Medicaid managed care contrasted sharply with turmoil in the Medicare and private health care sectors. The peculiar affinity of Medicaid for managed care may be more acceptable—and perhaps more successful—because state administrators, private health care providers, and beneficiaries all recognize that Medicaid's resources are limited.[31]

Congress rewrote the nation's welfare laws in 1996 to reduce cash assistance and encourage welfare recipients to seek employment.[32] Federal lawmakers acknowledged that many parents who found work would not receive or be able to afford health insurance. They therefore appropriated $500 million to help states identify and enroll children of former welfare recipients who might still be eligible for Medicaid. Although nearly half the mothers and nearly one-third of their children were uninsured within one year of leaving welfare, few states took advantage of the funding, leaving about $383 million unspent at the end of 1999.[33]

As part of the Balanced Budget Act of 1997, Congress also created the State Child Health Insurance Program (SCHIP) to provide health care coverage for children whose families earned too much to qualify for Medicaid but not enough to afford private insurance. States had three years, until the end of September 2000, to spend the first $4.2 billion installment of a ten-year, $40 billion appropriation. They could use their share of the money for new child health programs, expansion of current Medicaid programs, or a combination of strategies, but they were responsible for paying 16 to 35 percent of the program's costs.

Wisconsin decided to combine its federal allocations from SCHIP and Medicaid to serve entire families, reasoning that healthy parents could better support and care for their children. In order to cover parents, state lawmakers supplemented federal funds with general revenues and money from a national tobacco lawsuit settlement.[34] Wisconsin's program, called BadgerCare, provided the same benefits as its Medicaid managed care program, and HMOs already involved with Medicaid served BadgerCare beneficiaries. When enrollment began in the spring of 1999, the state based the cost of its premiums on federal poverty guidelines that considered, for example, a family of four to be poor if its annual income was $16,700 or less. Families earning less than 150 percent of the federal poverty level were entitled to receive free care. Families with incomes equal to 150 to 185 percent of the poverty level paid monthly premiums representing no more than 3 percent of their wages, and these families were allowed to remain in the program until their earnings reached 200 percent of the poverty level.[35] Several HMOs were concerned about reimbursement rates and resisted participation until the state made serving BadgerCare beneficiaries a requirement for keeping their Medicaid contracts.[36]

The Marshfield Clinic continued to serve Medicaid beneficiaries on a fee-for-service basis until 1997, when its Security Health Plan (SHP) contracted to serve them under newly revised reimbursement arrangements with the Wisconsin Medicaid Managed Care Program. Within two years SHP was one of only a few plans in the state to show a profit from its Medicaid contract. Many other health plans had reduced their participation or dropped the program entirely because they found reimbursement levels inadequate. SHP administrators attributed their ability to work within Medicaid's capitation to their emphasis on primary, prenatal, and preventive care; a twenty-four-hour "nurse line"; and an extensive education campaign targeting schoolchildren and adults. The education program included translation services and materials specially prepared for Hmong-speaking patients, who accounted for 20 percent of SHP's Medicaid enrollees.

When Wisconsin added BadgerCare to its Medicaid program in 1999, the Marshfield Clinic, its Family Health Center, and SHP mounted an aggressive campaign to identify, refer, and help as many eligible families as possible obtain coverage. Within five months SHP had 11 percent of the thirty-seven thousand state residents enrolled in BadgerCare. SHP expanded Marshfield's program for high-risk pregnant women, including those enrolled in the BadgerCare/Medicaid program, by helping local health departments and other prenatal care providers in twenty-three counties identify and provide outreach services to pregnant clients. In addition to prenatal care, the program offered these women transportation to obstetrical visits, emotional support, and assistance with drug, alcohol, and smoking addiction. SHP's approximately twenty-one thousand beneficiaries, who comprised one-sixth of its total enrollment, made it the largest Medicaid-BadgerCare provider in the state in 2000. As many as five hundred of those beneficiaries were pregnant at any one time. SHP received a "Friend of the Family" award from the Wisconsin Maternal and Child Health Coalition that year for its collaborative efforts to improve care for high-risk women and "for service beyond the duty of HMOs."[37]

Despite considerable enthusiasm for SCHIP among its supporters, its national record for its first three years was disappointing. Only ten states spent their initial allotments by the September 2000 deadline, and the program enrolled just 2.5 million of an estimated eleven million eligible children.[38] Some states facing forfeiture of their unspent allotment reported problems organizing programs or finding and enrolling eligible children. Other states were unable or unwilling to pay their share of program costs or were reluctant to deal with what they considered complex forms.[39] As of 2001, SCHIP involved few health plans that were not already serving Medicaid beneficiaries.[40] The refusal of states to promote SCHIP, and of many providers and health plans to participate in that program, seems socially unjustifiable. A study released in 2003 reported a strong relationship between public expenditures on health care for children and child outcomes across a wide range of indicators, including measures of child mortality, elementary school test scores, and adolescent behaviors. States in the Northeast and Midwest generally spent far more and had much better outcomes than those in the Deep South.[41]

BadgerCare enrollment greatly exceeded its annual projections, but Wisconsin did not receive formal federal approval to provide coverage for parents until its program was three years old. As a result the state spent only half its allocation before the 2000 deadline. Even after additional federal money became available, state legislators continued to cover Badger-Care's budget shortfalls because they recognized the value of the program and were eager to extend benefits to more low-income residents.[42] Eight other states and the District of Columbia were approved or already using SCHIP and Medicaid monies to care for parents by the end of 2000. However, the National Academy for State Health Policy and the federal Health Care Financing Administration considered BadgerCare one of the nation's most comprehensive Medicaid-SCHIP benefit programs.

An eleven-state survey of managed care plans participating in Medicaid or SCHIP or both in 2001 found participating plans were usually supportive of both programs and able to secure providers to care for beneficiaries. However, some analysts predicted that SCHIP participation in those plans and others not already involved in Medicaid was unlikely to increase while states face tight budgets. While prepaid capitated payments to managed care organizations were an important tool for controlling costs, respondents to the survey worried that states confronting serious financial crises in 2001 would reduce payments to HMOs, causing them to drop their Medicaid enrollees.[43]

Apparently in response to recommendations from the National Governors' Conference, the Center for Medicare and Medicaid Services, formerly known as the Health Care Financing Administration (HCFA), announced a demonstration initiative called Health Insurance Flexibility and Accountability (HIFA) in 2001. HIFA allows states to change their eligibility criteria for Medicaid enrollment and subsidizes the enrollment of beneficiaries in private insurance plans that offer more limited coverage than traditional Medicaid plans. Some observers feared that HIFA would move Medicaid toward the private insurance model, causing serious reductions in benefits for millions of individuals with chronic illness or disability. As of May 2004, however, only six states were involved in this experimental program.[44]

By 2002 the federal-state Medicaid program had become the nation's largest insurance program. It financed health care and social services for more than one in every seven Americans, including twenty-four million children, fourteen million adults, and thirteen million disabled and elderly people. It was the nation's largest purchaser of long-term care services, paying for more than half of all nursing home expenditures. It provided Medigap coverage to the low-income elderly and disabled enrolled in Medicare. It was the largest payer of medical care for people with HIV infections and AIDS. It provided major support to various institutions that treat mental disorders. It paid for a third of all births and through SCHIP served an additional 4.6 million children whose families earn too much to quality for Medicaid but not enough to afford private insurance. In 2002 the federal government provided 57 percent of $259 billion paid out by Medicaid, with the other 43 percent coming from state budgets. Despite the program's high costs, the low payments to physicians, dentists, and managed care plans discourage their participation. Because Medicaid represents the largest share of state budgets, it presents an easy target for cuts when the economy is poor, at the very time when more unemployed people need its services.[45]

When Congress revisited federal welfare reform issues in 2002 during a downturn in the economy that left many more families uninsured, some reformers hoped that Tommy Thompson, the former Wisconsin governor, would use his position as the secretary of the U.S. Department of Health and Human Services to advocate a Badger-style health care system nationwide.[46] But instead, Thompson outlined a Bush administration proposal in 2003 (reminiscent of Republican proposals from the mid-1990s) that would have given states sweeping authority to remake Medicaid by expanding, reducing, or eliminating the benefits of millions of people covered by the program. Administration officials said the initiative offered states under extreme financial pressure the opportunity to free up money for other programs. The proposal drew immediate objections from Democrats, who said it would jeopardize care to vulnerable citizens, and Ron Pollack, president of Families USA, who called the proposal a "green light to slash health care for people who desperately need it." And Congress refused to approve any reductions in Medicare spending that would add to the growing number of uninsured Americans.[47]

Within a few weeks, the Bush administration decided that states had the authority to tell HMOs and other managed care organizations that they could limit and restrict the coverage of emergency services for their Medicaid beneficiaries in order to facilitate more appropriate use of preventive and primary care. That policy change, disclosed in a letter to state Medicaid directors, contradicted standards established in the Balanced Budget Act of 1997, under which states can require Medicaid recipients to enroll in HMOs but must provide coverage in any situation that a prudent layperson would regard as an emergency. Bush withdrew this change shortly after the Democrats challenged its legality but then early in 2004 accused several states of gouging the federal Medicaid program to offset state deficits. The president said that the federal government would save $23.6 billion by 2014 if state Medicaid agencies restored fiscal integrity to their fiscal accounting procedures.[48]

Medicaid funding promises to be a contentious issue for many years to come. The Kaiser Family Foundation estimated that total Medicaid spending from 1992 to 2002 increased at an annual average rate of 8 percent. If that rate of increase were to continue at the same pace until 2030, Medicaid's annual costs will reach $2.2 trillion.[49]

Many low-income patients ineligible for Medicaid or SCHIP rely on community and university hospitals for charity care. The ability of a hospital to serve the poor was severely compromised, first in the 1980s by Medicare's prospective reimbursement system and later by insurers' demands for large discounts.[50] Revenue losses also forced the closure of four hundred hospital emergency departments between 1992 and 1997, mostly in inner cities and rural communities, where medically indigent patients used them as a regular and sole source of outpatient care.[51] Even with fewer hospital emergency rooms, the Centers for Disease Control reported that emergency visits increased from 95 million in 1997 to 108 million in 2000. Patients who needed care for nonurgent problems but lacked insurance coverage or primary care providers accounted for much of the increase. Although seriously ill patients were usually seen rather quickly, the time that people spent waiting for nonurgent care increased 33 percent during that three-year period.[52] Moreover, emergency department congestion routinely forced urban hospitals to reroute ambulances to other institutions.

Some rural hospitals formed cooperative alliances in order to remain financially viable and better serve their constituents. A prototype for many such groups was the Rural Wisconsin Hospital Cooperative, which was formed in 1970 and owned and operated by twenty-five rural acute care, general medical-surgical hospitals. The cooperative is nationally recognized as one of the earliest and most successful rural hospital networks.[53]

Federally subsidized community health centers, such as Marshfield's Family Health Center (FHC), continued to provide valuable safety nets for some low-income working Americans in medically underserved areas. During the 1990s the community health center program targeted inner city and rural residents, migrant and homeless populations, and public housing residents. Because of their locations many centers found themselves serving large numbers of Medicaid and low-income Medicare beneficiaries. Meager reimbursements from those two programs deprived the centers of adequate funds to serve their primary clientele—the poor who could not qualify for Medicaid.

Provisions in the Omnibus Budget Reconciliation Act of 1989 (OBRA) sought to remedy this situation by requiring Medicaid and Medicare to fully reimburse federally qualified community health centers for the cost of serving their beneficiaries. OBRA automatically qualified all community health centers that were receiving federal grants, as well as other community clinics that were not federally funded but performed similar functions, thereby enabling them to receive cost-based reimbursements for services to Medicaid and Medicare patients. Although federal funding for the health center program had stagnated by then, the infusion of higher reimbursements from Medicaid and Medicare enabled the centers to expand their services. By the mid-1990s approximately seven hundred organizations were managing eighteen hundred clinic sites and serving more than seven million patients.[54]

In states that awarded all their Medicaid contracts to HMOs, some community health centers converted to prepaid managed care in the early 1990s so they could serve Medicaid beneficiaries and receive steady revenue from capitation. Responding to concerns about these conversions, Congress asked the General Accounting Office (GAO) to investigate. The GAO found that while managed care was compatible with the health center mission, many centers lacked sufficient expertise and financial stability to deal with the prepayment mechanisms of managed care. By the time the GAO released its report in 1995, health center administrators in what was now called the Bureau of Primary Health Care, and members of the National Association of Community Health Centers, were offering training and technical assistance to centers that held or were considering prepaid contracts.[55] The Balanced Budget Refinement Act of 1999 preserved the safety-net function of the community health centers but left many other community health programs on the edge of financial disaster.[56] The health centers that survived are usually able to provide primary care, medications, and medical supplies to most of their uninsured patients on site. However, they are limited in their ability to provide diagnostic, specialty, and mental health services or to arrange for nonemergency hospital care.[57]

The Marshfield Clinic's federally subsidized Family Health Center, in partnership with the clinic and SHP, is responsible for serving the system's Medicaid and BadgerCare beneficiaries and thirty-one hundred other low-income patients. Medicaid and BadgerCare enrollees have access to clinic staff physicians, as well as all of SHP's affiliated physicians and affiliated hospitals in their area. FHC's low-income enrollees have access to the system's outpatient service but lack hospitalization benefits. FHC was serving twenty-six thousand people at the time of its twenty-fifth anniversary in 1999 but had another forty-four hundred eligible residents on its waiting list. Only $1.5 million of its $23.5 million budget came from the federal community health centers program; other funding sources included $1.1 million from enrollee income-adjusted premium payments; $16.9 million from Medicare, Medicaid, and other insurance reimbursements; and $4 million from clinic contributions.[58]

One-quarter of FHC's enrollees in 1999 were elderly or disabled Medicare beneficiaries, many with prescription drug bills that exceeded their Social Security checks. Pharmacy charges alone cost FHC more than $2 million a year.[59] With state and federal assistance Marshfield's FHC opened a state-of-the-art automated mail order pharmacy in 2000, enabling its patients to purchase their prescriptions at significantly discounted prices. The pharmacy's director predicted that the new service would produce an annual savings of $250,000 for patients and $1 million for the health center.[60]

The savings were much greater than anticipated. More than 90 percent of FHC's enrollees were using the pharmacy's mail order service by 2002 and no longer needed to pay $8 for each prescription they might otherwise have purchased from a community pharmacy. FHC's pharmacy receives large discounts on its drug purchases as a federally funded (340B) organization and, in some instances, obtains free drugs from pharmaceutical companies that sponsor programs for indigent patients. During fiscal year 2002–2003, FHC patients purchased about 147,000 prescriptions through the pharmacy and saved nearly $1.2 million in copayments, while FHC saved more than $2 million in prescription expenditures for its program.[61]

Marshfield's FHC also gave disadvantaged residents in central Wisconsin a powerful voice in the management of their health care services. A majority of the members of the center's governing board were FHC enrollees. Many had served on the board for several years and played a crucial role in helping the center develop appropriate programs for low-income residents throughout the region. Greg Nycz, who directed the program, often presented his board's views and requests to legislators in Wisconsin and Congress.[62] In 1995 the American Dental Association recognized his efforts to extend dental care to disadvantaged people.[63] And four years later the Wisconsin Rural Health Association honored him for his work on behalf of the state's rural population. In nominating Nycz for that award, Tim Size, director of the Rural Wisconsin Hospital Cooperative, said, "Greg's analytic and communication skills have been absolutely critical in getting leadership, both in Wisconsin and Washington, to understand the complex, often arcane, nature of how mind-dulling reimbursement formulas and data have consequences to people."[64] Also in 1999 the Clinton administration called Marshfield's FHC a model program for improving access to health care for uninsured workers.[65]

When FHC celebrated the thirtieth anniversary of the neighborhood health center program in 2002, it was the only continuously operating community health center in Wisconsin, one of fifteen centers in the state, and one of one thousand centers nationally that were providing care for uninsured patients at thirty-four hundred sites. While most programs limit their patients to particular sites, FHC's enrollees have many choices of where to obtain their care. "What we try to address is very simple: 100

percent access and zero health disparity," said Nycz. "The care of the poor, minorities, and those living in isolated rural areas should be no different than for those who are insured and live in urban areas."[66]

When FHC celebrated its own thirtieth anniversary the next year, the program was serving 3,900 enrollees from nine counties. All the enrollees earned less than 200 percent of the poverty level ($18,630 for a single person or $37,700 for a family of four) and paid premiums on a sliding income-based scale. The program continued to place a heavy emphasis on primary care and prevention but provided full access to specialty services as needed.[67]

According to Nycz, early in the new century community health centers achieved their highest level of federal and state support in their thirty-year history. President George W. Bush's proposal to expand and double the nation's community health centers had widespread bipartisan support in Congress. Despite budget shortfalls, many states continued to partner with the federal agencies in support of grant programs that enabled community health centers in their jurisdiction to provide more comprehensive primary care, emphasizing behavioral (mental) and dental health care services. Community health centers nationwide took advantage of such grants to establish small programs that addressed the refusal of dentists to treat Medicaid clients and other low-income individuals. Using state funding, Marshfield's FHC partnered with the clinic in the early 2000s to establish a $2 million, seventeen-chair dental clinic in a small, centrally located northern Wisconsin community. The facility initially had a staff of five dentists and five hygienists and was open to all residents on a sliding fee scale. During its first six months of operation it served residents from thirty-seven of Wisconsin's seventy-two counties. But within two years of opening, the dental clinic had a three-month backlog of appointments and a waiting list of more than 3,500 patients. Due to the unexpectedly high demand for services, the clinic could no longer accept new patients from outside the five counties in its original service area but would continue to serve patients from outside that area if they needed follow-up care on procedures already performed. The dental clinic implemented a triage system to help staff identify and accommodate patients with the most acute needs, hired more dentists and dental hygienists, and was working with the FHC to locate resources for establishing additional dental centers in the northern Wisconsin.[68] In 2003 Nycz was invited to the National Conference of State Legislators in San Francisco, where he spoke at a pre-conference program that addressed rural dental health issues.[69]

Community health centers are now also involved in a program called Disease Disparities Collaboratives, which encourages more intense efforts to identify high-risk patients, proactively manage their health care, and promote lifestyle changes and preventive services that will improve health outcomes. These collaboratives bring community health center teams together under the guidance of national experts for twelve months in order to generate rapid improvements in care by focusing on the management of a particular chronic disease. The initial testing and learning year is followed by disseminating their findings throughout the health care system. Partnerships formed at the national, state, and community levels have resulted in increased access to expertise, computer software, discounted pharmaceuticals and laboratory equipment, direct community resources for patients, health education materials, and community-level marketing and educational resources for the participating communities. Nycz said that this approach to health care, impossible under fee-for-service reimbursement systems, will eliminate health disparities among advantaged and disadvantaged populations within local health care systems. "That's how we improve health care," he said, "one community at a time."[70]

Changes in pricing and underwriting policies excluded many central Wisconsin residents from participation in the Marshfield Clinic's Security Health Plan during the 1990s, but the clinic's aggressive involvement in programs to assist economically disadvantaged residents in the northern half of Wisconsin remains unparalleled.

Managed Care for Medicare Beneficiaries

Medicare, the principal source of health care coverage for elderly and disabled Americans, covered more than forty million beneficiaries in 2002.[71] Medicare's enrollment is expected to reach nearly 79 million by 2035, when its spending will account for 5.3 percent of the gross domestic product.[72] In 2000 prescription drugs and Medigap policies (for services not covered by Medicare, such as long-term care) cost each beneficiary an average of $3,000, more than the annual stipend that many received from Social Security, their only source of income.[73] Beneficiaries who had Medicare+Choice policies, Medicare Part A Hospital Insurance, prescription drug coverage, and were in fair health saw their out-of-pocket costs increase 62 percent, to $2,432, between 2000 and 2002, while those with similar coverage but in poor health saw their costs rise even faster, to an average of $4,783.[74] The researchers who compiled these figures failed to address the even higher out-of-pocket costs incurred by chronically ill beneficiaries who were enrolled in substandard Medigap policies or lacked drug coverage. Medicaid protects very poor Medicare enrollees, but those who are near-poor suffer considerable financial hardship.[75]

Medicare's efforts to reduce federal spending by encouraging beneficiaries to enroll in HMOs failed during the 1970s and 1980s for reasons that I described in chapter 5. Enrollment in Medicare HMOs grew more rapidly in the late 1990s after Congress passed the Balanced Budget Act of 1997 and directed the Center for Medicare and Medicaid Services (CMS) to introduce new inducements for HMOs to enroll beneficiaries. One option, called Medicare Select, enabled preferred provider organizations (PPOs) to participate in Medicare risk contracts for the first time. Premiums for Medicare PPOs often cost less than some private Medigap policies, but beneficiaries had to pay extra fees if they sought nonemergency care from out-of-network providers. Medicare Select expanded HMO enrollment, but it had no effect on public costs because the CMS reimbursed providers on a fee-for-services basis, which encouraged them to deliver more medical services.

Another new option, called Medicare+Choice, allowed loosely structured managed care organizations, such as independent practice associations (IPAs) and PPOs, to participate in capitated risk contracts for the first time. Like the risk contracts described earlier, the capitation formula assumed that the prepaid health plans would provide more cost-efficient patient care so it was based on 95 percent of the adjusted average per capita cost of treating Medicare beneficiaries in each health plan's area. Nevertheless, government costs for Medicare+Choice and other Medicare risk contracts were usually higher than if beneficiaries had remained in traditional fee-for-service programs. The reason was that most of the risk-contract HMOs were from areas where their average costs for treating all beneficiaries and their reimbursement formulas were very high, but they enrolled only relatively healthy beneficiaries who required less than average amounts of care so as to make more money.[76]

Congress anticipated that Medicare+Choice would attract more beneficiaries to prepaid health plans, but CMS faced an uphill battle. One quarter of Medicare patients then enrolled in prepaid health plans would not recommend their plan to anyone with complicated health problems.[77] Moreover, a 1997 review of health care quality from fifteen peer-reviewed studies showed several instances in which Medicare enrollees with chronic conditions received worse care in HMOs than in fee-for-service settings.[78]

Several other studies in the mid-1990s, including one by the General Accounting Office, found no evidence that HMOs reduced government spending. Instead, these studies found that Medicare overpaid most HMOs by 5 to 20 percent because they enrolled only healthy beneficiaries requiring little care.[79]

The Balanced Budget Act of 1997 continued two other managed care models that were supposed to save money by keeping the frail elderly out of nursing homes. The Program of All-Inclusive Care for the Elderly (PACE) served low-income seniors and was funded by Medicaid and Medicare. The other program, Social HMOs, was funded by capitated payments from Medicare (Medicaid if eligible) and member premiums and copayments.[80] Neither program served enough beneficiaries to have a significant effect on public costs.

More significant provisions in the Balanced Budget Act of 1997 required CMS to address two issues regarding reimbursement formulas that had discouraged Medicare risk contracting for nearly two decades: low reimbursement levels in some regions of the country, and failure to account for beneficiary health status and treatment needs. CMS's adjusted average per capita cost (AAPCC) formula punished HMOs in areas where care was cost efficient while richly rewarding health plans where fees were high and care was inefficient. Relatively few physicians in low reimbursement areas were willing to enter Medicare capitation contracts, so seniors in those areas had to purchase Medigap policies that often were inadequate and rarely offered extra benefits. Conversely, seniors in high reimbursement areas usually had several HMOs to choose from, paid little or nothing for premiums, and received many extra benefits such as prescription drugs, eyeglasses, hearing aids, dental care, and even health club memberships.[81] Urban-rural enrollment figures for 1996 show a direct relationship to reimbursement disparities for Medicare risk contracting: 20.5 percent of Medicare beneficiaries living in major urban areas were enrolled in risk HMOs, compared to 8.6 percent in other urban areas, 1.4 percent in rural-urban fringe areas, and 0.7 percent in other rural areas.[82]

CMS's long-awaited formula revisions in 1997 raised Medicare payments to HMOs in low reimbursement areas and reduced the rate of capitation increases (though not the capitations) in areas where payments were perceived as overly generous. When confronted with the prospect of lower-than-anticipated revenues, some HMOs in high-paid areas charged monthly premiums for the first time or raised existing premiums, cut optional benefits, or simply dropped their Medicare enrollees.[83] As 1998 ended, forty-three of 347 Medicare risk-contracting HMOs announced plans to cancel their contracts the following year. Another fifty-four HMOs said that they would reduce their geographic service areas. For-profit Medicare HMOs that needed to satisfy investors terminated a disproportionately large number of beneficiaries.[84] Many of the abandoned senior citizens were profoundly distressed; nearly a quarter had to find new primary care physicians. Some were able to switch to other HMOs, but one-third had to return to a fee-for-service system where they received fewer benefits and paid more for premiums and much more for prescription drugs.[85]

President Clinton called the decline in Medicare+Choice enrollment "a trickle rather than a flood," but some of the nation's largest health plans left the program, including CIGNA, Aetna, Blue Cross–Blue Shield, Oxford, and Kaiser Permanente.[86] Karen Ignagni, president of the American Association of Health Plans, called the situation a crisis but predicted that Congress would shore up the financially strapped (and mostly for-profit) HMOs. Even after Congress made some concessions in the Balanced Budget Act of 1999 (described later in this chapter), the trickle increased to a steady stream when several more HMOs announced plans to reduce the enrollment in Medicare+Choice by about 10 percent in 2000 and still more in 2001.[87]

Large reimbursement discrepancies remained among various regions of the country even after CMS substantially raised capitation levels in low reimbursement areas. While monthly capitations jumped from $200 to a new minimum of $367 in rural Wisconsin counties, some Florida HMOs received nearly $800 a month.[88] In fact, Medicare capitation levels continued to short-change the entire state of Wisconsin in 2000. Most of the state's HMOs refused to participate in Medicare+Choice contracts because capitation rates were still unreasonably low, they said. As a result the state's elderly and disabled residents not covered by retirement or disability programs had to buy their prescription drugs and pay an additional $1,500 to $2,000 a year for Medigap policies. In the absence of risk-contract Medicare HMOs, Wisconsin's Medicaid program had to cover about seventy-five thousand recipients who were eligible for both Medicaid and Medicare. Wisconsin forfeited more than $5 million each year that eight other states with similar capitation rates collected.[89]

CMS was also supposed to revise Medicare's capitation formula so that it would adequately compensate Medicare HMOs that were serving seriously ill beneficiaries. Many health plans, which stood to lose money if they continued to enroll only healthy applicants, opposed risk-adjusted capitations. Following massive defections from Medicare+Choice because of earlier capitation revisions, CMS decided to spread implementation of its risk-adjusted formula over five years, with only minimal adjustments the first year.[90]

Policy analysts agreed that Medicare payments should not reward HMOs in high-spending states or plans that rejected unhealthy beneficiaries, but none of the solutions that they offered found widespread acceptance.[91] Many observers thought that CMS was too underfunded and overworked to address reimbursement issues. Since 1977, when Congress created HCFA, CMS's predecessor, to administer Medicare and Medicaid, the agency's fiduciary responsibility has increased tenfold but its workforce has declined from 4,961 full-time-equivalent employees in 1980 to 4,219 in 1999. Between 1996 and 2000 CMS was responsible for implementing about seven hundred provisions of five major laws, including the complex and controversial budget act of 1997. Many provisions in these laws required the agency to assume new tasks that fell outside the expertise of its staff. By 2001 CMS was the single largest health care purchaser in the world, and it controlled 15 percent of the federal budget. CMS's $476 billion budget financed health care services for seventy million disabled, elderly, and poor beneficiaries. However, the agency's administrative costs amounted to only 2 percent of claims payments because its small staff had no marketing expenses or private investors to satisfy. In contrast, administrative costs of private insurers averaged about 11 percent of their payments for medical services. The General Accounting Office concluded in 1999 that inadequate funding prevented CMS from performing its assigned functions. On the heels of that report, fourteen health policy experts from some of the nation's most prestigious institutions and influential organizations—and from across the political spectrum—urged the Clinton administration and Congress to increase CMS's administrative funding. Their request attracted little attention from the Clinton and Bush administrations or from Congress, where lawmakers found it more politically expedient to criticize the agency's inadequate performance than to properly fund its work.[92]

Congress restored $16 million for Medicare services in the Balanced Budget Refinement Act of 1999, but few providers were satisfied with the distribution formula or their reimbursements.[93] Legislative proposals to equalize Medicare payments over time, such as the Medicare Fair Payments Plan Act introduced by the bipartisan House Fairness Caucus in 1999, seemed doomed to failure. States receiving the highest payments had powerful lobbyists and representatives who chaired influential committees.[94] The views expressed by an administrator at PacifiCare, a large HMO in southern California, revealed the prevailing sentiment in high reimbursement states. Medicare enrollees accounted for only 25 percent of PacifiCare's membership in 1997, but Medicare capitation supplied 60 percent of the HMO's revenue. When faced with formula revisions, Craig Schub, PacifiCare's senior vice president of marketing, said, "You simply can't take away Medicare money. If that happens, we'll need to inform our members. They'll tell their representatives. Seniors vote."[95]

Legislative remedies for low reimbursement states seemed unlikely to win passage so Minnesota's attorney general and the Minnesota Senior Federation sued Medicare in November 1999. Wisconsin followed with a similar suit in March 2000. Both states sought to force the federal government to change its formula for calculating payments to Medicare HMOs. In announcing his suit, Attorney General James Doyle of Wisconsin said, "Wisconsin senior citizens paid just as much in Medicare taxes during their careers as the elderly in other states. It is unacceptable for the federal government to subsidize expensive health care benefits in some parts of the country while seniors in other areas are forced to choose between buying food and buying the medications they need to stay alive."[96] The U.S. District Court for the Eastern District of Wisconsin dismissed the state's suit for lack of standing, and a federal district judge in Minnesota dismissed the Minnesota Senior Federation's case. He said that the Medicare reimbursement system resulted in "gross unequal treatment of senior citizens" but was not unconstitutional and that Congress ought to correct the situation quickly.[97] The Minnesota Senior Federation decided to appeal the district court ruling.[98] Before the appellate court refused to reinstate the case, Congress made slight but significant adjustments to rural reimbursement formulas in 2001.[99]

Medicare risk HMO enrollment grew from 3.3 million beneficiaries in 1990 to 19.4 million in 2000, but several announced plans to drop nearly one million beneficiaries in 2001.[100] Tim McBride, a health panel member of the Rural Policy Research Institute, found the news particularly discouraging for rural HMO beneficiaries. Although few rural senior citizens belonged to HMOs, they were twice as likely to be dropped from Medicare+Choice plans as their urban counterparts and five times more likely to have to return to the fee-for-service system.[101]

The Marshfield Clinic had followed Medicare reimbursement issues closely since 1987 when it started the Senior Security Health Plan to accommodate Medicare beneficiaries dropped from a risk-contracting demonstration. In 1997 the clinic's staffers recommended that the Security Health Plan contract for capitated reimbursements under the new Medicare+Choice option because they hoped that such a contract would enable them to work with CMS in devising the diagnosis-based risk adjusters that the agency was supposed to incorporate in its reimbursement formula by January 2000. When CMS showed little interest in the clinic's offers to test formula revisions, the clinic decided to stay with the more generous fee-for-service reimbursements for a while longer. The Marshfield Clinic reevaluated the capitation issue again in 1999 and reached the same decision, this time because other health care providers had received Medicare+Choice so poorly and CMS had made little progress in its risk-adjusted formula.[102]

Marshfield revisited the Medicare+Choice option a third time in 2001 after Congress began to revise risk formulas and increased monthly minimum payments to rural health plans. By then Senior Security had the largest Medicare enrollment of any Wisconsin HMO. Medicare+Choice plans in high reimbursement states had successfully petitioned Congress to slow the pace for implementing risk-adjusted capitation. However, Marshfield staffers calculated that the new reimbursement formulas, with even a small amount of risk adjustment, would enable Senior Security to reduce its premiums by as much as 50 percent. In addition, greater flexibility under capitation reimbursement would allow the clinic to institute a number of new strategies for tracking the health status of enrollees with chronic conditions such as diabetes.[103]

The clinic's board of directors finally authorized the Security Health Plan to offer a Medicare+Choice option in April 2002. The new program, called Advocare, provides benefits typically covered by Medigap plans, including some drugs and medical supplies. Applicants are not denied membership because of existing conditions, except for end-stage renal disease, which is covered by a special Medicare program. Unlike Senior Security, SHP's standard Medicare supplemental program, Advocare premiums do not increase with age, but enrollees are charged copayments for office and emergency room visits and hospital admission. Advocare Plus offers a point-of-service option with higher deductibles and copayments for individuals (such as retirees who travel south in the winter) who want to see unaffiliated providers in or out of the SHP service area.[104] While other health plans in Wisconsin and elsewhere were closing their Medicare accounts, the Marshfield Clinic embarked on an aggressive marketing campaign to enroll as many elderly patients as possible in its new risk-contract program. Despite additional federal funding for Medicare+Choice and more generous payments to rural areas in the late 1990s, most health plan administrators found risk contracting to be an unprofitable experience.[105]

Marshfield's careful monitoring and support of elderly patients with chronic conditions stands in sharp contrast to other HMOs, which frequently offer chronically ill Medicare beneficiaries care inferior to that in the fee-for-service system. A study of health care services in Australia, Canada, New Zealand, the United Kingdom, and the United States revealed that sources and types of barriers varied widely, but all the countries could do a much better job if they used tracking systems, shared electronic medical records, and carefully monitored medications to prevent adverse interactions, side-effects, and prescription errors. Such efforts to improve care coordination, the authors noted, could be particularly fruitful in the United States.[106]

HMOs generally have a poor track record with chronically ill seniors, but two policy analysts concluded that capitation payment might be the most logical way to finance the case management of such individuals. These authors noted that the fee-for-service reimbursement system does not lend itself to providing many of the nonmedical support services needed to deflect potentially serious problems. Because the widespread involvement of HMOs with chronically ill Medicare beneficiaries seems unlikely in the near future, the analysts recommended that the government make special payments to fee-for-service physicians who take on additional case management responsibilities.[107] Ironically, the Marshfield Clinic's Medicare-HMO programs already provide many case management services recommended by the authors because such services help patients stay healthy and reduce their use of expensive medical services.

In fact, many observers have suggested that CMS could realize substantial savings if the agency were to focus the attention of health care providers on the approximately 5 percent of beneficiaries who consume nearly half of Medicare's spending. Although approximately one-fifth of the patients in this group who die each year may receive too much inappropriate and expensive end-of-life care, most of the patients suffer from chronic conditions such as congestive heart failure, diabetes, or cognitive impairment that would clearly benefit from improved case management. Saving money in this way is difficult, however, because of the need to first identify those beneficiaries who will account for high spending and then intervene with case management practices before their care becomes inordinately expensive.[108]

A federal study found Medicare patients in the fee-for-service system were getting better treatment in 2000–2001 than in 1998–1999 for heart attacks, pneumonia, breast cancer, and diabetes, but the quality of care varied widely by region and remained poorest in the South. Furthermore, Dr. Stephen Jencks, director of quality improvement at CMS, noted that all health care systems were ignoring many opportunities to use well-proven, low-cost preventive measures like flu shots, mammograms, and eye exams for diabetics because the attention of providers continued to be more focused on treating acute illness than on prevention.[109]

In the Balanced Budget Act of 1997 Congress had directed CMS to revise fee-for-service payments to physicians serving Medicare beneficiaries but for entirely different reasons: to reduce payment disparities rather then improve services. Those revisions are relevant to this discussion because they influenced CMS's reimbursement formula for HMOs. For its payment revisions CMS used a resource-based relative value scale devised in the 1980s by Dr. William C. Hsaio of the Harvard School of Public Health. The value scale considered cognitive effort, training, time required to perform services, practice costs, malpractice premiums, and local circumstances. The effect of the formula was to reduce reimbursement disparities by lowering payments to specialists and urban doctors while raising payments to generalists and rural practitioners.[110] When CMS first tried to implement a new fee-for-service formula in January 1992, many physicians in procedure-oriented specialties were so angry about the compensation revisions that they refused to treat Medicare beneficiaries or required senior citizens to pay the doctors directly and recover what they could from Medicare.[111]

Despite opposition from some specialists, public and private health care administrators found several applications for the value scale system. Many states used it to calculate their Medicaid reimbursements, and private insurers found it to be a rational tool for pricing and analyzing claims, as well as for negotiating HMO contracts with physicians.[112] The issue was far from settled, however. Researchers at Harvard, Johns Hopkins University, and elsewhere continued to evaluate payment systems that placed even more value on cognitive services and less on procedures.[113] While sbattles raged among medical specialties, a CMS actuarial team reported in 1998 that efforts to reduce physicians' charges to Medicare were ineffective. When faced with reduced fees, physicians simply increased the amount of services to each patient and submitted claims for slightly higher levels of service so that they could continue to earn as much money as they had in the past.[114]

In January 2002 CMS implemented its new, long-dreaded fee schedule for physicians, which included an across-the-board reduction in Medicare fee-for-service payments that averaged 2.9 percent. In 2003 Congress mitigated these payment reductions in the face of vociferous opposition from surgeons and other doctors who perform expensive procedures. Agreeing to their demands significantly increased Medicare's budget, but refusal to do so might have resulted in wholesale defections from approximately 550,000 doctors who still provide care to Medicare's 39 million disabled and elderly beneficiaries, and created even more access problems for beneficiaries in underserved areas.[115] The solution to these problems will not come by addressing them in a piecemeal fashion or by throwing only money at them. Solving these problems requires a major change in physicians' attitudes about standardized treatment protocols, regardless of where they practice; a willingness among high-priced specialists to accept less money for their procedures, given that much of their training was financed by taxpayers; and less reliance on costly, unproven drugs and surgical procedures. The solution also requires a major overhaul of Medicare's reimbursement formulas so that physicians who practice in underserved areas that typically are considered "low cost," or who treat seriously ill patients in managed care systems, are adequately rewarded.

The decision by Congress to promote enrollment of Medicare beneficiaries in HMOs during the 1980s had been hailed by economists for the potential cost savings and by geriatricians for the potential improvements in patient care in a more highly integrated system.[116] Neither expectation was fulfilled by the end of the century. The Congressional Budget Office (CBO) reported that Medicare spending declined by 1 percent in 1999 because of slower-than-anticipated growth in the number of Medicare beneficiaries, a successful antifraud campaign, and greater-than-expected reductions in the use of home health services. Although the much-vaunted Medicare+Choice program and CMS's various reimbursement revisions for HMOs and physicians played no role in those spending reductions, the CBO predicted that program costs for the subsequent five years would be $62 billion less than originally forecast.[117]

Congress had many opportunities to enact meaningful reforms in the 1990s, but it failed to address quality of care issues or to adequately reimburse health plans that enroll public beneficiaries who have substantial health care risks and most need services. Federal lawmakers eventually and halfheartedly reduced regional variations in reimbursements to risk-contract HMOs, but they ignored two fundamental problems: the enormous regional variations in Medicare's fee-for-service spending that help determine HMO reimbursements and the well-documented evidence showing that health outcomes and satisfaction with care are no better for Medicare enrollees who receive more care in higher spending regions than for those who receive less care in lower spending regions.[118]

The number of Medicare beneficiaries enrolled in prepaid care increased in the 1990s with the introduction of Medicare+Choice, peaking in 2001 with 14.7 percent of eligible beneficiaries. However, enrollment dropped to 8.8 percent in 2003 because HMOs were withdrawing from the program, or reducing their benefits and increasing premiums to the extent that seniors were voluntarily leaving the plans.[119] In fact, the exodus from Medicare+Choice was so great by the end of 2001 that HHS secretary Thompson declared a "special election period" in December when Medicare beneficiaries could switch from Medicare+Choice to Medigap policies without fear of being denied coverage because of preexisting medical conditions.[120]

Rather than deal with underlying problems in the nation's health care system, the Bush administration and Congress increased the complexity of government programs with another round of ill-conceived stopgap measures euphemistically packaged as the Medicare Prescription Drug Improvement and Modernization Act of 2003. Bush said the legislation would bring Medicare into the twenty-first century, but detractors saw it as a giant windfall for drug companies and commercial insurers that promised to destroy a health care safety net that serves forty million elderly Americans.[121]

Provisions in the prescription drug act enabled Medicare beneficiaries to purchase drug benefit discount cards for a $30 annual fee in 2004 and 2005. Low income seniors (singles seniors with an annual income of less than $12,123 and couples living on less than $16,362) were entitled to a free discount card and up to $600 of free drugs.[122] Beneficiaries were locked into the discount card of their choice for a full year but sponsors of the drug cards could change their prices and the list of covered drugs as often as weekly, if they chose to do so. CMS did not mandate what drugs ought to be offered at discounted prices but companies issuing discount cards were required to offer discounts on at least one drug in each of more than 200 categories of medications commonly needed by Medicare beneficiaries.[123] Such controls could adversely affect seniors who must avoid many drugs within a specific category because of interactions with other medications they use.

Beginning in 2006, the act requires private firms to administer Medicare's drug benefit on a regional basis. It calls for beneficiaries to purchase drug coverage policies from private health plans that provide the rest of their care or from other private companies for a monthly premium of about $35. Employers are entitled to tax subsidies if they offer equivalent drug coverage to their retirees or pay all or part of the premiums when their retirees enroll in Medicare drug plans. When implemented, these plans will involve a $250 annual deductible and a three-phase coverage system much too complicated to describe here. [124] For seniors with drug coverage through their Medigap policies, provisions in the new law may decrease their coverage. For those without coverage, generic drugs sold in the United States and Canada may offer the best buy. Provisions buried within the seven-hundred-page drug law may also limit the discounts that insurers and pharmacy benefit managers can get from drug makers, further reducing the benefits that seniors will derive from the new law. Some analysts believe that the law will offer little relief to the two million chronically ill, elderly Medicare beneficiaries who failed to take drugs prescribed for them in the past because of high out-of-pocket costs. Others suggest that the Bush administration and those members of Congress who voted for the drug bill may not fully comprehend its meaning, consequences, or social costs for several years.[125]

The "Medicare modernization" provisions in the 2003 law allow workers younger than 65 who receive employer health benefits the option of buying medical policies with deductibles of at least $1,000 for a single person and $2,000 for a family in order to establish tax-free "health savings accounts." Unlike the current use-it-or-lose-it health savings accounts offered by some employers, workers could invest the unused money in these accounts to pay for their medical expenses in retirement. The new accounts and high-deductible insurance policies would replace, not supplement, existing coverage from employers. This provision is expected to cost the federal treasury $6.4 billion in lost revenue during its first ten years. Conservatives argued that allowing participants to keep unspent money in their accounts encourages them to use fewer medical services. Bush said the new plan, which promotes the privatization of Medicare, is an important part of Medicare reform. Opponents say the new accounts will appeal mainly to the wealthy as a tax shelter and to the healthy because they do not expect to have any expenses. Health care analyst Marsha Gold argues that privatizing Medicare further stigmatizes Americans who are already disadvantaged by their income, race or ethnicity. "Overriding the questions of how to finance Medicare," she said, "is the broader question of Medicare's social obligation for beneficiaries."[126]

CMS had promised to increase payments to Medicare risk-contract HMOs by an average of 10.6 percent in 2004, but areas in Wisconsin and other Midwestern states that offer cost-efficient services to elderly residents were once again short-changed. CMS payments for Wisconsin's twelve thousand seniors who were enrolled in Medicare Advantage (formerly called Medicare+Choice) HMOs increased a mere two percent. Providers serving Wisconsin's other 690,000 Medicare beneficiaries in the fee-for-service system receive slightly better compensation and were unaffected by this particular rate change. The small reimbursement increase was particularly disappointing for Marshfield's Security Health Plan, which served half of the Medicare risk-contract enrollees in the state, many of whom were seriously ill. Security's administrators were presumably consoled by the fact that CMS's new health-risk adjusted formula (which had been mandated by Congress in 1997 to provide higher reimbursements to plans that enrolled beneficiaries with health problems) would be fully implemented in 2007.[127]

Dismal results at the national level with HMO enrollment of Medicaid and Medicare beneficiaries contrasted sharply with the situation in central Wisconsin, where enrollment of public beneficiaries in Security Health Plan was at an all-time high in 2004. SHP lost many of its direct-pay families who most needed care when competition forced it to abandon community rating and the private subsidies that system afforded in the 1980s. But the clinic capitalized on new initiatives in the 1990s and early 2000s, bringing many of those families back into its health plan with public subsidies from Medicaid and BadgerCare. In one instance after another, clinic administrators showed how public programs that finance care for disadvantaged residents can be cost efficient and very good. Such victories were rare indeed.

Chapter 12

HMO Enrollment Growth in the Private Sector in the 1990s and Early 2000s

It makes no sense to have a health care system in which the name of the game
is to avoid caring for sick people.

Jerome P. Kassirer and Marcia Angell, 1998

Congress rejected President Clinton's health reform legislation in the
early 1990s, but debate about his proposals for managed competition and
provider accountability had enormous influence on the employers who
purchased most of the nation's private health care insurance. Employee
benefit costs for manufacturers had increased more than ninefold between 1970 and 1990, reducing their ability to compete in international
markets where overhead costs were relatively low. Unlike their foreign
competitors, Detroit automobile makers spent more on each car for health
benefits for employees than they did for steel.[1]

Employers' demands for less expensive health care coverage brought
large, usually for-profit, insurance companies into a race for national markets. Private sector enrollment in prepaid care grew at unprecedented
rates. In the process, rapid commercial growth transformed HMOs from
organizations that assumed responsibility for financing and delivering comprehensive health care into businesses that developed and sold prepaid
insurance packages to corporate purchasers and sold "managed care" by
contracting with physicians, hospitals, and others to provide required

services at discounted rates. Not a single piece of evidence suggests that commercialization of managed care slowed the rate of health care inflation or increased the quality of care.

The Marshfield Clinic expanded considerably during the 1990s and acquired the more grandiose title of Marshfield Clinic Health Care System. The clinic diverged further from mainstream trends in the health industry because its motives were often vastly different from those that guided other nonprofit and for-profit corporations. I start this chapter by describing how the growth in for-profits and competition in the insurance, pharmaceutical, and hospital industries changed the practice of medical care in the 1990s. I end the chapter by comparing the Marshfield Clinic's system with other strongholds of nonprofit care.

The Growth of For-Profit Health Care

Large corporations controlled almost every aspect of health care in the United States by 2000, from HMOs and doctors' practices to hospitals, nursing homes, home care services, and pharmaceutical companies. For-profit corporations operated nearly three-quarters of the nation's health plans and covered two-thirds of managed care enrollees.[2] In addition, many workers and their families were enrolled in plans operated by corporate employers that contracted directly with providers.[3] As managed care enrollment grew during the 1990s, the proportion of workers with traditional indemnity insurance policies fell from one-half to one-quarter.[4]

The proliferation of HMO mergers and buyouts in the 1990s motivated A. M. Best, a leading insurance company analyst, to evaluate the financial status of HMOs for potential investors.[5] Because of mergers and decisions by several carriers to discontinue their health insurance products, the number of major national companies selling health care policies dropped from about two dozen to six between the late 1970s and late 1990s. During that same period independent local and regional HMOs declined in number and lost national market share. Many independents were nonprofit plans operated by group practice physicians, medical society foundations, hospitals, community cooperatives, and university health centers.[6] Some independents, such as the Ross-Loos Clinic in Los Angeles, which had served as a model for many physician-operated plans like Marshfield's, sold out to large insurance corporations. Others remained fiercely self-sufficient in a sea of growing commercialization.

In retrospect, the intense competition in the HMO movement during this period marked the turning point in the American health care revolution. Capitalizing on a growing need for medical services, our nation's quintessential zeal for entrepreneurial success quickly transformed an assortment of localized health plans, private practitioners, and community hospitals into a massive impersonal industry.

Aetna, which had previously acquired U.S. HealthCare and NYLCare, merged with Prudential Insurance Company of America in 1998, becoming the nation's largest health insurer with 21 million enrollees. The other big players were CIGNA HealthCare with 14 million policyholders, United Healthcare with 8.6 million, Kaiser Permanente with 8 million, Well-Point-UniCare with 7.5 million, and Humana with 5.9 million. Of these, only Kaiser was nonprofit. The Blue Cross and Blue Shield Association (BCBSA) covered more policyholders than any other insurer, but its affiliates operated independently.[7] According to the *Wall Street Journal,* not a single major HMO merger in 1997 was able to integrate its financial and medical management or live up to earning expectations. Financial experts faulted the new conglomerates for devoting too much attention to premium collection and claims payments and not enough to service.[8]

Some plans encountered serious financial problems when they tried to extend their operations too rapidly. These included Maxicare Health Plans, touted as the industry's best-managed HMO in 1986; the fifty-year-old Health Insurance Plan of Greater New York; and Kaiser Permanente, which posted losses of $270 million in 1997, its first deficit in more than fifty years of operation.[9] Kaiser Permanente remains dominant on the West Coast, where it established an early lead with a fairly rigid group practice model. While it was able to capture and hold a market share (often through acquisition of other plans) in some metropolitan areas like Cleveland, Ohio; Washington, D.C., and Hartford, Connecticut, it did not do well in other markets, including Dallas; Raleigh-Durham; and Kansas City, Kansas, where loosely organized networks of managed care physicians already had a strong foothold.[10]

Aetna was still trying to integrate five million customers acquired from Prudential two years after their merger. The company eventually sold its financial services division, ousted its chief executive, cut five thousand jobs, raised premiums 11 to 13 percent, and dropped two million customers in unprofitable markets, including 340,000 seniors enrolled in its Medicare HMOs.[11] By the early 2000s, a much smaller but more profitable Aetna had abandoned it mission of cost-conscious managed care in favor of a sales strategy that offered consumers more information about quality, a variety of choices at higher prices, more responsibility for costs, and a range of insured and self-insured funding mechanisms that further eroded the HMO concept of pooling risk to provide implicit subsidies for patients who are chronically ill.[12]

Several BCBSA plans that reorganized as for-profit corporations encountered similar problems with overextension.[13] The failure of a West Virginia plan in 1990 prompted federal regulators to investigate other affiliates as well. U.S. Senate hearings on the Blues' business practices revealed gross mismanagement, misappropriated premiums, irresponsible expansion, fraud, and CEOs with inordinately large salaries and expensive perquisites. One observer at the hearings thought that several Blue Cross officials resembled mafia leaders, carving the country into territories. The Blues, he reported, had become commercial insurers in the guise of public interest, nonprofit institutions.[14] The General Accounting Office called for more effective state oversight in 1994 after finding that 25 percent of all BCBSA policyholders were in financially ailing plans.[15]

The Wisconsin Blues, the Marshfield Clinic's former health plan partners, were notably aggressive in their efforts to expand within and beyond the state's borders. Thomas Hefty, president and CEO, told a reporter in 1995, "Our goal now is not to be the biggest, it is to be the best," but his actions suggested quite the opposite. Convinced that universal health care was imminent, Hefty announced plans to convert his United Wisconsin Services to for-profit status and reorganize its five divisions so that they would be in a better position to capture government contracts.[16] When company stock prices fell from $44 to $21.25 a share a few months later, Hefty blamed the decline in part on the failure of Congress to enact Clinton's health reforms.[17]

While waiting for the Wisconsin commissioner of insurance to approve conversion of all components of United Wisconsin Services, the parent company of several Blue Cross and Blue Shield plans, to for-profit status in 2000, Blue Cross Blue Shield United of Wisconsin (BCBSU) expanded its managed care coverage to two million enrollees in the other forty-nine states. After the company posted losses for the sixth consecutive quarter and its stock price tumbled to $4.44, the Blues dropped their unprofitable Medicaid and Medicare beneficiaries.[18] United Government Services, another subsidiary of United Wisconsin Services, became the nation's largest processor of Medicare claims for hospitals and nursing homes upon signing a $40 million West Coast contract at the end of 2000.[19] Shortly after converting to for-profit status, BCBSU merged with United Wisconsin Services to form a new company called Cobalt Corporation.[20]

The Wisconsin Blues were not unique in their zeal to shed nonprofit status and responsibility to the communities they served. An executive from WellPoint Health Networks, a for-profit California Blue Cross plan, acknowledged at a meeting with the San Mateo County Medical Association that his company believed that it had no social responsibility in the community. WellPoint's presence in one county or another was purely a business decision. Moreover, there were no "fair" provider contracts, only signed and unsigned contracts. Stockholders mattered because they expected a yield on their investment, he said. The next day's *Wall Street Journal* reported that WellPoint's net income rose 17 percent in 2000 because membership growth and premium increases had outpaced medical costs. According to that article, WellPoint kept 24.5 percent of its premium dollar, more than any other California health plan, for overhead and profits. WellPoint CEO Leonard Schaeffer, whose annual compensation exceeded $3 million and accumulated stock options topped $20 million, earlier told a *Wall Street Journal* reporter that he advised doctors who complained about his plan to "just drop out."[21]

WellPoint Health announced its intention to buy Cobalt for $906 million in 2003, thereby increasing its combined assets to $13 billion and 14.3 million subscribers. Schaeffer apparently thought that the Cobalt purchase would fit well with his firm. Ignoring both companies' decisions to drop thousands of public beneficiaries, he noted that "Cobalt has an outstanding customer-focused culture and demonstrated excellence in providing superior service and value to the people of Wisconsin."[22]

Just a few months after acquiring Cobalt, Leonard Schaeffer, thought by some to be one of the most successful chief executives in health care (and certainly one of the best paid), announced that he was relinquishing the helm of WellPoint Health Networks and selling it to Anthem. The merger created the nation's largest managed care provider, with Blue Cross plans in thirteen states from Maine to California. Despite numerous requests to block the merger on antitrust grounds, the Department of Justice approved it in February 2004. The new corporation kept the WellPoint name but consolidated operations at Anthem's headquarters in

Indianapolis; Schaffer was to serve as chair, and Larry C. Glasscock of Anthem became the new firm's CEO.[23]

Mergers and Competition in the Pharmaceutical Industry

The urge to merge also consumed many pharmaceutical companies and hospitals. Such mergers usually raised the cost and sometimes limited the supply of products and services. Antitrust watchdogs were relatively sanguine about drug company mergers. However, the Federal Trade Commission reacted quickly, filing suit against Mylan Laboratories, the nation's second-largest drug manufacturer, after it cornered the market on a key ingredient for two generic antianxiety drugs and suddenly raised prices from $11 to $377 per bottle for one and from $7.30 to $190 per bottle for the other.[24] In November 2000 a U.S. District Court found Mylan Laboratories guilty of conspiring with other pharmaceutical companies to unreasonably restrain trade in the markets for lorazepam and clorazepate tablets and active pharmaceutical ingredients. The court ordered the company to pay, within three days, nearly $72 million into an escrow fund for consumer claims and more than $28 million into an escrow fund to satisfy state agency claims. The court also ordered Mylan and the other defendants to avoid such pricing agreements in the future.[25]

Spending on prescription drugs was a major reason for the double-digit rise in health plan premiums during the late 1990s and early 2000s. About one-fourth of the increase in total prescription drug spending between 1997 and 2000 was the result of price increases. Shifting from older, less expensive drugs to newer, higher-priced drugs was responsible for 28 percent of the increase, and the remainder resulted from greater use of prescription drugs.[26] Total spending for prescription drugs jumped from $140.8 billion in 2001 to $162.4 billion in 2002.[27] The number of prescriptions written rose because the elderly population was larger, and doctors had come to rely more on drug therapy. Nearly half the increase in retail drug spending went for treating just eight conditions: high cholesterol, arthritis, chronic pain, depression, ulcers and other stomach ailments, high blood pressure, diabetes, and seizures. Major drugs for these conditions were extensively advertised to both physicians and consumers. Indeed, ten drugs with the heaviest direct-to-consumer advertising accounted for more than 24 percent of the total increase in prescription spending.[28]

Some observers argue that newly developed drugs are expensive but reduce overall medical expenses because they enable people to stay healthy, live longer, and avoid expensive hospital stays and surgical procedures. For example, a year on anticoagulant medicines might cost a little more than $1,000, but the lifelong cost of caring for a patient who suffers from a severe stroke averages about $100,000. Researchers also report that Medicare saves $7 in hospitalization costs for every dollar spent on better medicines for heart disease and safer surgeries to unclog or repair arteries.[29] Others question the use and value of new drugs that are invariably expensive and have not yet demonstrated their superiority to older medications and other forms of therapy.[30] The Institute for Health Care Management Foundation, a leading research group, found that nearly half the prescription drugs introduced between 1989 and 2000 were not much different from their predecessors. Companies reintroduced drugs with minor variations and new names so they could protect their patents for another three years and dissuade patients from using less expensive generic drugs that might be equally effective. Drug industry representatives called the new report a "politically and financially motivated cheap shot" because eleven of the institute's twelve board members were Blue Cross–Blue Shield executives critical of drug industry pricing.[31]

Several prestigious medical journals from Western nations issued a joint statement in 2001 after learning that many highly favorable papers that they had published about new drugs were based on incomplete evidence or inaccurate conclusions. Their editors warned that drug companies had gained too much control of medical research and publication of experimental results. The editors blamed revenue losses from managed care contracts and Medicare reimbursements for forcing researchers at university medical centers to rely on drug company funding, which accounted for 70 percent of the clinical trials performed in the United States. All too often, the editors said, drug companies tried to influence how researchers examined and reported on their products.[32] As one of the most profitable industries in the world, American drug companies can buy a lot of influence. The $13 billion that they spent on self-promotion in 1999 included hiring one drug "detail" salesperson for every ten doctors, $2 billion for direct-to-consumer advertising, and $7 billion for "free" drug samples.

After the Food and Drug Administration (FDA) relaxed rules governing pharmaceutical advertising in 1997, direct-to-consumer advertising created a patient demand for many drugs that had yet to show an advantage over older, less expensive treatments. The industry's claims that its advertising educated the public without increasing costs defied the facts: Advertising created a huge patient demand for brand name drugs that sometimes cost five to six times more per month of therapy than equally effective generic products.[33] A bill before Congress in 2000 sought to control pharmaceutical advertising to consumers because such marketing practices deludes the public, adversely influences physicians' prescribing decisions, increases health care costs, and leads to unnecessary injuries and deaths, according to its sponsor, Rep. Pete Stark, D-Calif. Indeed, the inordinate fanfare surrounding some new products causes many patients to believe that physicians who refuse to prescribe such drugs are withholding the best available treatment. Fear of a malpractice claim clouds professional judgment. In 2002 the FDA reported that 69 percent of patients who asked doctors for a drug that they saw advertised on television received a prescription for that drug.[34] According to the latest information available, dollars spent on prescription drug promotion more than doubled from 1997 to 2000. Although television, radio, billboard, magazine, and newspaper ads seem pervasive, they accounted for only 12 percent of the nation's more than $21 billion pharmaceutical advertising bill in 2002. Drug companies spent most of their marketing dollars, more than $18 billion, on visiting doctors' offices and distributing "free samples."[35] While prescription drugs expenditures doubled from 5.8 percent of the nation's total health expenditures in 1992 to 10.5 percent in 2002, hospital expenditures dropped from 36.5 percent to 31.3 percent.[36]

Mergers and Competition in the Hospital Industry

During the late 1990s payer-driven competition and evolving technologies reduced hospital occupancy rates and the average lengths of stay. Some community hospitals closed, and others converted their acute hospital beds to less intensive types of care or developed an array of profitable outpatient services. Most community hospitals retained their nonprofit status, but the discounts that they had to give in order to win contracts from employers and insurers greatly reduced their ability to meet their obligations for serving indigent patients and promoting medical education.[37]

According to the American Hospital Association (AHA), nearly two-thirds of the nation's five thousand community hospitals were part of multihospital systems in 1998, up from one-third two decades earlier. The nation's two largest hospital corporations each owned more than two hundred institutions. The AHA argued that mergers were necessary in order to compensate for falling occupancy rates and to meet demands from health plans for greater cost efficiency.[38] But financial analysts concerned about antitrust violations suspected that many mergers were designed to reduce competition so that hospitals could negotiate higher prices with managed care organizations.[39] Indeed, the conversion of hospitals to for-profit status, often in the process of merging with other institutions, usually led to higher insurance premiums.

After reviewing two decades of peer-reviewed literature, the authors of an editorial in a 1999 issue of the *New England Journal of Medicine* concluded that for-profit hospitals delivered inferior care at inflated prices and cost Medicare an extra $5.2 billion annually.[40] In 2002 other researchers conducted a meta-analysis of fifteen studies involving more than thirty-eight million patients treated at twenty-six thousand hospitals in the United States between 1982 and 1995. They found that patients in private proprietary hospitals were more likely to have insurance and less serious conditions than patients in private nonprofit hospitals, but the risk of death was greater in for-profit institutions because they had lower staffing levels of skilled personnel.[41]

Fallouts from Mergers and Competition

Corporate reorganization throughout the health care industry created a great demand for specialty lawyers. Nathan Hershey, a professor of health law at the University of Pittsburgh, recalls that only a couple of lawyers made their living in the health care field when he developed a legal manual for hospitals in 1956. By the 1990s health care institutions required legal experts who understood antitrust law, tax law, insurance law, the regulation of employee benefits, and reimbursement under Medicare and Medicaid. According to Gerald R. Peters, a health care lawyer at Latham & Watkins in San Francisco, "We're in the midst of one of the largest industrial reorganizations in history, and it's a viciously competitive environment."[42]

Three legal scholars observed in 2003 that "competition continues to reshape the manner in which medicine is practiced and purchased in America and law can take considerable credit for this transformation. Indeed, it is only a slight exaggeration to view antitrust law as the engine that powered the emergence of a competitive market in health care."

However, managed care has increased judicial skepticism of the motives of insurance companies that claim to be agents of consumers. As a result, the authors suggested, courts may become more willing to accept the medical profession and nonprofit hospitals as patient representatives. Furthermore, they noted that "the bottom-line orientation of some managed care plans has forced the question of whether a market model is compatible with traditional social objectives in medicine, such as compassion, charity, and trust."[43]

Competition, growth, and profit-driven management practices pervaded every facet of health care in the 1990s. The economist Robert Samuelson expressed considerable skepticism about the motivation of corporate management practices across a full spectrum of industries, but his comments seem particularly appropriate for health care:

Management is one of our most overused, least understood and most expedient concepts. We visualize it as the means by which companies mold themselves into our desired Good Corporations, combining economic efficiency and social enlightenment. . . .

The idea of management is a myth: a figment of our collective imaginations. It projects business (especially big business) as we would like to see it, not as it actually is. . . . It certainly is not a precise set of skills, a body of knowledge, or a bundle of business techniques that apply to all companies. . . . What works in one company, in one industry, or at one time may not work at another company, in another industry, or at another time.

Not only did the cult of management underestimate the power of personal ambition and vision, it exaggerated the efficiency and stability of the large organization. . . . The Peter Principle afflicts many big companies: they expand to their level of incompetence. Success sows the seeds of failure. It fosters overconfidence, waste, and insularity. Corporate bureaucracies expand, and executive privileges increase.[44]

Samuelson conceded that big companies have inherent strengths: economies of scale, the opportunity to serve customers as they move, the ability to transfer lessons from one market to another, and ample capital. But, he said, "Good ideas become bad ideas because they are overdone."[45]

Nonprofit Health Care in Central Wisconsin and Elsewhere

The population of the city of Marshfield never exceeded twenty thousand in the three decades after the clinic started its Greater Marshfield

Community Health Plan in 1971. However, Marshfield Clinic Health Care System's service area grew to include 1.5 million residents in thirty counties throughout central, northern, and western Wisconsin. Its physician staff expanded from about ninety doctors working at a single facility in Marshfield to more than seven hundred doctors located in Marshfield and at forty primary care and regional specialty centers. Several health care institutions in the western part of the state joined Marshfield's system in 1996, and the Wausau Medical Center and its subsidiary clinics merged with the clinic in 1997. During the fiscal year ending in September 2003, the system's treatment facilities reported 1.8 million patient encounters, $695 million in net revenues and $30 million in net earnings.[46]

The Accreditation Association for Ambulatory Health Care awarded the Marshfield Clinic its fourth consecutive certificate of accreditation in 1997. Dr. Jon Stenseth, who chaired the accreditation team, told clinic leaders, "I don't know if you are the best clinic in the nation, but I don't know the name of one that is better. You are the model of how health care should be delivered to a rural population."[47]

The clinic had established its nonprofit tax-exempt Marshfield Medical Research and Education Foundation in 1959. Three years after the Internal Revenue Service granted the clinic nonprofit tax-exempt 501(c)(3) status in 1987, the clinic and foundation merged in order to increase opportunities for research, education, and charity care.[48] Since the clinic was organized in 1916, its doctors have, as a matter of policy and pride, treated all patients equally, regardless of their ability to pay. For nearly eight decades the clinic business office implemented that policy by reducing or forgiving charges to low-income patients unable to pay or (in later years) qualify for public assistance. In 1995 the clinic created Community Care, a program designed to identify and assist patients too poor to pay for care. Patients already in the clinic system were informed of their eligibility and encouraged to seek medical attention as soon as they needed it.[49] Community Care distributed nearly $7.7 million in charity care in 1999 but only about $5.4 million in 2000 after many former recipients enrolled in BadgerCare.[50]

One patient who benefited from this program was a grandmother who raised seven children to adulthood on her own and had not seen a doctor in six years. When she became ill and lost fifty pounds in a relatively short time, an area hospital refused her care because she lacked insurance. Taking her daughter's advice, she visited the Marshfield Clinic's Patient

Assistance Center, where a counselor found that she was eligible for Community Care and arranged for her to see a board-certified internist, who diagnosed breast cancer, diabetes, and acid reflux disease. During the next several months this woman received regular attention from her internist as well as an endocrinologist, a gastroenterologist, a physician's assistant who specialized in diabetes, and an oncologist. She also received services from an orthopedic surgeon, diagnostic radiologist, and surgical oncologist. When she was back on her feet, she said, "I couldn't believe these people. I thought there was never any hope until I came here. No matter what I needed, they made it happen. They got me my first new glasses in seven years and all the prescriptions I needed. . . . My only bill for all my care was a $400 co-payment. My son helped some and I used my tax refund for the rest."[51]

The Security Health Plan (SHP) was organized as a nonprofit 501(c) (4) corporation in 1987 after the Greater Marshfield Community Health Plan partnership dissolved. In 2004 SHP's coverage extended to approximately 117,000 enrollees in twenty-seven counties throughout central, western, and northern Wisconsin. Group subscribers represented only 57 percent of SHP's enrollment, a figure that was low compared to the group enrollments for all other for-profit and nonprofit health plans nationally. Conversely, SHP's proportions of direct-pay enrollees (8 percent), Medicare beneficiaries (15 percent), and Medicaid/BadgerCare beneficiaries (20 percent) were each unusually high. SHP spent 92 percent of its premium income on medical services.[52] That meant its administrative costs were lower than those of any other HMO in Wisconsin and the national average for all non-profits, and much lower than the national average for commercial health plans.[53]

The clinic, SHP, and the Family Health Center aggressively recruit low-income individuals and families into their Medicare/BadgerCare and FHC programs, which charge no copayments for medical services and, in the case of FHC, base premiums on a sliding scale. SHP's coverage options for private-sector consumers resemble those of most insurers to the extent that they all rely on deductibles and copayments for office and emergency room visits and hospital admissions in order to reduce premium cost and resource use. SHP offers several options to large and small employers, self-funded employers, and individual subscribers that may or may not include prescription drug coverage, behavioral health services, maternity care, and other services.

SHP's policies regarding premiums, copayments, and benefit coverage are the result of intense insurance competition in northern Wisconsin and reflect the needs of employers and direct purchasers for affordable coverage. They are a far cry from the idealistic principles that gave birth to its predecessor, the Greater Marshfield Community Health Plan. The clinic had to make some compromises with its health plan, but its commitment to cost-efficient quality care and its compassion for the patients its serves remain unchanged. When SHP anticipated a need to increase premiums as much as 17 or 18 percent for fiscal year 2000–2001, clinic physicians voted to take $4 million less in earnings (an average of about $6,000 per doctor) and allocated $9 million to SHP for reduction of premium rate increases.[54]

Taken as a whole, the Marshfield Clinic Health Care System stands in stark contrast to the commercial health plans that shed their nonprofit status to avoid community obligations and show little regard for the people they serve. Unlike other businesses, success in health care should not be measured by investment ratings and profits. Patients are more than customers; their dependence on providers is often a matter of life or death. Health plans that want to satisfy their investors must limit their enrollment to healthy subscribers. Such practices deny access to patients with serious health and financial problems and place a tremendous burden on providers that are more socially motivated.

The health care writer Robert Kuttner reported that many of the nation's nonprofit health plans were forced to compromise their principles during the 1990s. For example, the Group Health Cooperative of Puget Sound accepted only individual members from the time it was organized as a consumer cooperative in 1945 until the 1950s, when it began to contract with large employers. By the late 1990s Group Health had 660,000 members and was the largest health plan in the Northwest. As a result of increasing economic pressures, the plan modified its community rating for age and then, in 1997, formed an alliance with Kaiser Permanente. Despite those changes, Group Health continued to cover whatever physicians ordered and awarded physician bonuses according to three criteria: patient satisfaction; screening, immunization, and other performance goals; and overall budgetary targets. Kuttner regarded Group Health as a leader in the type of integrated case management that the entire industry professed to offer.[55]

Kaiser Permanente, the nation's largest nonprofit HMO with nine million subscribers, also had to make compromises in its quest to become a national company. In the 1990s Kaiser acquired widely scattered groups of affiliated physicians, built too many hospitals, and encountered problems with performance quality. Although physicians in Kaiser's Permanente Medical Groups controlled clinical decisions, the company could not maintain the core standards of its West Coast plans as it expanded.[56]

Competitive pressures and expansion into neighboring states caused the nonprofit Harvard Pilgrim Health Care to drift away from the 1969 founding principles of its predecessor, Harvard Community Health Plan. In the late 1990s less than a quarter of the Harvard plan's 1.3 million subscribers were in the original plan, which had changed its name to Harvard Vanguard Pilgrim. Harvard Vanguard devoted more than 90 percent of its premium to patient care, but its physicians were at greater financial risk and generally had more controls than those who worked at Group Health or Kaiser. According to Kuttner, the Group Health Cooperative of Puget Sound, Kaiser Permanente, and Harvard Vanguard Pilgrim Health Care all showed more concern for the welfare of their enrollees than other plans.[57] However, none of them approached Marshfield in its enrollment of disadvantaged populations.

In 1997 Kaiser Permanente and Harvard Vanguard administrators explained why their organizations favored nonprofit health care: "Health care that is structured to accommodate the sensitivities and demands of human biology will look different from health care that is organized to meet the requirements of stockholders. . . . A health plan constructed for financial profit measures success quarterly. A health plan created to accommodate the needs of human biology, on the other hand, adopts the perspective of a life span; its success is expressed in health outcomes and quality of life."[58]

Nonprofit HMOs must also be measured by how well they treat nonenrollees in their communities. The Internal Revenue Service introduced community benefit as a rationale for awarding tax-exempt status to nonprofit hospitals in the 1960s and later used similar incentives to hold nonprofit HMOs accountable for their tax benefits. A pair of researchers studied a group of large and well-established HMOs with nonprofit status and found considerable variation in social responsibility. Some partnered with community agencies that helped disadvantaged groups; provided medical services in schools, homeless shelters, and other local venues; or engaged in community philanthropy. Only a few addressed environmental issues or participated in public health activities.[59]

In the late 1990s several other researchers studied community participation among health care groups. One study involved eight nonprofit metropolitan health care systems that had been singled out by industry experts as having strong reputations among their peers for involvement in public health services. Administrators in all eight organizations acknowledged that changes in the health care environment had motivated them to "give back to the community." However, the activities at each study site were "a portfolio of standalone efforts," generally unconnected to each other or to any organizational strategy. Moreover, these organizations showed little interest in environmental health issues and poor cooperation with local public health agencies regarding communicable disease control.[60]

Another study reported in 2001 that HMOs were more likely to collaborate with public health agencies when they had nonprofit status or enrolled Medicaid beneficiaries. However, their range of activities was relatively narrow and their community participation rates were substantially lower than those of hospitals, state and local agencies, universities, nonprofit organizations, and private physicians.[61]

Unlike most of the nonprofits described earlier in this chapter, the Marshfield Clinic has greatly enhanced the lives of countless Wisconsin residents, regardless of their affiliation with the clinic or its health plan, through countless programs too numerous to mention here (but described in appendix 1). However, Marshfield and other nonprofits need government funding far in excess of the benefits derived from tax exemption in order to provide effective community service. Expecting private systems to provide services to nonenrollees is probably unrealistic unless the entire industry shares such responsibilities and receives adequate government support. Increasing commercialism in the health care industry clearly robbed most nonprofits of their important roles in protecting community health.

Chapter 13

Demands for Accountability

How unfortunate that it took the jolt of managed care to prod medical schools into doing what many knew they should have been doing all along.

Kenneth Ludmerer, 1999

Concerns about provider accountability increased during the 1990s among employers, managed care administrators, and legislators who wanted top value for their money and patients who worried that cost cutting could harm them. Their demands led to the development of better methods of evaluating HMOs and treatment outcomes and profoundly changed the practice of medicine in the United States.

Consumer-Driven Demands

Reports of patients' claiming to have suffered serious injuries when their HMOs denied them care substantially amplified consumers' fears about managed care. Despite a great deal of negative publicity, a 1996 Harris poll found that 55 percent of its respondents had never heard of managed care and did not know what the term meant. Even more surprising at that late date was that a third of the respondents were unfamiliar with the terms *health maintenance organizations* or *HMOs*.[1] However, when another poll the following year asked people to rate job performance in twelve industries, respondents ranked health insurance carriers and managed care organizations second and third from the bottom, just above tobacco companies.[2]

Allegations of poor performance and patient mistreatment spawned hundreds of consumer protection bills.[3] California lawmakers passed eighty-nine laws pertaining to access, disclosure, mandated benefits, patient billing and claims practices, and provider contracting and solvency between 1990 and 1997, and they introduced ninety bills in 1997 alone.[4] Congress and legislators in several states passed laws with such requirements as minimum hospital stays for postpartum mothers and postoperative mastectomy patients, although the laws were inappropriate in many circumstances.[5] All too often lawmakers based their actions on anecdotal reports or personal bias rather than scientific evidence.[6] For example, testimony from one couple whose two-day-old daughter died of an infection the day after hospital discharge led to federal and state laws requiring minimum stays of forty-eight hours for all newborns and their mothers.[7]

Consumer discontent generated a great deal of research as well. A California task force studying consumer backlash against managed care in the mid-1990s found that 42 percent of consumers surveyed experienced one or more problems with their health plans during the previous year. Researchers were unable to evaluate what effect those problems had on quality of care. They suggested, for example, that difficulty obtaining referrals to specialists might have been appropriate, given a well-documented overreliance on specialists. Also, complaints about a lack of specific services may have stemmed from limitations placed on health plans by employers rather than providers' austerity.[8]

Consumers in the California study reported many problems, but only 8 percent were dissatisfied with their health plan. Group practice HMOs requiring enrollees to use their staff physicians received much higher satisfaction ratings than loosely organized plans offering patients a wide choice of providers.[9] (Several other surveys in the 1990s yielded similar results.)[10] The health economist Alain Enthoven, who headed the California task force, and his associate Sara J. Singer concluded that the managed care backlash would not relent until HMOs were held to strict standards of service and Americans reconciled their competing demands for lower costs and unlimited care.[11] Such reconciliation might have occurred quite rapidly if health care consumers were responsible for selecting their own plan, instead of being removed from decisions and costs, as so many are, by third-party payers.

Many patients would find less fault with their health plans if they understood their physicians' explanations and instructions. A study released in 2004 by the Institute of Medicine reported that approximately 90 million Americans are unable, for example, to understand the significance of their diagnosis or their drug labels. This problem extends far beyond individuals with limited reading, language, or cognitive skills to many well-educated people who fear they will appear ignorant if they ask questions or find their circumstances so complex that they cannot find the words to ask appropriate questions. The institute's videotaped sessions documented many misunderstandings that could lead to serious consequences. Its report recommended that the federal government investigate ways to improve health literacy. The institute also encouraged health care educators to teach their students how to communicate with patients, and urged public and private insurers to develop creative ways to clearly explain health information.[12]

In the late 1990s one group of researchers faulted negative news reports for public and legislative reactions against HMOs. They reviewed eighty-five articles about managed care published in several leading newspapers. Most of the stories selected (which excluded survey reports, editorials, letters to the editor, and nonclinical articles) dealt with patients' concerns and issues of quality and costs. The researchers concluded that only 8 percent of the articles were likely to encourage readers to join or remain in an HMO, whereas fully two-thirds portrayed managed care so unfavorably as to discourage HMO membership.[13]

Some observers thought that health plans were morally obligated to provide information about their performance and benefit options so that purchasers and patients could make intelligent choices.[14] But only half of Americans with employer-based coverage were given a choice of plans, and only one-third of those could select from among more than two options.[15] Moreover, some workers were limited to products from one insurer's portfolio.[16] Despite all the discussion about choice, researchers in the late 1990s acknowledged that they knew very little about the consumer decision-making process or how choice affected the quality of patient health care and health status.[17]

The issue of health plan accountability attracted many ethicists. Norman Daniels, a professor of philosophy at Tufts University, and James Sabin, a clinical professor of psychiatry at Harvard Medical School and codirector of the Center for Ethics in Managed Care, identified several elements of an ethics policy for HMOs. They said that health plans should have patient care standards that "fair-minded people" would agree were appropriate under necessary budget constraints. Consumers should have a right to expect certain services from their HMOs: reasonable access to providers, including specialists; well-planned continuous care; emergency care when symptoms suggested a medical emergency; exceptional drugs when medically necessary; and an external independent review process when denial of services might cause death within two years. Last, HMOs should have clearly defined, fair, and consistent procedures for explaining denial of service to enrollees and providers.[18] While these guidelines have great value, decision makers who purchased health benefits for workers rarely considered such issues.

Health plans sometimes denied care inappropriately, but they also paid for too much unnecessary care. A presidential commission concluded in 1999 that procedures lacking scientific justification accounted for as much as 30 percent of the nation's medical spending. Commenting on the commission's report, the health economist Enthoven warned, "The country risks making a terrible mistake if it overreacts and treats every denial as an assault on patients. Denials are a necessary feature of a well-run plan."[19]

Consumer Protection Rulings, Regulations, and Legislation

The U.S. Supreme Court seemed to agree with Enthoven in June 2000 when it ruled in *Pegram v. Herdich* that patients could not use existing federal law to sue HMOs for rewarding doctors who held down costs. Writing for the unanimous court, Justice David H. Souter said, "The fact is that for over twenty-seven years the Congress of the United States has promoted the formation of HMO practices. The federal judiciary would be acting contrary to congressional policy . . . if it were to entertain claims portending wholesale attacks on existing HMOs solely because of their structure." Souter said that such lawsuits could mean the end of HMOs, which need to have financial incentives to operate effectively. But, he added, the ruling did not bar patients from filing lawsuits against HMOs in state courts.[20] Some observers thought that such ambiguity reflected "a central tension in the justices' treatment of health care between their generally favorable stance toward market-driven change and their support for shifting regulatory authority over the health sphere from federal to state government."[21]

State oversight of HMOs varied widely. Some states merely collected information about health plans. Others conducted site visits to inspect

HMO records and facilities, specified standards of service, required licenses, and mandated processes for dealing with peer review and consumer grievances.[22] Seven states had laws in 2000 that allowed patients to sue their HMOs, and state courts elsewhere permitted lawsuits in the absence of such legislation when patients believed that they had been harmed by their insurer. Lexington Insurance, the nation's largest malpractice reinsurer for managed care organizations, experienced a 2.5-fold increase in lawsuits against its clients between 1990 and 1997.[23] That increase was enormous, considering that half the nation's workers and their families were covered by employer-owned health plans that can deny patients' claims with impunity because the federal Employee Retirement Income Security Act (ERISA) exempts those plans from certain provisions in state insurance laws.[24] Organized labor was working through Congress and the federal courts to remove such exemptions so that workers could seek legal redress from irresponsible plans.

"Patients' Bill of Rights" legislation, promoted by the Clinton administration, and supported by George W. Bush during his 2000 presidential campaign, would have allowed disgruntled patients to sue their health plans in federal court.[25] The economist Robert J. Samuelson believed that the debate about patients' rights treated managed care "as an all-purpose ogre that is defeating the promise of modern medicine." Much of the backlash against managed care, he noted, came from doctors who felt that their incomes and independence were threatened.[26] The political columnist David Broder thought that it was absurd for patients' rights proponents to assert that only doctors could make medical decisions. "If cases go to court," he said, "decisions will be made by judges and juries, laymen struggling with an inevitable welter of conflicting expert medical testimony."[27] Broder and other critics also warned that such a bill would drive up health insurance costs and increase the number of uninsured.[28] Many employers polled in late 1999 feared that patients' rights legislation would expose them to litigation; one-third said that they would probably eliminate employee health benefits if such legislation were enacted.[29] Clive Crook of the *National Journal* called Clinton's proposal "a bill of goods" that would undermine rather than extend the principles of managed care.[30] Perhaps because of such opposition, the bill's proponents had not yet garnered sufficient votes to enact such legislation in 2003. Even without federal mandates, many HMOs had already improved their services by giving physicians more latitude in treatment decisions and offering patients better grievance procedures.[31]

In 2001, 80 percent of Americans said that they supported some type of patient protection law with the right to sue, but they were less certain about that issue when confronted with the possibility that premium costs would rise or more workers would lose their health benefits.[32] That same year the Consumers Union teamed up with the Kaiser Family Foundation to produce a free online guide to handling health plan disputes. It describes specific grievance procedures for each of the forty states that have such measures in place for their residents.[33]

Such laws do not increase the frequency of complaints, but grievances made in those states are more effectively resolved. In Wisconsin, for example, an Associated Press report found that the Commissioner of Insurance Office intervened in only about one of every ten complaints from patients who believed that they were inappropriately denied medical services. In response the state organized and authorized three independent review organizations to examine health insurance grievances. During their first year of operation the review boards overturned 42 percent of the discussions for which they had received complaints.[34] The crusade to enact a national patients' bill of rights lost momentum and dropped from view in the fall of 2003, but many Americans, particularly members of racial minorities, are unaware of grievance procedures and other measures that are available for their protection.[35]

Some observers saw the AMA's effort to promote its patient protection bill in Congress as a carefully crafted attempt to protect economic prerogatives of fee-for-service providers at the expense of managed care organizations. Key features in that bill would have required all HMOs to become federally certified, accept any willing providers into their plan, and offer all enrollees a fee-for-service option.[36] HMOs argued that the "any willing provider" clause undermined their ability to control use by forcing them to hire or affiliate with all qualified provider applicants, regardless of their practice patterns. Many states had enacted laws requiring HMOs to accept willing providers, but provisions in ERISA seemed to preempt the application of those laws to employee benefit plans. The U.S. Supreme Court upheld Kentucky's "Any Willing Provider" law in 2003, ruling that state laws can "regulate the business of health insurance" within the meaning of ERISA and are thus saved from preemption. Henceforth, managed care plans and other insurance companies must accept out-of-network health care providers—physicians, pharmacists, and specialists like nurse-practitioners—who agree to the insurer's reimbursement rates and contract terms. The ruling will benefit providers who seek to have their services covered by more insurers, consumers who believe that they were denied access to qualified providers, and rural patients who previously had to travel great distances to see someone associated with their health plan. However, insurers will have a harder time monitoring the cost and quality of a provider's services.[37]

Organized medicine was also responsible for laws in nearly forty states that gave HMO enrollees the right to seek independent medical opinions whenever they were denied treatment or tests. Legal experts hoped that the Supreme Court would eventually resolve conflicting rulings from state courts on the constitutionality of those laws.[38] In 2002 the Supreme Court upheld an Illinois law that allowed patients to bypass health plan gatekeepers who refuse to pay for procedures. Writing for the majority, Justice David H. Souter said that when an HMO guarantees "medically necessary" care, states can allow an independent review to look at the necessity. This ruling does not apply to the estimated fifty-five million people in self-insured plans. Patients' rights advocates hailed the ruling, but analysts predicted that it would drive up health insurance costs, forcing many employers to reduce workers' benefits. In 2004 the U.S. Supreme Court ruled that states can allow the 140 million Americans covered by employer-funded health plans to sue for reimbursement of treatments that their doctors deemed medically necessary but not for damages resulting from a denial of benefits. The insurance industry called the decision a "victory for employers," but the AMA said the decision would allow health plans to practice medicine without a license and without the malpractice accountability that physicians face every day. In response to recent state laws and regulations and federal court decisions, many health plans continue to back away from aggressive cost management, further increasing premium costs.[39]

James C. Robinson of the School of Public Health at the University of California School in Berkeley concluded that managed care had achieved considerable economic success but was a social and political failure. He said, "Health plan managers are rapidly moving in the direction of traditional health insurance by broadening physician panels, removing restrictions and reverting to fee-for-service payments." That shift has created a proliferation of insurance products that rely on the expectation that consumers will make informed, price-sensitive choices based on personal preference and budgetary constraints. But such expectations are unreasonable when patients lack the ability to predict their future needs or evaluate the proficiency of health care providers (or lack the ability to shop for their own health plan). For Robinson, "a consumer-driven health care system would be grossly inefficient as well as grotesquely inequitable."[40]

Employer/Purchaser Demands for Managed Care Accountability

More employers purchased managed care policies or adopted managed care strategies for their self-funded plans during the 1990s because they believed that such systems did a better job of controlling costs than fee-for-service care. Nevertheless, health insurance premiums rose about 35 percent between 1996 and 2000. At the end of the decade the average annual health insurance premium cost $2,655 for single coverage and $6,772 for family coverage. More employers were offering health benefit coverage at the end of the decade because of a tight labor market, but coverage for employees dropped to 59 percent and coverage for retirees older than sixty-five fell to less than 11 percent in 2001.[41] In an effort to get better value for their benefits dollars, employers turned to the HMO industry and physicians for methods that they could use to measure and evaluate medical services.

HMO advocates invariably reported that the quality of managed care was equal to or better than fee-for-service care.[42] Although such conclusions may have been appropriate in the 1980s, objective studies in the 1990s usually identified strengths and weaknesses in both systems. Patients usually had better coverage and fewer out-of-pocket costs with prepaid care but experienced fewer organizational hassles in the fee-for-service system. HMOs did a much better job of coordinating patient care, but patients reported more satisfying interpersonal relationships with fee-for-service caregivers. Patients in independent practice associations (IPAs) and other fee-for-service settings sometimes had better access to specialists than enrollees in staff model HMOs. However, researchers were unable to determine whether greater access to specialists improved quality of care.[43] Most patients fared equally well in either system, but the poor, elderly, and chronically ill tended to do better under the care of fee-for-service providers.[44]

HMOs offered slightly more prevention services than fee-for-service insurers, and group practice HMOs were better than other prepaid models in this regard.[45] The U.S. Preventive Services Task Force demonstrated the value of such services in 1989 when it issued *A Guide to Clinical Preventive Services,* featuring information about nearly two hundred diagnostic tests, vaccines, and medical services used to prevent or monitor diseases. A second edition released in 1996 covered many more procedures.[46] The guidelines gave providers, employers, and insurers economic justification for using certain tools to prevent or identify the onset of serious illness; they also enabled physicians to focus physical examinations on the health risks of individual patients.[47]

Evidence that preventive services were cost effective increased employers' interest in promoting health and preventing disease in their workers and fueled demands for health plans to implement such services. The Business Health Care Action Group in Minnesota's Twin Cities attracted national attention in the 1990s when several large companies worked with major health care providers to develop standards for measuring accountability.[48] By 1997 nearly a quarter of the nation's companies, including many small businesses, were participating in coalitions that enhanced their ability to bargain with providers.[49]

A growing demand for managed care organizations to demonstrate the worth of their services prompted the Group Health Association of America (GHAA) to assist major employers in turning the National Committee for Quality Assurance (NCQA) into a highly respected private agency for HMO evaluation and accreditation. GHAA and the American Managed Care Review Association had created NCQA in 1979 in order to establish standards for their industry and evaluate their members' performance.[50] NCQA lacked credibility during its early years because its reviews were invariably favorable. Moreover, many people still believed that health care quality was impossible to define or measure. The highly credible Joint Commission on Accreditation of Health Care Organizations decided to accredit HMOs as well as hospitals in 1988 but gave up on HMOs in 1990 when its results were largely ignored. That same year the Robert Wood Johnson Foundation awarded NCQA a $400,000 grant to help it become a quasi-independent nonprofit organization serving the needs of corporate health care purchasers.[51]

NCQA spent five years and $2.1 million developing sixty performance indicators for companies to use in selecting health plans for their employees. After a second, more workable version of the Health Plan Employer Data and Information Set (HEDIS 2.0) was approved by eight large national companies and thirty HMOs, NCQA evaluated twenty-one health plans in 1995.[52]

Some observers continued to question NCQA's credibility because that organization was dominated by large employers and health plans whose evaluation criteria differed from those of patients. These critics would have preferred an independent accreditation body empowered to correct or punish unsatisfactory behavior.[53] Others faulted features in HEDIS that failed to address how plans performed when patients were seriously or chronically ill.[54]

In order to address its concerns about the value of HMO services for Medicare beneficiaries, the federal government developed the Consumer Assessment of Health Plans Study (CAHPS). All Medicare HMOs were eventually required to report certain types of HEDIS and CAHPS information so that beneficiaries could select a health plan appropriate for their needs.[55] Recognizing that people with chronic health conditions have difficulty evaluating the care offered by various health providers, a group of providers and consumers, spearheaded by the HMO promoter Paul Ellwood, had formed the Foundation for Accountability (FACCT) in 1995. This nonprofit organization complements the federal government's provider evaluations and distributes information through its website and other outlets that helps patients with chronic conditions and their families assess the performance of their health care provider.[56]

At the end of 2003, fifteen prominent health care analysts and administrators noted in an open letter to their peers that the human and financial costs of medical error and substandard care were well documented. And private and government agencies like the National Committee for Quality Assurance and Agency for Healthcare Research and Quality had taken significant steps toward measuring quality. However, inertia within the health care system could easily overwhelm efforts to raise average performance levels out of mediocrity. They said that Medicare, as the biggest purchaser in the nation's health care system, had the fiscal leverage to take the lead in assuring that health care providers adopt widely accepted best practices. The cosigners called upon the Bush administration and congressional leaders to equip Medicare with reimbursement formula tools that would make "pay for performance," a bedrock principle in most industries, into a national strategy for improving health care quality.[57]

Other critics noted that none of the tools for performance assessment recognized socioeconomic, racial, or ethnic disparities in health care. Compared with other Americans, the poor and members of minority groups have more illness but receive less care, even when they have access to health insurance. Their advocates chided HEDIS for giving HMOs favorable ratings even when those plans ignored populations with high health risks. Such concerns appear to be well founded. Although most health plans are not required to submit reports to NCQA, evidence published in 2002 showed that mandatory reporting mechanisms for physicians and hospitals inevitably gave providers the incentive to decline to treat more difficult and complicated patients.[58] NCQA commissioned a study to identify and measure such health care disparities, and a subsequent report issued in 1999 recommended that performance data furnished by HMOs include social and economic determinants of outcome. In addition, the U.S. Department of Health and Human Services adopted a policy requiring all its data collection and reporting systems to include racial and ethnic categories. Reformers hoped that such steps would eventually promote greater accountability for the quality of care provided to disadvantaged groups.[59]

Ironically, some information that NCQA and its HEDIS data uncovered about managed care performance came back to haunt the American Association of Health Plans (AAHP), which was formed when GHAA merged with the American Managed Care Review Association in 1995. AAHP's membership included more than one thousand managed care organizations, many of which were profit-making enterprises. AAHP generally portrayed for-profit and nonprofit health plans as providing care of similar quality, but some observers questioned whether such comparisons were accurate. Information collected by NCQA and other groups unequivocally gave higher marks to nonprofit HMOs, which usually devoted about 90 percent of their premiums to patient care. On the other hand, commercial plans spent 80 percent, but sometimes as little as 60 percent or 70 percent, of their premiums on medical care, devoting much of the remainder to high earnings for investors and top administrators.[60]

U.S. News and World Report compiled the 1997 NCQA data on prevention services, access to care, accreditation, and physician and member turnover and satisfaction, and the magazine's results showed that thirty-three of thirty-seven top-scoring HMOs were nonprofit. Others who analyzed that data reached similar conclusions.[61] A 1996 *Consumer Reports* survey of HMOs found that all top-ranking health plans were nonprofit, whereas twelve of the thirteen lowest-ranking plans were investor owned. A 1997 report of HCFA data from all Medicare HMOs revealed that nine of ten plans with the fewest voluntary membership losses were nonprofit, whereas seven of ten plans with the most membership losses were proprietary.[62] Patients' assessments of health plans were similar in 2002. Enrollees in nonprofit plans were more likely to be very satisfied with their overall care than enrollees in for-profit plans. Moreover, patients who said that they were in fair or poor health gave higher scores to nonprofit than to for-profit plans.[63]

Marshfield's Security Health Plan regularly topped many HMO report cards for membership satisfaction: NCQA, Central Surveys, and Wisconsin state employees ranked it best in 1997; the National Research Corporation said that it was fifth best in the United States in 1998; and NCQA named it first in the nation again in 1999.[64] Three years later NCQA ranked SHP as one of the four best HMOs in Wisconsin and among the fifteen best plans in the country. The three other Wisconsin HMOs were Touchpoint Health Plans in northeast Wisconsin (ranked best in the nation), Group Health Cooperative of South Central Wisconsin, and the Madison-based Physicians Plus Insurance Corp.[65]

Wisconsin's four top plans showed an interesting contrast in corporate structure, size, Medicaid enrollment, percentage of premiums spent on medical expenditures, and profits. Touchpoint is a for-profit corporation that covers 140,350 members (11 percent Medicaid) in sixteen counties, spends 89 percent of its premium income on medical care, and reports a 1 percent profit. Group Health Cooperative is a nonprofit cooperative that covers 52,140 members (5 percent Medicaid) in five counties, spends 88 percent on medical care, and reports a 3 percent profit. Physicians Plus is a for-profit corporation that covers 102,325 enrollees (none on Medicaid) in eight counties, spends 86 percent on medical care, and reports a 3 percent profit. Security Health Plan is a nonprofit service corporation that covers 117,780 enrollees (20 percent Medicaid) in twenty-eight counties, spends 92 percent on medical care, and reports a 1 percent profit.[66] These differences suggest that NCQA's criteria for determining excellence pay little attention to the portion of premiums used for administrative costs or the willingness of health plans to serve Medicaid beneficiaries.

NCQA's influence grew rapidly because of increasing interest in its published results and eagerness among some HMOs to prove their superiority. Participating plans showed significant improvements from year to year, but the gap between HMOs that were providing high-quality and poor-quality care remained enormous. NCQA-accredited plans outperformed unaccredited plans, and HMOs that publicly reported their performance information generally outperformed those that did not.[67] While NCQA's ratings were published widely, even on the Internet, no such information was available anywhere for half the HMOs that did not submit performance information or for fee-for-service providers, who had no comparable accountability process.[68] In fact, NCQA reports covered only 28 percent of insured Americans in 2002. Margaret E. O'Kane, NCQA's president, acknowledged that "we have work to do—a large part of the health care system still doesn't measure anything." Added Nathaniel Clark, vice president for clinical affairs of the American Diabetes Association, said, "To manage health care, you have to measure it, and measurement has not been a part of medicine."[69]

NCQA and the HEDIS scorecards are still imperfect, but employers and health industry leaders involved in developing these tools deserve credit for providing a way to encourage accountability and evaluate HMO performance.[70] But as late as 1999 only 9 percent of employers required NCQA accreditation for the health plans that they offered to their employees. Instead, most companies ignored the ratings, remaining more concerned about cost than quality, despite growing evidence that high-quality care could save money.[71] Bruce Bradley, who directed General Motors's $3.6 billion managed care program, which covered more than a million employees, retirees, and dependents, warned a group of employers, "We're the customers. If we don't [demand quality], it's hard to complain about our providers. There is a business case for improving quality, but the ethical incentives are just as important. . . . If our health care providers don't show us a sense of values, ethics and commitment, we ought to call them on the carpet."[72]

Employers' interest in quality health care had gathered more steam by 2002. The ten-year-old National Business Coalition on Health (NBCH) boasted a membership of nearly ninety employer-led coalitions, representing more than seven thousand employers and approximately thirty-four million employees and their dependents. NBCH said that its members were committed to improving the value of health care provided through employer-sponsored health plans and to making the coalition movement a vehicle for meaningful change in the U.S. health care system.[73]

The Chicago-based Midwest Business Group on Health reported that low-quality health care in the United States was costing nearly $400 billion a year, about 30 percent of the $1.3 billion spent annually on medical expenditures. Using dozens of studies and previously published reports, as well as interviews with business and health industry executives, the new research suggested that medical errors, unnecessary treatments, misused drugs, and bureaucratic waste cost employers $1,700 to $2,000 a year for each insured worker. The report urged employers to scrutinize doctors, hospitals, and health plans for quality performance rather than choosing the least expensive option, which would cost them more money in the long run.[74]

Changes in the Practice of Medicine

Many observers faulted the medical profession for failing to develop criteria by which to judge the efficacy and value of medical treatments or to recognize how often human errors or inappropriate treatments lead to preventable deaths. Some researchers estimated that 50 to 85 percent of the treatments that doctors ordered in the 1990s were inadequately tested.[75] In 1999 the Institute of Medicine's Committee on Quality of Health Care in America reported that "medical errors" cause 44,000 to 98,000 hospital deaths annually—claiming more lives than car accidents, breast cancer, or AIDS.[76] Inadvertent deaths in other treatment venues, such as nursing homes and doctors' offices, add to that toll. Health care writer Michael Millenson reported "almost random variations in how different doctors treat patients with the same clinical symptoms. Variations show up in the therapy the doctor chooses and in how that therapy is provided . . . across regions of the country and among doctors at one hospital."[77]

Demands for accountability and cost-efficient care from employers and managed care organizations eventually goaded doctors into working with one another and with public and private agencies to develop practice guidelines for the diagnosis and treatment of specific diseases.[78] In his history of U.S. medical education in the twentieth century, Kenneth Ludmerer reported that medical school faculties waited until the 1990s to re-examine how they taught and practiced medicine and to emphasize more scientifically appropriate uses of medical resources.[79]

In 1989 the newly created federal Agency for Health Care Policy and Research initiated many new research projects designed to reduce Medicaid and Medicare expenditures by promoting evidence-based practice of medicine in everyday care. The agency's reports and technology assessments gave clinicians, health system managers, consumer organizations, and policy makers valuable tools for improving and assessing quality.[80] In 2000, the renamed Agency for Healthcare Research and Quality used a $205 million appropriation from Congress to fund research projects at several institutions, including Marshfield Medical Research and Education Foundation, Kaiser Triangle Institute, and Cornell University's Weill Medical College in New York City. The contract with the Marshfield Medical Research and Education Foundation and its Center for Health Services Research established Marshfield as a member of the agency's newly created "rapid response network." The role of this network was to evaluate the cost effectiveness of clinical and technological innovations, organizational structures, and care payment strategies; develop new approaches for rapidly translating research into practice; and assess information gaps and research needs. Marshfield was partnered with CODA, Inc., a social and biomedical survey research company, and Project HOPE's Center for Health Affairs. Their first grant was to assess the effects of four organizational changes in the Marshfield Clinic's system with regard to quality and efficiency of care.[81]

The AMA belatedly endorsed the concept of practice guidelines at its annual convention in 1996. That action represented an about-face for organized medicine, which had consistently fought efforts to recommend or evaluate how its members practiced medicine. Many old-guard doctors refused to accept what they called "cookbook medicine" because they believed that their training and experience enabled them to do what was best for their patients. Moreover, they feared that insurers, regulators, and malpractice courts might use practice guidelines to discredit their judgment or withhold payment.[82]

Other physicians believed that widespread acceptance of practice guidelines would enable them to better protect their patients' interests from overly zealous utilization managers. They also hoped that such standards would reduce the need for the defensive medical practices so common and costly in the past. The standard of care traditionally accepted in malpractice lawsuits—more care is better care—ignored reality: Defensive medicine provides many more opportunities for physician-induced harm than does conservative care.[83] In the late 1980s the AMA estimated that doctors spent more than $15.4 billion (17 percent of their earnings) on liability protection: $3.7 billion for insurance premiums, $1 million for time in court, and $11.7 billion for defensive medical practices.[84] No comparable estimates are available for 2004, but medical malpractice insurance premiums have doubled or quadrupled in various parts of the country since the last figures were compiled.[85]

Liability insurance rates increased ever more rapidly in the early 2000s, forcing doctors in some states, particularly those in high-risk specialties like obstetrics, emergency medicine, general surgery, surgical specialties, and radiology, to switch to less risky forms of practice or move to less litigious states. Insurers attributed the higher premiums to staggering increases in the size of payouts to successful plaintiffs and a noticeable increase in the frequency of claims. Physicians and hospitals blamed trial lawyers for promoting public expectations of perfection in medicine, noting that unsuccessful health outcomes often had nothing to do with negligence or malpractice. Trial lawyers argued that lawsuits are an important means of motivating providers to practice more safely.[86]

Legal scholars fault the courts for refusing to establish standards for appropriate care. The 1993 U.S. Supreme Court ruling in *Daubert v. Merrell-Dow Pharmaceuticals* ordered trial judges to ensure that testimony by scientific experts is relevant and reliable. But six years later a review of appellate court decisions found that most judges had failed to rule on the scientific veracity of evidence. To complicate matters further, physicians cautioned the legal profession that evidence-based medicine may reflect the best treatment options but that such guidelines should not be applied to every patient's circumstances or used as the sole legal standard.[87]

The tort system clearly requires reform. In 2003 Philip K. Howard, an attorney and founder of the Common Good, a bipartisan coalition dedicated to legal reform, told attendees at the annual meeting of the American College of Obstetricians and Gynecologists that he was "genuinely horrified by what my profession has done to your profession." A petition signed by seventy prominent health care leaders called upon Congress to create a new medical justice system that would consider the judgments of medical experts because few, if any, judges have the expertise to distinguish between good and bad medical care.[88]

In 2004 the U.S. Senate killed Republican stopgap measures that would have limited malpractice damages because the Democrats argued that large damage awards to victims of medical malpractice were often justified.[89] One result of allowing large damage awards is that millions of Americans have to pay much higher insurance premiums and countless patients had far less access to obstetrical and surgical services and emergency room care in 2003 than they had in the past.

Evidence-based medicine did not force doctors to conform to widely recognized standards, but it did hold them more accountable for their actions.[90] As the twenty-first century began, medical centers throughout the Western world were engaged in developing practice guidelines and publishing treatment protocols in textbooks, journals, and on the Internet. While great strides had been made, the process was far from complete.[91] The three greatest challenges facing guideline developers were keeping their information current, making it easily accessible, and motivating providers to incorporate such standards into everyday practice.[92]

A study of patient care in twelve metropolitan areas in the United States, based on telephone interviews with patients and examination of their medical records reported, in 2003 that only 55 percent of the participants received care that is generally recommended for their condition. Among the remaining participants, nearly half did not receive enough care, nearly half received too much care, and 11 percent received care that was not recommended and was potentially harmful. In order to close the gap between what is known about best practices and what is actually done, the research team recommended a major overhaul of current health information systems in order to automate the entry and retrieval of key data for clinical decision making and for quality measurement and reporting.[93] Another study found striking variation in the resources devoted to end-of-life care, even among U.S. medical centers with good reputations for clinical care. On average, regions where hospitals allocated fewer resources to dying patients tended to have lower mortality and do better on other measures of quality for all their patients. A reviewer who commented on this report in the *British Medical Journal* noted that the study's findings "should come as no surprise to observers of the National Health Service and other health care systems. They are neither unique nor confined to the Untied States. It is an iron law of health policy that supply determines utilization and demand . . . [and] the power to determine what happens within health services resides firmly with clinicians based in acute hospitals."[94] Michael Millenson observed in 2003 a persistent refusal within the health care community to confront providers responsible for several quality problems. The failure to take corrective actions or to discuss openly the true consequence of that inertia has undermined the moral foundations of the medical profession, he said.[95]

The Marshfield Clinic has a reputation for practicing high-quality, conservative medicine. In order to promote that philosophy among all providers throughout its rapidly expanding system, the clinic began in the mid-1990s to develop standardized clinical practice guidelines. Those responsible for coordinating this effort encouraged physicians and other clinical providers to participate in the process by using the clinic's internal website. As guidelines were developed and posted on the website, they were linked to other internal documents, such as standards for laboratory tests, and external sites like that of the Centers for Disease Control and Prevention in Atlanta. Physicians were not required to follow the guidelines, but compliance rates were high because the doctors were involved in the process and the guidelines were readily available.[96]

In the 1990s the locus of medical care shifted rapidly from private office to group practice settings staffed by salaried physicians. By the end of the decade half of all doctors were employed by health care organizations, and 80 percent of newly trained doctors were taking salaried positions. Nearly all physicians received some portion of their income from managed care contracts, but such contracts accounted for only half of all medical practice revenues in the United States. With less than 8 percent of all physician earnings derived from capitation, traditional fee-for-service reimbursement remains a dominant force in the U.S. health care system.[97]

Managed care organizations intent on promoting the value of their services to consumers are ideally situated to help physicians improve the quality of their care by providing them with protocols and educational services and supporting appropriate treatment. However, most health plans do not effectively exploit these opportunities.[98] Instead, they use capitation to dissuade doctors from ordering inappropriate services or they provide financial incentives to reward physicians for practicing cost-effective medicine. Little is known about how such incentives influence physician behavior and quality of care. The effect of bonus payments on physician practices is unclear. Placing individual physicians at financial risk seems to be effective in reducing resource use, but researchers have found no evidence to suggest an optimal level for risk bearing.[99]

Physicians working in most managed care environments were generally satisfied with their patient relationships, but many believed that their increased workload reduced the time that they could spend with patients

and compromised the quality of care.[100] Researchers found that office visits usually lasted somewhat longer than in years past, but doctors may have
felt greater time pressures because protocols required them to treat complex cases in their office rather than in a hospital setting. Doctors also had
to evaluate more treatment options and offer more advice about smoking,
obesity, domestic abuse, and other health dangers.[101]

Some physicians reported feeling ethically compromised by limitations placed on their treatment decisions. More than a third of doctors responding to a nationwide survey in 1998 admitted having deceived insurance companies in order to help patients get care that they needed, and
more than half of those doctors reported being more deceitful than in the
past.[102] Karen Ignagni, president of AAHP, suggested that health plan denials of prescribed treatments might be appropriate in light of the scientific evidence. In addition, she said, provider problems could be the result
of physicians' lack of experience in managed care plans.[103] AAHP's chief
medical officer, Dr. Charles M. Cutler, warned that doctors who deceived
insurers to get treatment coverage for their patients increased premium
costs because they "allowed people to get benefits for which they had not
paid."[104]

More recently, some physicians have stopped asking patients to pay
the $10 or $20 fees that insurers, including Medicaid and Medicare,
sometimes require them to collect in an effort to cut down on the number
of office visits a patient makes. While some physicians may be waiving the
copayments in order to attract patients who would otherwise use other
doctors on their health plan's preferred list, other practitioners may be trying to reduce their billing and collection costs or help people with limited
financial resources. Insurers discourage the waiving fees on a regular basis, and in many jurisdictions it is against the law. However, the American
Medical Association's Council on Ethical and Judicial Affairs has decided
that physicians should forgive or waive copayments if they pose a financial
barrier to the patient's obtaining care that she or he needs.[105]

Physicians were particularly aggravated by "gag rules" that prevented
them from discussing with their patients the negative aspects of a health
plan or treatment options not covered by their policies.[106] The General
Accounting Office warned Congress in 1990 that such restrictions could
reduce services inappropriately and threaten the quality of care.[107] Subsequent federal regulations limited how managed care organizations could
reward doctors for controlling utilization and costs, and these rules pre-

vented health plans from restricting physician-patient discussions. While those rules applied only to HMOs serving Medicare and Medicaid beneficiaries, they set new standards for the entire industry.[108] AAHP's Ignagni insisted that complaints about gag rules were "largely a red herring created by a sensationalist press. . . . Given the historical sanctity of the doctor-patient relationship, it would be hard to imagine how health plans could contemplate—let alone perpetrate—such an obvious and severe breach of ethics."[109] In fact, major HMOs, including Humana, U.S. Healthcare, and a Kaiser Permanente plan in Ohio, engaged in such practices and gave them up only when pressured to do so by federal regulators and intense media scrutiny.[110] A subsequent GAO review of 529 HMO contracts in 1997 found no specific gag rule provisions. Although some contractual clauses could be construed as limiting communication, the GAO concluded from interviews with physicians that such clauses had little effect on their activities.[111]

Nearly all doctors felt overburdened by the increasing amount of paperwork required of them by public programs and private insurers and by an overwhelming variation in the benefits available to each patient. Medical ethicists far removed from the scramble of daily practice advised physicians to become familiar with their patients' health plan policies so that they could use their "gatekeeper" role to their patients' best advantage and refer them to specialists when appropriate.[112] Restricting referrals was generally thought to save money, but researchers who participated in the Rand Health Insurance Experiment found no significant difference in overall expenditures for specialists and primary care physicians when they compared various models of HMOs. In fact, only 3 percent of patients who were free to self-refer in loosely organized HMOs sought services from specialists without first obtaining a referral from their primary care doctor.[113] Security Health Plan's experience in central Wisconsin confirmed Rand's findings. Even though SHP enrollees had access to all the specialists within the clinic's system, the health plan's medical service costs were comparable to those of HMOs that limited specialist referrals.

The AMA tried to remain neutral on the issue of managed care in order to protect its well-entrenched preference for fee-for-service care. As a result, managed care physicians were poorly represented by organized medicine. Doctors also lost much of their former bargaining power in the 1990s because their supply far exceeded the demand for services, especially where working conditions were attractive. A survey of twelve thousand internal medicine residents on the day that they finished their training in 1996 found that 11 percent had not yet found jobs and 7 percent had agreed to take part-time jobs or to work in a less desirable area of medicine. Such conditions would have been quite unusual just one decade earlier.[114]

Physicians who found themselves in a weak bargaining position with their employer occasionally followed the example of other workers and unionized. The AMA established its Division of Representation in 1997 to defend doctors whose authority was challenged by their health plan. Two years later the association voted to form a doctors' union called Physicians for Responsible Negotiations. By then, about 35,000 of the nation's 1 million practicing doctors belonged to unions, including 15,000 who had recently established the National Doctors Alliance, a local of the Service Employees International Union.[115] The U.S. Supreme Court ruled in 2001 that nurses could not unionize because they were supervisors. But using the court's definition of supervisory responsibilities, the National Labor Relations Board ruled in 2002 that doctors who are employed by health plans and other organizations can organize and are protected by the National Labor Relations Act.[116]

Self-employed physicians who contracted independently with HMOs were unable to unionize under labor laws. Furthermore, the AAHP and Federal Trade Commission opposed their joining with other private practitioners to negotiate fees and managed care contracts.[117] Some doctors considered litigation the only appropriate alternative when contract negotiations with HMOs failed. For example, the California Medical Association filed a federal lawsuit against the three largest national for-profit health plans in its state, alleging that their reimbursement policies forced doctors to provide less than adequate health care. The AMA urged other state affiliates to file similar class-action suits whenever insurers denied or delayed payment for legitimate claims. Calling the AMA's directive misguided, an AAHP spokesperson said, "There are many other and better avenues for problem-solving that don't involve sending things to courts."[118]

In fact, physician discontent with working conditions and loss of decision-making prerogatives engendered many constructive responses. Doctors sought training to prepare for administrative positions in managed care organizations where they could effectively promote good medical care.[119] Others formed independent medical groups that contracted directly with HMOs and employers but used their own medical directors and physician committees to monitor usage and clinical decisions.[120] Some medical groups sold their practices to or signed agreements with practice management companies. The growth of such companies slowed substantially when owners and investors found that buying physicians' practices was easier than changing the way that they delivered care.[121]

Physicians everywhere were probably less satisfied with their practice in the early 2000s than before the HMO movement began in the 1970s. The close monitoring of their treatment patterns altered the way that they practiced medicine. They lost a great deal of independence, their workload felt heavier, and their income was lower.[122] They also had far more paperwork. Nevertheless, most physicians retained extraordinary power among their own patients, even as patients became more assertive, more suspicious of health plan interference, and better informed about health care issues. And the medical profession still retains considerable influence among business and political leaders.[123] Some doctors approaching retirement held fast to their old ways, refusing to join the managed care movement. However, younger physicians had accepted many of the revolutionary changes in medical practice and were looking to the future, wondering how they could improve the system in the new century.

Private and public sector enrollment in HMOs grew from 2.8 percent of the U.S. population in 1976 to 13.4 percent in 1990 to 30 percent in 2000 and then decreased to about 26 percent in 2002. Most of the expansion during the 1990s was attributable to the proliferation of for-profit plans and gains in the private sector. Rapid changes in financing and delivery arrangements often seemed to favor the interests of health plan administrators and investors but increased the discontent among patients, providers, and their legislators. HMO enrollment also declined in 2002 because Prudential closed many of its plans and because of drops in Medicare+Choice enrollment.[124]

A few bright spots afforded hope. The U.S. health care industry made great progress in developing and promoting standards and measurements for quality care during the 1990s. The proliferation of practice guidelines and promotion of evidence-based medicine will surely decrease the use of new and invariably costly treatments until they have proved their worth. Consumers enrolled in HMOs that report to NCQA seem to be getting progressively better care. Scorecards for measuring HMO services offered employers who purchased workers' benefits, and patients who had a choice of plans, the ability to make rational decisions based on quality of care, an opportunity unavailable in the fee-for-service system. Because many health plans still do not report their information, the new scorecards pertain to only the one-quarter of Americans who have health care coverage.

Wider use of measurements that compare and evaluate health plans could have negated the need for patients' rights legislation. Still broader application of those measurements to include all providers in the managed care and fee-for-service sectors would undoubtedly improve the quality of care for all patients. That may be too much to ask. Physicians have boasted about scientific medicine for at least a century but seldom applied scientific criteria to their treatment decisions until competition and demands for accountability forced them to do so. Many physicians still rely on commonly used but unproven treatments and ignore carefully crafted practice guidelines that could save many lives.

Chapter 14

Critics and Would-be Reformers

We are the only major nation where people are refused health care because they cannot pay. In the United States, access to health care in time of need is a privilege, not a right.

Vincente Navarro, 1994

HMOs covered less than a third of the U.S. population in 2002 and their enrollments were dropping, but concepts of prepaid and managed care permeated nearly every corner of the health insurance industry. Criticism of the U.S. health care system grew louder at the turn of the century as concerns about health care costs, access, and quality increased. Surprisingly few knowledgeable observers blamed managed care. Instead, they faulted the employment-based financing of private health care, failures in the marketplace, myopic legislators, greed, insatiable appetites for new technology, and lack of concern for the disadvantaged.

Dr. Frank Davidoff of the American College of Physicians–American Society of Internal Medicine and Dr. Robert D. Reinecke of Jefferson Medical College in Philadelphia called the U.S. health care system "an embarrassing, world-class mess." They said, "Our deep distrust of central government control, coupled with our profound faith in the moral precepts of commerce and the market, our driving need for personal autonomy, and our occasional spasms of intense partisanship, have frustrated our best efforts at system improvement."[1] Their views were echoed by Mark A. Goldberg and Theodore R. Marmor of Yale University and Joseph White of the Brookings Institution, who noted that "the combination of diminishing coverage and spiraling costs is not some law of nature.

It is a peculiarly American disease, inculcated by ignorance and worsened by political failure."[2]

David Mechanic argued that inappropriate criticism of managed care by politicians and the media had detracted from efforts to meet the needs of uninsured and underinsured people. Mechanic, who directs the Institute of Health, Health Policy and Aging Research at Rutgers University, acknowledged that managed care "remains an imperfect, unfinished, and evolving product." But, he said, "managed care strategies offer the best potential for increasing population coverage while controlling costs" and improving patient care. Achieving universal coverage would address a fundamental flaw in the nation's health care system while "building social capital and a stronger and more cohesive community."[3]

Critics of the existing system often promoted universal health care. According to the policy analyst Robert Kuttner, "Many enthusiasts of market reform suspect—but cannot quite bring themselves to conclude—that the superior approach would be to cut the increasingly convoluted knot and move to a universal, unfragmented system of health insurance."[4] The health care sociologist Donald W. Light of the University of Pennsylvania Health System concurred. "What enlightened managed care needs, and what every other industrialized country provides, is a universal health insurance system for everyone," he said. "Efficiency and quality of good clinically managed care for whole populations can be attained only in a system that provides universal, stable coverage."[5]

The National Roundtable on Health Care Quality, convened by the Institute of Medicine in 1996, examined how rapid changes in the health care industry were affecting the quality of health and health care in the United States. The roundtable's 1998 report concluded that serious and widespread quality problems existed everywhere. Moreover, problems of underuse, overuse, or misuse occurred about as often in managed care and fee-for-service systems. Quality of care was the problem, not managed care.[6] In response to its roundtable's report, the Institute of Medicine organized the Committee on the Quality of Health Care in America to develop a strategy that would substantially improve the quality of health care in the next ten years.

The committee's 2001 report, *Crossing the Quality Chasm: A New Health System for the Twenty-first Century*, envisioned a health care system that was evidence based, patient centered, and systems oriented. It contained thirteen ambitious recommendations designed to make health care more effective, timely, efficient, equitable, and safe. The report also called upon patients and their families to demand a health care system appropriate to their needs. While perfect health care was a long way off, committee members believed that new information technologies provided a catalyst for greatly improving the present system.[7]

Equity is a serious problem. Forty-five million Americans were uninsured in 2003, but Families USA, a private advocacy group, found that 82 million people—one third of the U.S. population younger than sixty-five—lacked health insurance sometime during 2002 and 2003 and most were uninsured for more than nine months. The numbers were especially high for minorities, who are disproportionately represented in low wage job that offer no benefits. Nearly 60 percent of Hispanics and 43 percent of blacks were uninsured, compared to 23.5 percent of whites. According to Risa Lavizzo-Mourey of the Robert Wood Johnson Foundation, which sponsors "Cover the Uninsured Week" each year, "being uninsured is a very common and very risky experience. Being insured for even a short time puts people in jeopardy."[8] Being uninsured is particularly common and risky for minorities. The annual National Healthcare Disparities report issued by the Agency for Healthcare Research and Quality in July 2003 found a continuing broad array of differences related to access, use, and patient experience of care by racial, ethnic, socioeconomic, and geographic groups. The six priority areas of concern are cancer screening and treatment, cardiovascular disease, diabetes, HIV infections and AIDS, immunizations in children and adults, and infant mortality. The federal government, academic community, and private sector all have programs underway to address these persistent problems.[9]

Social justice demands that all people have access to good health care. According to the ethicist Norman Daniels, the central moral importance of preventing and treating disease and disability with effective health care services (including public health, environmental measures, and personal medical services) derives from how such services allow individuals to function normally. That ability affords people the opportunity to participate as fully as possible in the political, social, and economic life of their society.[10]

Uninsured Americans received about $35 billion worth of uncompensated care in 2001 through patchwork funding from hospitals, clinics, government programs, and private sources. Total government spending for the uninsured accounted for 80 to 84 percent of their treatment that year. According to the health care analysts Jack Hadley and John Holahan, the additional money needed to provide medical care coverage for the uninsured in public programs would amount to $44.9 billion and in private insurance plans to about $68.7 billion. The differences between public and private costs reflect payment rates rather than use of services. They noted that the yearly cost of additional medical care for a fully insured population is considerably less than the annual revenue loss of almost $179 billion from federal tax cuts enacted since 2001.[11]

Attacking the nation's health care crisis from a financial perspective, the Health Policy Consensus Group, a coalition of eighteen leading health economists with widely varied political views, blamed tax exemptions for workers' benefits for many problems in the private health care sector.[12] The economists John Sheils and Paul Hogan calculated that the federal and state governments lost nearly $125 billion in 1998 by exempting from taxation employee and other health benefits, health spending under flexible spending plans, and personal health expenses. They noted that families with annual incomes of $100,000 or more received an average tax benefit worth at least thirty-three times more than families with incomes of less than $15,000. They said, "These results raise important equity issues concerning the current distribution of tax benefits."[13] According to John Iglehart, editor of *Health Affairs,* a journal devoted to health care policy issues, this tax exemption cost the U.S. Treasury about $141 billion in 2000, making it the third-largest federal health program on the basis of expenditures, after Medicaid and Medicare.[14]

Analysts found other reasons to oppose job-related benefits as well. They said linking something as vital as health insurance to the vicissitudes of the job market was ill-conceived public policy. Too often, employers selected worker coverage on the basis of cost rather than quality. Self-insured companies seldom provided workers with adequate grievance procedures. And the system forced many people to make employment decisions based on the availability of health benefits rather than potential career opportunities. Concerns about employer-financed health care increased as the number of workers with benefits dropped in the 1990s, leaving many more breadwinners and their families without insurance.[15] "Sooner or later," wrote the health care researcher Victor R. Fuchs of Stanford University, "the inequities and inefficiencies associated with employment-based health insurance will become so apparent as to dictate disengagement."[16]

The Commonwealth Fund, a private foundation supporting independent research on health and social issues, found that the percentage of workers with health insurance coverage slipped from 66 percent in 1979 to 54 percent in 1998. When sorted by hourly wage, 80 percent of workers in the highest brackets had health benefits in 1998, whereas only 26 percent of the lowest-wage earners were so fortunate. The foundation viewed the federal budget surplus at the end of 2000 as an opportunity to improve care for vulnerable populations such as children, the elderly, low-income families, and minorities. Approximately 22 percent of the projected federal surplus for the forthcoming decade came from lower-than-anticipated Medicaid and Medicare expenditures after passage of the 1997 Balanced Budget Act. Rather than do away with tax subsidies for employers, as many economists advised, the foundation proposed using the surplus health care funds to increase incentives for employers to insure more workers and expand Medicaid and Medicare coverage to more uninsured Americans.[17] However, the new administration of President George W. Bush distributed the surplus as tax rebates to all Americans, whether they needed an extra few hundred dollars or not.

Insurance companies argued that favorable tax treatment for employment-based coverage enabled insurers to pool risks for 168 million working Americans. Moreover, they said, many employers were sophisticated purchasers who had played an important role in developing managed care, reducing costs, improving quality, and maximizing worker benefits.[18] Although benefit costs rose in the late 1990s, the proportion of workers with coverage increased slightly as businesses tried to attract and retain employees in a tight labor market.[19] But the shift was temporary. A study released by the Health Insurance Association of America in December 2000 predicted that the ranks of uninsured nonelderly Americans might reach forty-eight million (1 in 5) in 2009 if the economy remained stable and sixty-one million (1 in 4) if the nation entered a recession.[20]

In fact, many Americans lost their jobs and insurance during an economic recession in 2001 after they had already spent their tax rebates. According to a National Institute of Medicine report issued in May 2002, "Care without Coverage: Too Little, Too Late," individuals experiencing only a relatively short interruption in coverage suffer a decline in their health. Uninsured patients get poorer care than the insured: They are less likely to get screening for cancer and other life-threatening diseases; they are admitted to hospitals less often; they receive fewer services when admitted; and they are more apt to die. Uninsured patients who are hospitalized for a heart attack have a greater risk of dying during their hospital stay or shortly after discharge. The study estimated that more than eighteen thousand Americans died prematurely in 2000 because they lacked insurance.[21]

Most of the nation's biggest insurers (Aetna, CIGNA, Humana, the United Health Group, and WellPoint Health Networks) announced in 2002 that they would shortly introduce new plans featuring a complicated menu of premiums, copayments, and deductibles. Designed to reduce employers' benefit costs, these plans encourage workers to use medical savings accounts in combination with catastrophic illness insurance. According to Fuchs, "One of their major effects will be to shift the burden of health care costs from employees who use little care to those who use more. Thus, the new plans will be another nail in the coffin of health insurance as a form of social insurance." The U.S. Bureau of Labor Statistics reported that the percentage of covered employees in private industry dropped from 63 percent in 1993 to percent to 45 percent in 2003, while employee contributions grew an average of 75 percent to $229 a month for a family and $60 for an individual. Workers earning less than $15 an hour were half as likely to be covered by their employers as workers who earned more than $15 an hour. Fewer than half of private industry retirees had employer-sponsored health coverage; retired union workers had higher rates of coverage, and the likelihood of nonunion retirees' having health benefits declined with the size of the company. The analysis did not cover government employees, who are more apt to have coverage, or employees in the agricultural sector and self-employed individuals, who are less likely to find affordable coverage. Most people consider it fair to charge good drivers or homeowners who install smoke detectors less for their insurance policies, and these policies promote socially desirable behavior. But Fuchs argued that "the actuarial model applied to health care conflicts with a sense of justice and collective responsibility: it attacks a core element of what it means to be a society."[22]

John Iglehart believed that many employers and insurers who have been burned by the backlash against HMOs wanted to remove themselves from the patient-physician relationship and place patients in charge, armed with information and financial incentives for using health care resources more prudently. But, he said, findings of the twenty-five-year-old Rand Health Insurance Experiment are still relevant. That study showed that insured people generally seek medical attention less often when they pay a portion of the costs out of pocket, and far less often if they are a low-wage earners. Moreover, he added, Rand's research suggested that cost sharing is a rather crude instrument for matching health care services with individual health care needs.[23]

Alain C. Enthoven and Sara Singer of the Stanford Graduate School of Business stressed the need to address broader social goals. They noted that competition in the health care market had left many people with insufficient health care resources:

Market failure in health insurance is an important public policy problem because health care has a special moral status. Most people consider it unacceptable for people to suffer, to be disabled, or to have shortened lives because they cannot pay for care. . . . In a sense, universal access to necessary health care is a public good. Thus, any realistic discussion of regulation of health insurance and health services must be in the context of widely supported social goals: insurance should be wide-spread if not universal, affordable and distributed equitably. Because of moral imperative, collective action at some level is needed to make access and coverage widespread, and to make the market work with tolerable efficiency.[24]

Although Enthoven and Singer were not enthusiastic about government regulation, they acknowledged that government might need to have a role in motivating or requiring the healthy to subsidize the sick. Under a system of "managed competition," described at the end of chapter 8, the federal government would help consumers evaluate differences among plans and assess the value of add-ons, encourage insurers to enroll all applicants, and provide subsidies to compensate insurers for the additional costs of caring for patients with serious health problems.[25]

The legal scholars William Sage, David A. Hyman, and Warren Green-berg believe that competition law (which includes concern for antitrust as well as consumer protection) plays a valuable role in helping consumers weigh the cost and quality of health care providers. With the rise and subsequent fall of managed care, they note that the courts are now less inclined to view insurance companies as agents of consumers and more willing to accept the medical profession and nonprofit hospitals as patient representatives. And, given the profit-driven orientation of some managed care plans, the authors question whether a market model is compatible with such traditional social objectives in medicine as compassion, charity, and trust. The authors conclude that "Congress, enforcement agencies and the courts will need to decide whether and how considerations such as charity, access for the uninsured, and therapeutic trust between patients and providers—atypical subjects for economic analysis—should be incorporated into competition policy. . . . The challenge for competition policy in the twenty-first century is to move beyond its traditional focus on price competition and explicitly address the complexities raised by non-price competition in all its various manifestations."[26]

The Marshfield Clinic's experience with open enrollment and community risk–shared premiums demonstrated that health plans cannot serve seriously ill patients at affordable costs if the market playing field is uneven and insurers engage in predatory practices. When about 5 percent of the population consumes 58 percent of the nation's health care budget each year, public policy must support those health plans willing to serve the sick.[27] In the early 2000s about thirty states operated high-risk pools that offer policies to people who are not eligible for group coverage and have been denied individual policies because of their health status. High-risk policies in most states were very expensive, required long waiting periods before they covered preexisting conditions, and offered limited benefits. People who are seriously ill should not be forced to purchase exorbitantly expensive policies from high-risk pools or go without care but few states adequately fund their programs. The health care sociologist Odin Anderson said it best: "The private profit and private nonprofit sectors are not capable of assuring services to all segments of society. In the final analysis, only a government responsible to the electorate can assume that task."[28] Judging from what has happened to our nation's health care system since the early 1970s, our governments have been more responsible to their powerful and affluent constituents.

Many people want Congress to overhaul the nation's health care system, but federal lawmakers would rather patch the current system. Bills that include tax credits to help the uninsured buy policies on their own resurface during each session. Their proponents argue that such tax refunds would complement the job-based system by providing more choices to workers in small businesses. The problem with giving people tax credits to buy their own insurance is that the high administrative costs of individual policies and inevitably high premiums for individuals with serious health problems would require too much funding to meet the needs of the very poor.[29] While Congress considers underfunded tax credits for people who are unemployed or work in low-paying jobs, it ignores—for obvious political reasons—the billions of tax dollars lost each year from tax exemptions to employers who finance health benefits to workers (who are often already well paid) and to workers who receive as untaxed income health benefits valued at thousands of dollars.

Many federal lawmakers are eager to privatize Medicaid and Medicare and encourage greater enrollment in managed care organizations but refuse to acknowledge the inability of such organizations to serve the needs of the nation's poor, chronically ill, and rural populations in a highly competitive market. They would rather reduce reimbursement to providers and services to beneficiaries than examine the reasons why they have not been able to equitably control costs. After three decades Congress still ignores widespread regional spending variations that benefit the pockets of providers more than the health of their patients. Health care researchers say that Medicare could save as much as 30 percent of its costs—more than $120 billion a year—if all areas in the United States were to achieve spending levels comparable to those of the lowest-spending regions. Such savings would provide the resources to fully fund prescription drug and other benefits or extend the life of the Medicare Trust Fund for future retirees.[30]

Why this resistance to wholesale reform? The answer is the money—campaign contributions that protect the interests of large employers, insurers, providers in high spending areas, and pharmaceutical companies—that buys influence and helps win elections. According to John Kitzhaber, the Oregon governor whose state Medicaid program I describe later in this chapter, "One of the real problems with politics today is the growing number of people in public life for whom there is nothing so important as winning an election."[31]

Although many policymakers believe that managed care is capable of controlling public and private health care inflation, several factors work against any spending rate reductions in the foreseeable future. The aging population of the United States requires progressively more medical care. The current surplus of doctors and hospital beds increases demand for services.[32] The use and cost of new drugs are rising, and consumers' expectations have made expensive procedures, like joint and organ replacement, coronary bypass surgery, and in-vitro fertilization, commonplace.[33]

The American public apparently acknowledges no bounds for health care spending. In the early 1990s half the individuals responding to a Harris poll refused to set a monetary limit—even $5 million—on what should be spent to save a life. Ninety-one percent thought that "everyone should have the right to get the best medical care—as good as the treatment a millionaire gets." Yet three-quarters agreed that "all health insurance plans will have to make tough choices about what they will and will not pay for."[34] The Harvard Community Health Plan formed the LORAN Commission (named for the long-range navigational device) in 1992 to establish guidelines for the use and coverage of new medical technologies. The commission urged the federal government to evaluate expensive new therapies and insurance companies to delay coverage until such treatments are proved to be more effective than those they would replace. That and other of its recommendations have been largely ignored.[35]

Recent studies of certain popular prescription drugs and surgical procedures have shown them to be of questionable value, although they consume millions of health care dollars each year. One example is the randomized study by the Women's Health Initiative of female hormone replacement therapy, which was stopped before completion when researchers found fewer benefits than expected and some contraindications for use.[36] Another elaborately contrived, double-blind, randomized study of arthroscopic knee surgery for osteoarthritis found that patients who actually had the surgery experienced the same degree of relief as patients who *thought* they had the surgery.[37]

There are other ways to control, or ration, the allocation of medical resources. Many legislators refused to utter the word *ration* in the context of health care for fear of damaging their political career.[38] Policymakers prefer to use the term *priority setting* because it implies public involvement in a decision-making process about the redistribution of resources. The health economist Uwe Reinhardt argues that, regardless of what it is called, a pervasive system of health care rationing, based on income and ability to pay, already exists in the United States. That inequity, he said, is not lessened by using "judicious code words" or by pretending that rationing does not exist: "The nation has not been able to avoid rationing in the past and will not be able to avoid it in the future. The nation has merely lacked the courage to admit rationing forthrightly, and to debate the merits of alternate forms of rationing in good faith."[39]

Per capita health care spending in the United States exceeds that of all other nations. Dr. David Eddy, a senior adviser for health policy and management at Kaiser Permanente, thinks that Americans need to accept, once and for all, that health care resources are limited. Resources wasted on ineffective treatments are resources taken from other patients, not from insurers and administrators. Providers have an obligation to help patients understand the societal consequences of limited resources and the need to restrict unnecessary or unproved services. Rather than offering expensive treatments that carry potentially small benefits, providers must learn to evaluate therapies in terms of what offers the greatest good to the most patients. For physicians, Eddy said, that means "when in doubt, don't."[40]

Such advice creates an ethical challenge for physicians who refuse to acknowledge the growing scarcity of money for health care or the ways in which limited resources ought to influence their treatment decisions. Nearly all physicians feels a primary responsibility to the welfare of their patients, but some still believe that more care is always better than less care or are hesitant to acknowledge how financial incentives influence their practice. Such forms of denial deter essential efforts to limit consumers' direct and indirect health care costs and to develop more equitable resource allocations for the good of all citizens. Physicians are in a privileged position to promote policies for the fair allocation of health care resources both locally and nationally, but they can do so only if they examine their own practices and those of the health care systems in which they work.[41]

The growing trend among private insurers to relax restrictions on consumer access to providers and services may expose more patients to unnecessary services that are potentially harmful. Equally worrisome to many policy analysts is the threat to the private health care system from the increasing use of genetic testing and therapy. The health care writers Philip J. Longman and Shannon Brownlee reported in the *Wilson Quarterly* in the fall of 2000 that a collision of genetic testing and "right to privacy" laws could make private-sector health insurance unworkable and universal health care increasingly difficult to avoid. If privacy laws enable patients to purchase health care coverage without revealing unfavorable genetic test results, their subsequent medical care would cause private insurance costs to rise beyond the means of still more employers and individual buyers. But if insurance carriers are given access to test results in order to keep their policies affordable, they would have to deny coverage or dramatically increase policy costs for those likely to suffer from inherited diseases. The authors questioned whether Americans would be willing to preserve their private health insurance system if the price was loss of privacy and genetic discrimination.[42]

Some have suggested replacing the patchwork U.S. system with a national single-payer program like other Western countries have. In 2003 the Physicians' Working Group for Single-Payer National Health Care System called for the elimination of all for-profit hospitals and private insurance plans and the creation of a single-payer national health care system that would cover every American and be financed entirely with government funds. The doctors said the efficiency of such a plan would save enough to pay for health insurance for all citizens who lacked coverage. Under their proposed system, modeled after the Medicare system, the government would pay private doctors to provide services and would cover all medically necessary services, including long-term care, mental health and dental services, and prescription drugs and supplies. Panels of medical experts and community representatives would determine what services were medically necessary and effective. By eliminating the high overheads and profits of private, investor-owned insurance companies, the new system would save at least $200 billion a year. An increase in taxes to fund the new system would be fully offset by the elimination of insurance premiums and out-of-pocket costs.[43]

Robert Moffit, director of the Center of Health Policy Studies at the Heritage Foundation, the conservative think tank, said that the physicians' proposal for free health care would lead to "unlimited demand," forcing the government at some point "to make the decision about who is going to get care, when they get care, and how they get care." Instead, he proposed a system of tax credits or subsidies that would force providers to compete for services by providing better services at lower prices. The doctors contend that market-based reforms have not worked in the past, leading instead to higher costs, lower quality, and more uninsured people.[44]

Two-thirds of the physicians who responded to a 2003 survey conducted in Massachusetts, a state with high managed care market penetration, favored a single-payer system. The same proportion said they would take a 10 percent reduction in fees in return for a very substantial reduction in paperwork. A slightly smaller number said they would agree to a salary system if their incomes were reduced by no less than 10 percent. A resounding 89 percent felt that society has the responsibility, through its government, to provide everyone with good medical care, whether they can afford it or not.[45]

Oregon offers an American model for distributing health care resources equitably and broadly among the economically disadvantaged. In the early 1990s Oregon expanded its Medicaid program to provide basic medical services to all residents at or below the federal poverty level. Before the implementation of this innovation a state-appointed commission composed of professionals and laypersons consulted with experts and community groups to determine what benefits the program would cover. The commission recommended that the Oregon Health Plan, which is funded by Medicaid, Medicare, general revenues, and, more recently, funds in the State Children's Health Insurance Program) cover several hundred preventive, curative, and palliative treatments of proven worth. It planned to review services as new information became available and allow physicians to prescribe treatments beyond the basic package when warranted by extenuating circumstances.[46]

The beneficial results of Oregon's decision to broaden its recipient base while limiting costly, unproved remedies soon became apparent. Between 1993 and 1996 the nation's Medicaid enrollment increased 11 percent and program costs climbed 30 percent. During that same period Oregon's Medicaid population grew 39 percent, but expenditures rose only 36 percent.[47] Although Oregon reduced its number of uninsured residents from 17 percent in 1992 to 11 percent in 1997 and 1998, the nation's uninsured population grew from 14 percent to more than 16 percent.[48] Like its counterparts in many other states, the Medicaid program in Oregon was in fiscal crisis in 2003, not because of the program's generous benefits but because Oregon's unemployment rate during the recession was the highest in the nation.[49]

Some researchers criticize the Oregon Health Plan because they find little evidence of rationing health services or substantial savings. The plan excludes relatively few services of medical value, and its mental health and dental care services are superior to those offered by the state's original Medicaid program or Oregon's commercial insurers. Coverage of transplants is also more generous and comprehensive than when the Oregon Health Plan was enacted, and physicians take advantage of loopholes to provide uncovered medical services. Rather than rationing services, the Oregon Health Plan has received additional revenues from higher cigarette taxes and reduced costs by moving Medicaid recipients into managed care plans, the critics say. Moreover, these critics charge that political concessions and constituency pressures have severely compromised the Oregon Health Plan's original formula for determining coverage based on a cost-benefit analysis and outcomes data. Oregon has not been able to ration its services enough to satisfy some critics, but its experience shows that public participation in coverage determinations builds support and raises revenue for expanding insurance for the poor. More significant is that the Oregon Health Plan has provided coverage to an additional 600,000 people for relatively little extra money.[50]

More recently, a few other states have enacted legislation to make health care coverage more affordable to more of their residents. For example, Maine led the nation in per capita health care spending for more than a decade beginning in the early 1990s and accumulated about $275 million in unpaid bills and charity care each year because 1 of every 8 residents lacked coverage. In 2003 newly elected governor John Baldacci assembled a sixty-member health action team representing business, government, consumers, providers, and purchasers to advise him. Acting upon their recommendations, he created an independent state agency to run a health care program targeted initially at small businesses, self-employed people, and other individual consumers. Subsidies are available for families and individuals with incomes equal to as much as 300 percent of the poverty level. The new agency determines eligibility, and services are funded through a combination of employer and employee payments, Medicaid dollars for eligible beneficiaries, and a tax on the gross revenues of health insurers. The system still has many details to resolve but is well on its way.[51] In 2003 Wisconsin legislators created five regional health insurance purchasing cooperatives through which Wisconsin farm families, small business owners and self-employed workers will be able to negotiate collectively with health insurance providers for affordable coverage. However, implementation was delayed when a U.S. Senate subcommittee decided in 2004 to exclude funding for that project from a key bill.[52]

Most other industrialized nations try to distribute health care resources equitably among their citizens, choosing to restrict certain services to everyone rather than limiting access to some.[53] In Sweden, for example, the government sets priorities by balancing health care spending with revenues from taxes. Its priorities are based on core principles that recognize the equal value of its citizens; an obligation to offer special protection to those who are weakest and most vulnerable; and a need to allocate resources for the greatest good. Swedes sometime chafe at having to wait for particular procedures. But they generally regard methods of distributing medical services morally unacceptable if they sacrifice the well-being of the poor, elderly, dissolute, or prematurely born or allow better treatment for the wealthy, socially prominent, or politically powerful.[54]

News reports in the 1990s frequently predicted the impending demise of Canada's government-operated health care system, which still has considerable support among physicians and residents. Iglehart and *Health Affairs* revisited Canada in 2000 after a decade's absence. He found physicians there were greatly dissatisfied with their system's deterioration. They were also remarkably supportive of the principles on which it is based and skeptical of claims that the country would be better off with a private, market-based model.[55]

Problems with the Canadian system developed when the federal government tried to stem deficit spending in the early 1990s by combining and reducing total allocations to the provinces for health care, higher education, welfare assistance, and other social programs. When services declined, the percentage of Canadians who ranked their health care as "excellent" or "good" fell from 61 percent in 1991 to 24 percent in 1999. Iglehart attributed Canada's health care problems to inadequate funding and its unique and long-standing ban on private insurance for publicly insured services. In 1998 Canada spent just 9.3 percent of its gross domestic product (GDP) on health care, compared to 14 percent of GDP in the United States.[56] Colleen Fuller, author of *Caring for Profit: How Corporations Are Taking Over Canada's Health Care System,* also blamed funding reductions for Canada's health care problems and for other growing social inequities. She reported that 80 percent of Canadians wanted their government to be chiefly responsible for health care, whereas only 6 percent preferred to have private enterprise in that role. Nevertheless, private corporations were slowly intruding into the system, often with the open collaboration of federal or provincial governments.[57]

In Great Britain, where the National Health Service spends only about 7 percent of the GDP (compared to a European average of 9 percent) on health care, debate rages about which services should be offered and which should be denied, beyond those that are clearly ineffective.[58] Some observers blame perceived deficiencies in the program on the self-serving interest of professionals who sometimes feel overworked and underpaid and who are unwilling to acknowledge publicly that some disease processes are inexorable, not a reflection of inadequate health service.[59]

A study comparing the National Health Service with California's Kaiser Permanente did not support the widely held belief that the National Health Service is efficient and that underinvestment explains its poor performance in certain areas. Instead, the authors claimed that Kaiser had achieved better performance at roughly the same cost as the National Health Service because of better integration throughout its system, efficient management of hospital use, greater investment in information technology, and the benefits of competition. Seventy-five readers of the *British Medical Journal,* where this report was published, fired back with immediate and often emotional letters. By a 2 to 1 margin health care providers on both sides of the Atlantic faulted the report's assumptions (which were based on entirely different patient and public health care responsibilities) and called its data, analyses, and conclusions misleading or simply wrong.[60]

Despite widespread reports in the medical literature that the British fear inappropriate rationing, surveys find that the British public and 86 percent of British doctors support the founding principles of their centrally funded system.[61] A British Medical Association report, prepared with help from a wide variety of health care industry representatives and published in early 2001, confirmed that the national program needed more resources to improve. However, it emphasized that private-sector funding mechanisms would be no more successful than the present system of taxation in narrowing the affordability gap. Rather, the amount of money that can or ought to be devoted to health care is finite, and some degree of rationing is invariably inevitable.[62] In fiscal 2002–2003 British prime minister Tony Blair's government raised the National Health Service budget 10 percent to bring its spending in line with that of other members of the European Union. The move is part of a long-term strategy to increase the number of medical personnel, resources, and services and make the service more consumer oriented. Although some details are unresolved, the biggest challenge will be to devise a structure and set of incentives that ensure efficient use of the new resources and achievement of the consumer-oriented goals.[63]

As Robert J. Samuelson observed in his 1995 book, *The Good Life and Its Discontents:*

Equity of care, an appealing ideal, becomes less so in practice. Paradoxically, health care was the most equal when there was less of it—say, in the nineteenth century—because it couldn't do much for anyone, regardless of their income. Ethical and economic dilemmas have emerged only as better and more expensive medicine created opportunities to cure diseases and repair injuries. . . . Somehow, limits have to be set; otherwise, unlimited insurance will mean unlimited spending. "Equality" is unattainable in the sense that all "needs" can be met.[64]

David Kindig argued in *Purchasing Population Health: Paying for the Results* that merely controlling the cost of health care services will not result in an optimal allocation of societal resources. In order to achieve the best possible health for the greatest number of people, money spent on health care must be balanced with the nonmedical factors involved in producing good health, including nutrition, housing, and education.[65]

Americans who expect high-quality medical care are often dissatisfied with what they get. Avedis Donabedian, who created the conceptual framework for quality assessments used by health care systems at the end of the twentieth century, was interviewed shortly before his death in November 1999. Donabedian described the health care problems that he had encountered during his nearly three-decade battle with cancer:

I have tried to choose doctors who work together reasonably well [but] there are areas where no one takes responsibility, where planning is weak, where I am left on my own. . . . The view of quality taken in the hospital is really limited to technical competence. . . . The ideal that patients should be involved in their own care is not really practiced in a responsible way. Today people talk about patient autonomy, but often it gets translated into patient abandonment.

HMOs today are good at measuring costs but pay little attention to measuring effects. The failure to look at outcomes undercuts all the reasons that so many of us were interested in the prepaid group practice model to begin with. . . . Sooner or later we are going to have to develop a national health care plan. The design and implementation of such a plan will be an exciting task of the fairly near future, I believe. This country has tremendous wisdom and tremendous goodness. Eventually it will triumph in health care.[66]

After the Clinton administration failed to enact meaningful health care reforms in 1994, David Blumenthal of Massachusetts General Hospital compared the dismal results of that federal initiative with the passage of Medicare legislation three decades earlier. He identified two significant differences between conditions prevailing during the Medicare debate in the early 1960s and the health care reform debate in the mid-1990s. Blumenthal noted that President Lyndon Johnson's legendary political skills and Wilbur Cohen's experience in drafting health insurance legislation were far superior to the talents available on Clinton's team. More significantly, a powerful voting bloc of elderly Americans and younger voters with aging parents supported Medicare because Democrats and organized labor had spent at least five years generating grassroots support for Medicare legislation. In contrast, the uninsured populations that Clinton tried to help constituted a weak and much less cohesive voting bloc. Moreover, Blumenthal argues:

Meaningful health care reform will only become a reality when it gathers a political constituency so strong and committed that neither special interests nor the inevitable bumps and detours of the congressional process can block it. For that to happen, our health care system's problems will have to affect the personal lives of many voters who have not yet been touched by its deterioration. Millions of additional Americans will have to lose their health insurance, believe strongly that such loss is possible at any time, experience major erosion of their existing insurance benefits, or become dissatisfied with the health care they are receiving. Advocates can continue to press for major changes in the health care system, but they will have to wait for Americans to conclude from personal experience that health care reform is worth some undeniable risks.[67]

Powerful lobby groups representing the interests of organized medicine, pharmaceutical corporations, and the insurance industry stand ready to challenge any meaningful reform of the U.S. health care system. The strength of that challenge increased perceptibly when the American Association of Health Plans merged with the Health Insurance Association of America in 2003. In announcing the merger, AAHP president Karen M. Ignagni said the new organization, America's Health Insurance Plans, would form a huge lobby that would speak with one voice on Medicare and industry regulation.[68] The merger of the two organizations, whose original components represented widely diverse views on the nature of health care financing and delivery of services—prepaid care on one hand and traditional insurers on the other—confirms the death of the HMO movement. Intent on greater profits, nearly all insurers now combine the health care management practices of prepaid care with commercial insurance's preference for risk-adverse underwriting and cost sharing. The insurance industry now has a much more powerful voice, but who speaks for the millions of uninsured and underinsured Americans? Does this history of the HMO movement provide any lessons that can help promote more socially responsible goals?

Conclusion

Lessons from Marshfield

The central question is whether the efficiency and fairness problems that exist [in our health care system] can be addressed by imperfect government or by imperfect markets.

Bryan Dowd, 1999

The Marshfield Clinic was a successful, well-regarded multispecialty clinic with a strong sense of community orientation long before the HMO movement began. It accomplished much of what HMOs, reinvented as new public policy in the early 1970s, were supposed to do. Ham-fisted federal and state government efforts, supposedly designed to promote HMOs, and a poorly conceived ethos of market competition battered the clinic and nearly destroyed it. Despite its rural setting, opposition from insurers, lawsuits, and problems with Medicare and Medicaid, it survived and continues to flourish in an increasingly competitive health care environment.

Marshfield experienced all the problems that other sponsors encountered when trying to organize HMOs in the early 1970s. Area physicians greeted the idea of prepaid care with hostility, believing that it would detract from their practices. None of the three insurance companies initially contacted by clinic physicians was willing to participate in such a venture for fear of losing policyholders. Although the insurers were not averse to prepaid care, they thought that the doctors' social goals for their plan would be financially disastrous. Indeed, all three companies started their own plans at about the same time as Marshfield did. Milwaukee's Blue Cross Associated Hospital Plan, which approached the clinic with a partnership proposal, was willing to tolerate the doctors' insistence on open enrollment, community rating, and other actuarially unsound ideas in order to gain an early foothold in central Wisconsin's prepaid market. The clinic accepted the Blues' legendary accounting problems because it needed their insurance expertise.

The Greater Marshfield Community Health Plan grew rapidly during its early years because of its liberal enrollment policies and the clinic's reputation for quality care. The doctors' refusal to heed Blue Cross's actuarial advice would have doomed the plan if the carrier had been less cooperative. The Blues brought considerable financial help and expertise to the venture. But GMCHP's ability to survive on very low returns during its early years was the result of the clinic's cost-efficient delivery system, uniform salary plan for physicians, and long-standing commitment to charity. The participation in the partnership by Saint Joseph's Hospital was halfhearted because its administrators were afraid of losing money. Blue Cross and the clinic were more willing to make financial sacrifices in order to prove that prepaid care could work in a rural setting. Judging from Marshfield's experience, providing health care to rural populations is rarely more than marginally profitable, even with a very efficient system.

The struggle in central Wisconsin to start a health plan in the early 1970s was repeated at dozens of sites around the country while Congress debated its role in promoting prepaid care. The long-awaited HMO Act of 1973 failed to resolve the nation's health care crisis and nearly derailed the HMO movement. Fearing that prepayment would cause providers to stint on services, both political parties loaded the legislation with regulations. Congressional Democrats expected HMOs to solve all the nation's health care problems, but the Republican administration responsible for implementation arranged to fund as few plans as bureaucratically possible. Almost immediately, health care reformers and providers began to draft amendments designed to weaken the Democrats' open enrollment and community rating mandates so that federally funded HMOs could compete more equally with other insurers.

Using evidence published shortly after Congress debated those amendments, officials of the Marshfield Clinic argued that requiring all insurers to use open enrollment and community rating would enable millions of Americans to have better access to health care. Instead, Congress restricted access by acceding to the powerful insurance lobby and the Group Health Association of America, whose members, including Kaiser

Permanente, marketed almost exclusively to employers and rejected community-wide rating. In health care, as in so many other sectors of the U.S. economy, federal legislation to protect special interest groups often harms the public good.

HMO sponsors started three times as many plans in the four years before passage of the HMO Act of 1973 as in the four years afterward. Subsequent federal and state legislation intended to facilitate prepaid health care often had the opposite effect. Federal funding gave prepaid health care a legitimacy long denied by the medical profession, but the federal requirements for HMOs deterred many potential sponsors. Widespread HMO development did not begin until employers demanded lower health care costs during the economic recession of the early 1980s. Although the federal government had withdrawn financial support by then, competition among insurance companies willing to invest in prepaid care quickly transformed health care into a corporate industry.

That industry showed little interest in serving rural populations for several good reasons. Sparsely settled areas offered relatively few opportunities to market group contracts to large firms. Farmers and other workers were often self-employed and poor. Many rural residents had serious medical problems. Health care providers and facilities were widely scattered and often substandard.

Instead of ignoring underserved populations, Marshfield sought federal and state grants to train and attract skilled caregivers, create new facilities, and provide a wide variety of improved medical and mental health services to residents of northern Wisconsin. GMCHP's affiliation with primary care providers in outlying communities linked thousands of northwoods people to comprehensive health care benefits for the first time. Federal subsidies enabled Marshfield's Family Health Center to deliver to thousands of local low-income families the same benefits that other Greater Marshfield subscribers received, as well as extra dental, pharmaceutical, and social services.

Marshfield's outreach programs increased the clinic's referral base and the demand for GMCHP coverage. But those programs also helped the patients and policyholders of competing providers and insurers to gain access to better and sometimes free screening, diagnostic, immunization, and dental services. While government programs continue to meet a variety of health care needs in northern Wisconsin and elsewhere, the federal bureaucracy that controls them lacks coordination and is hopelessly complex. Moreover, the pursuit of government grants requires a tremendously dedicated and persistent staff. Such work provides a livelihood for countless public and private-sector employees but wastes money better spent on basic medical care for disadvantaged populations.

Just as Marshfield developed a broad network of affiliated providers to meet the primary care needs of subscribers in outlying communities, federal policy allowed HMOs to assume a wide variety of forms in order to accommodate the needs of potential sponsors. During the 1970s physicians, sponsors, and investors favored independent practice associations (IPAs), which were relatively inexpensive to organize and allowed physicians to practice in their own office, where they could serve other patients as well. These loosely structured IPAs had more difficulty controlling usage, costs, and quality of care than group practice HMOs did. GMCHP's rural setting compounded the problems of dealing with affiliates because some areas had few, if any, qualified providers. In addition, health plan officials had to be diplomatic when criticizing its affiliates' costly and inappropriate treatment practices because the clinic's growing team of specialists depended on the affiliates for referrals. Unlike urban HMOs, neither the clinic nor GMCHP had the luxury of dismissing providers who failed to meet professional standards or health plan expectations.

Such problems offer still more reasons why so few HMOs started or expanded into rural areas. Still, Marshfield's commitment to improving its affiliated providers' medical skills shows yet another way in which HMOs can indirectly improve health care for all residents in their communities. Further, the clinic's willingness to work with affiliates demonstrates its determination to link rural people with specialized services so that their medical care could be just as good as, and perhaps even better than, what their urban counterparts received.

Clinic leaders started GMCHP as an experiment to assess the cost of providing high-quality prepaid care to all segments of a rural population, including Medicaid and Medicare recipients. In the mid- to late 1970s GMCHP became the first HMO to hold a prepaid Medicaid contract in Wisconsin and one of the first in the nation to participate in a Medicare "risk-contract" demonstration with the federal Health Care Financing Administration (HCFA). Greater Marshfield's contracts with the state and HCFA nearly depleted its operating reserves and were financially disastrous.

Reimbursement from the state and federal contracts were based on a percentage of the average fee-for-service costs for serving beneficiaries. Local charges in central Wisconsin were unusually low because of the influence of the cost-efficient clinic, so GMCHP's Medicaid reimbursements were a great deal lower than what HMOs in two of Wisconsin's urban counties received a few years later. Marshfield's insistence on accepting all applicants, regardless of health status, compounded its losses in the Medicare demonstration project because HCFA refused to adjust its reimbursement formula for serving unhealthy beneficiaries.

HCFA's stated goals for that demonstration were to test new incentives for increasing the enrollment of Medicare beneficiaries in HMOs and to find a way in which to incorporate patient health status into HCFA's reimbursement formula. Other HMOs in the demonstration project received higher payments than Marshfield did, some nearly twice as much, even though they rejected applicants with health problems. Congress had hoped to save money by increasing enrollment of Medicare beneficiaries in HMOs, but HCFA wasted money by paying HMOs much more than they deserved for enrolling only relatively healthy applicants. In addition to working at cross-purposes, these federal policies showed a shameful disregard for seriously ill beneficiaries, who were forced to go without supplemental coverage or to pay much higher premiums for traditional Medigap policies offering fewer benefits.

GMCHP finally fulfilled the vision of the clinic's founders in the early 1980s when it was able to offer coverage to poor, sick, and elderly residents in its marketing area. Its prepaid Medicaid program was serving the very poor. The Family Health Center was subsidizing health plan premiums for poor working families. And senior citizens were flocking to GMCHP's Medicare demonstration program. Although that utopia was short lived, it was not a pipe dream. Marshfield could have covered the expenses of its Medicaid and Medicare programs if its reimbursements had matched those of HMO demonstration projects elsewhere, even without adjustments for serving the very sick. Instead, impossibly low reimbursements, the withdrawal of hospital benefits from all participants in federally funded family health center programs, and an economic recession crushed GMCHP's grand aspirations.

The character of the HMO movement changed significantly as it entered its second decade. The first crop of prepaid care administrators began to emerge from programs that Congress had funded in 1978 to improve the quality of the management of prepaid health plans. Like GMCHP, many HMOs hired some of the new graduates to help reorganize or improve the efficiency of their management systems. Commercial insurance carriers hired others to strengthen their marketing of prepaid care to employers hurt by the recession. These new administrators introduced much-needed organizational expertise to the health care industry, but they also brought profit-driven management practices more appropriately applied to manufacturing than to health care. When they talked about the quality of product and service, they were speaking in the context of profits, especially when they represented commercial enterprises, which had to answer to investors. The heavily reliance of the new managers on data-processing systems improved the efficiency of prepaid care but also created inappropriately rigid benefits standards that HMO administrators often used to identify and dismiss patients and physicians who made frequent use of services and to reject treatment requests. Consumers revolted when low-level staffers armed with computers in distant offices tried to replace the judgment of physicians at the bedside.

The desire for profits radically increased health care competition during the 1980s. Ignoring national trends and efforts by Blue Cross to compete with other central Wisconsin providers, physicians at the Marshfield Clinic hooked up with Employers Insurance, which operated the North Central Health Protection Plan for Marshfield's neighbors forty miles away in Wausau, to offer more convenient service to residents in both marketing areas. The peer review process that was part of their cooperative agreement provided a forum for questioning inappropriate treatments and costs. Because all the cooperating doctors also were serving residents not enrolled in either prepaid plan, that process improved medical care and reduced costs for patients and insurers throughout central Wisconsin. Competition has the same effect in some industries but seldom works in health care.

Evaluating medical care and prepaid services was in its infancy during the first fifteen years of the HMO movement. Commonly used measurements included accessibility of care, availability of benefits, and consumer satisfaction. Most health plans failed the accessibility test from a social perspective because they marketed group contracts to companies, ignoring small businesses, workers in service jobs, and those who were self-employed or unemployed. GMCHP and a few health cooperatives that sold memberships to individual subscribers were exceptions. Member satisfaction was directly related to accessibility of services, benefit coverage, and relationships with caregivers. Consumers were generally happy with any kind of coverage until they had an opportunity to evaluate their system as a patient. Researchers found compelling evidence in the 1970s and early 1980s that prepaid health care was equal to or better than traditional fee-for-service care. When comparisons of the two systems eventually produced different results, some researchers attributed the change to improved measuring tools. However, I suspect that, as HMOs grew larger and more competitive, the quality of prepaid health care diminished relative to traditional care.

Predatory insurance practices forced the founding physicians at GMCHP to abandon some of their most cherished principles after the 1981–82 recession. The loss of group contracts, especially when other insurers encouraged ailing workers from these groups to remain with GMCHP, burdened its risk pool with a progressively sicker population. Eventually, the health plan was unable to sustain its community-rated, one-price-fits-all premium for groups and direct-pay subscribers. When the health plan increased premiums for its direct-pay program to reflect the greater medical needs of that population, many farm families moved into GMCHP group policies offered by their dairy cooperatives, which were suddenly more attractive to the price-conscious. That shift of high-risk patients to its group pool forced Greater Marshfield to abandon its single comprehensive benefits package. Instead, it began offering a variety of "products" with a selection of benefits, premiums, and copayments designed to meet the cost constraints of individual employers.

After GMCHP revised its rating and marketing strategies to more closely resemble those of other insurers, the health plan proved too successful for its own good. Blue Cross was unable to tolerate GMCHP's expansion into markets that it had staked out for Compcare, its own prepaid plan. The two organizations were destined to split after the clinic decided to use the health plan as a vehicle for increasing its referral business, and the insurer decided that it was time to expand its own prepaid operations. The GMCHP partnership lasted fifteen years but became more tenuous during its last five, as younger and more aggressive physicians and administrators replaced the founding partners in positions of power.

For about a year the clinic and Blue Cross offered one another a series of self-serving proposals for reorganization that sparked increasing frustration within both camps. Then, in the fall of 1986, Blue Cross announced its fifth straight year of losses and inability to meet state insurance reserve requirements. When the clinic refused to accept a lower capitation or smaller advertising budget for its health plan, Blue Cross pulled out of what it claimed was a money-losing partnership. Saint Joseph's Hospital had not favored dissolution during these negotiations but hoped to play an active role if the clinic developed another plan. When the clinic organized its own plan late in 1986, disgruntled hospital administrators balked at giving discounts. The hospital was in an ideal bargaining position because it had no local competition and its employees constituted one of the health plan's largest group contracts. Moreover, the Sisters of the Sorrowful Mother expected their Marshfield facility to support less profitable activities elsewhere.

Marshfield's attempts to keep the direct-pay program affordable for patients with serious health problems failed in 1988, forcing the clinic's two-year-old Security Health Plan (SHP) to refer those individuals to Wisconsin's high-risk health insurance program. The state requires all insurers operating within its boundaries to contribute to that program. Marshfield had contributed to the fund since GMCHP was organized in 1971, but neither GMCHP nor SHP referred anyone to the program until 1988. In fact, SHP was serving more high-risk patients than the entire state program at the time of its first referrals. During the preceding seventeen years the state never acknowledged Marshfield's exceedingly large high-risk population or reduced Marshfield's obligation to the state fund. Ironically, many of SHP's former enrollees could not afford the state's high-risk premiums and had to rely on charity from the clinic.

Marshfield's experience with predatory insurers in the 1980s shows how inequities in the nation's employment-based health insurance system affect disadvantaged groups. Current tax law allows tax exemptions for employers who contribute to workers' health care benefits and for workers who receive benefits in lieu of extra income. Health insurance for the self-employed is now 100 percent tax deductible, if they earn sufficient income, but no such exemptions are available for individuals and families who must purchase policies for themselves, unless their health care expenditures exceed 7.5 percent of their adjusted gross income. Inequities compound for direct purchasers because they are likely to be poorly paid or self-employed and often have health problems that make their premiums much more expensive than those for workers covered by group contracts. No wonder so many who lose their jobs or coverage are forced to do without insurance.

Despite losing some members after GMCHP's dissolution, the Security Health Plan still had nearly sixty thousand enrollees in 1990 when the average size of semiurban and rural HMOs in the nation was less than sixteen thousand. Blue Cross returned to Marshfield at about that time, seeking an arrangement whereby the insurer would market its own Compcare Plan and SHP in the same area, while the clinic provided medical services for both and a generous discount for Compcare. Marshfield refused to accept the terms of the various Blue Cross proposals, so Blue Cross filed an antitrust lawsuit against the clinic and its health plan.

Since 1975, when the Supreme Court decided that physicians could be subject to antitrust violations, judges, lawyers, and antitrust enforcers have been scrambling to interpret how federal regulations and legal rulings affect the health care industry. *Blue Cross v. Marshfield Clinic* raised more questions than it answered, but three points are certain. First, while the outcome of this case does not have broad application, it represents a major victory for health care providers trying to serve patients in rural areas where returns on investment are notably low. Second, the millions of dollars spent on this case could have provided Wisconsin's disadvantaged populations with a great deal of medical care. And last, the Blues' financial gamble, financed by higher rates for its policyholders, failed to weaken the clinic's bargaining power or SHP's territorial expansion. After the suit was settled, Blue Cross withdrew its demand for "most-favored-nation" discounts (a bargaining chip commonly used by the Blues' plans) and agreed to terms similar to those offered by the clinic five years earlier.

For the clinic the money, time, and energy devoted to defending itself from Wisconsin's insurance Goliath, and the legal vultures who sought battle scraps afterward, was a terrible waste and disheartening experience. Perhaps the greatest irony of this entire episode was a lawsuit against the clinic brought on behalf of Medicaid while the clinic was still reeling from the expense of the Blue Cross suit. At a time when many Wisconsin physicians and HMOs in relatively high reimbursement areas were refusing to serve Medicaid beneficiaries because payments were low, this suit accused the clinic and other northern Wisconsin providers in low reimbursement areas of charging "excessive, noncompetitive and unreasonable" prices. Rather than incur additional legal fees, the defendants settled out of court. Even before these suits were finished, the Marshfield Clinic began to merge with other providers, spreading its service and health plan coverage farther to the east, west, and north in Wisconsin and repackaging itself as the Marshfield Clinic Health Care System.

During the late 1990s new federal efforts to expand prepaid health care to more Medicaid and Medicare beneficiaries, and to children who had lost coverage because of earlier welfare reform legislation, met with little success. After its earlier experiences with state HMO contracting, the Marshfield Clinic had returned to serving Medicaid beneficiaries on a fee-for-service basis. SHP did not sign a new prepaid contract with Wisconsin until the state increased its reimbursements to HMOs in 1997. Two years later SHP jumped at the chance to enroll even more disadvantaged families when Wisconsin combined federal allocations from the new State Children's Health Insurance Program (SCHIP) with state funds to form BadgerCare, a program covering low-income children as well as their parents. Health plans in Wisconsin and elsewhere were initially attracted by higher payments from Medicaid and new funds from SCHIP, but many soon reduced their population of or entirely dropped low-income subscribers as money losers. Bucking that trend, SHP showed a small profit from these programs by emphasizing primary, prenatal, and preventive care.

Congressional attempts to increase the HMO enrollment of Medicare beneficiaries in 1997 were less successful than for Medicaid patients. Marshfield had operated its own health plan for the elderly since leaving Medicare's budget-breaking demonstration project in the 1980s. That plan, called Senior Security, combined monthly premiums from members with fee-for-service payments from Medicare to finance their care. In 2000 SHP was serving more Medicare beneficiaries than any other health plan in Wisconsin. The clinic resisted all opportunities to become involved in another prepaid Medicare contract until 2002, when the federal Health Care Financing Administration increased reimbursements to rural areas and added a minor payment adjustment for HMOs willing to accept seniors with preexisting medical conditions. SHP calculated that it could use the additional money to cut the monthly premiums for seniors by half while also providing them with many extra outreach services. Although Americans everywhere had contributed equally to the Medicare fund during their working lives, the benefits that they received from that program largely depended upon their health status and where they lived. Except in northern Wisconsin, rural beneficiaries with chronic health problems fared worst of all.

After three decades of wasteful federal spending, fewer than 9 percent of Medicare beneficiaries belonged to risk-contract HMOs in 2003. Although almost half of Medicaid recipients are enrolled in HMOs, that statistic is not encouraging because many counties and states require enrollment in a prepaid plan as a condition for receiving benefits. Even more distressing was the growing number of providers who believed that government reimbursements were inadequate and refused to serve Medicaid and Medicare on a fee-for-service or prepaid basis. Thus the failure to adequately reimburse providers diminished access and quality of care for all who were poor, sick, and elderly. The United States has not lacked the resources to serve such populations. Rather, the federal and state governments have squandered resources on inefficient overlapping programs that ignored large groups of disadvantaged people while rewarding providers who refused to serve those most in need.

In the private sector, employers' demand for less expensive health care services during the 1990s promoted rapid growth of for-profit health care dominated by multistate conglomerates. The for-profit strategy of rewarding investors by reducing medical costs prompted heath care purchasers and patients to call for more provider accountability. The public sector quickly adopted the performance indicators that had been developed for private-sector purchasers. Medicare, for example, has used some of these indicators to help beneficiaries choose the plan best suited to their needs if they had the luxury of such a choice. Calls for greater accountability also forced physicians to take more responsibility for developing meaningful scientific standards for their tests and treatments. Some researchers claimed that as many as 90 percent of the tests, medications, and other treatments that doctors ordered in the 1990s were not subjected to sufficient scrutiny. Greater use of evidence-based protocols in everyday practice will almost certainly reduce costs and improve the quality of medical care in the prepaid and fee-for-service systems.

Physicians' roles and responsibilities also changed considerably during the health care revolution. Doctors now spend more time in their office and less in the hospital. They are more likely to be an employee than an independent entrepreneur. Health plan and hospital personnel track doctors' practice patterns and sometimes question their professional judgment. Unless they practice in a physician-controlled organization like the Marshfield Clinic, doctors often have to mediate between their patients' needs and insurers' benefit constraints. The future holds hope that young physicians trained in the concepts of conservative cost-effective care will find ways to refuse their patients' inappropriate requests while helping them become more enlightened health care consumers.

HMOs have changed considerably in form and function since 1970, but they covered only about one-quarter of the U.S. population in 2004. However, precepts of managed care permeated a health care industry more intent on satisfying investors' interests than patients' needs. Initially, HMOs employed their own physicians and were closely involved with subscriber care, offering an array of benefits designed to keep patients healthy and treat them well when they were sick or injured. Enrollees usually had primary care physicians who coordinated their care and ordered special services as needed. Competition among insurers and providers drastically revised that model. Today, HMO administrators in distant offices contract with networks of providers to serve subscribers in various localities. As a result many HMOs have lost touch with their patients as well as the communities that they serve. Centralized management of local franchises scattered about a county may work well in some markets but not health care.

Health care markets are unique for many reasons. Unlike other sectors of the economy, health care consumers have little control over what services they can receive, who will provide them, or when they may use them, because employers or governments that purchase health care coverage make those decisions for employees. Consumers can decide when they need to buy a house but not when they need to be treated for pneumonia or rush to an emergency room for treatment of a heart attack. Health care is one of the few markets where sellers turn away those consumers who need too many of their goods and services. For-profit competition, the basis of capitalism, fosters better, less costly computers; it does not reduce the cost or improve the quality of health care. It merely reduces access for unprofitable patients.

The health care crisis facing the United States may be more serious than that which precipitated the HMO movement and ignited the revolution. Compared to the 1970s, health care today is relatively more expensive than other goods and services, and a greater proportion of people lack adequate coverage and care. Managed care has many desirable attributes that would make it an appropriate vehicle for delivering health care if the nation could resolve the unjustifiable financing inequities in the public and private sectors.

The Marshfield Clinic's experiences during the last three decades of the twentieth century offer many lessons. Today's employer-based system for funding private health care is grossly inequitable and unfair to workers who receive no coverage. Government funding for a befuddling array of health care programs for special groups—mothers, children, senior citizens, active and retired military personnel, government employees, Native Americans, migrant workers, other minority groups, the poor, and the institutionalized—is wasteful. No amount of money for special programs can provide adequate care for uninsured and underinsured populations. Insurance companies, which administer the distribution of most payments for private health care in this country, claim as much as 20 percent of those resources for their own operating costs. The United States spends twice and sometimes three times as much as other industrialized nations on health care, yet the returns on that investment, in terms of longevity, infant survival, and other measures of public health, are comparatively meager.

When the HMO movement began in the early 1970s, prepaid health plans assumed full responsibility for funding and providing carefully coordinated preventive, diagnostic, and treatment care to their subscribers. As the movement grew, HMOs underwent many permutations that involved progressively looser networks of independent providers whose services were difficult to coordinate and monitor with regard to quality. Economic pressures and competition forced these plans to offer options that were increasingly less comprehensive and required subscribers to pay often substantial out-of-pocket costs in order to use certain services. By the end of the century HMOs had few features that differentiated them from other insurers. Both contracted with networks of preferred providers but allowed their policyholders to shop elsewhere if they were willing to pay for the privilege. Administrators of these new plans often placed more emphasis on the financial management of provider services than on the medical management of subscriber care. The HMO movement, which created a revolution in the delivery and financing of health care, is dead, but the revolution continues under the rubric of *managed care*. While I make no attempt to predict what form our nation's health care will take in the twenty-first century, I do wonder how much longer we who live amid such affluence can tolerate a misguided, wasteful system that leaves so many disadvantaged Americans groveling for scrapes of care.

Appendix 1

The Meaning of Community Service
at the Marshfield Clinic

Marshfield Clinic physicians and their staff have devoted considerable time and energy to improving the quality of medical care for all residents in central, western, and northern Wisconsin. They have helped public health departments improve the performance of their duties; provided extensive mental health services; sponsored a variety of educational programs for patients, professional, and community groups; and used the products of their medical research for public good. In 2003 the Marshfield Clinic divided the functions of their Marshfield Medical Research and Education Foundation, splitting it into the Marshfield Clinic Research Foundation and the Marshfield Clinic Education Foundation in order to better manage its growing number of research and education programs. The following is a sample of their many activities:

Improving the Quality of Medical Care in Northern Wisconsin

- Many HMOs dismiss physicians who practice substandard care with seemingly little concern for how such doctors treat their other patients. Despite great cost, difficulty, and embarrassment, the Marshfield Clinic kept nearly all GMCHP's affiliated practitioners in its plan so that clinic physicians could help them improve their treatment standards and monitor their activities in order to protect all patients who were under the care of these providers.
- The clinic developed and continues to support a network of more than forty well-equipped regional and local centers that attract highly quali-

fied physicians and paraprofessional health care workers to northern Wisconsin communities.

- The clinic's medical student and residency programs have served hundreds of young doctors, many of whom have established rural practices.
- Clinic specialists regularly visit several communities and provide free telephone consultations to area practitioners.
- Grants from the U.S. Office of Rural Health Policy and its Office for the Advancement of TeleHealth in the late 1990s and early 2000s helped the clinic expand its specialty consultation services to remote treatment centers with two-way interactive teleconferencing and videoconferencing networks. As part of its continuing effort to educate its physicians and support staff, the clinic introduced a network video-streaming system that enables health care providers at its regional sites to "attend" lectures and conferences at the Marshfield Center as these events are taking place. The system does not allow two-way communication between viewers and presenters, but it is accessible from any personal computer within the system.
- TeleHealth's two-way interactive teleconferencing and videoconferencing networks provide many direct benefits as well. In 2000, for example, the clinic joined forces with a rural school district in a pilot program that linked the school's staff with a Marshfield triage nurse or pediatrician when students were ill or injured at school. The TeleHealth network also enables cancer patients at various clinic sites to talk to a Marshfield-based nurse, who helps them understand the various treatment plans available for their type of cancer, including potential benefits, risks, and side-effects, so that they can make more informed treatment choices. Patients who decide to enroll in protocol research studies can also avoid significant amounts of travel by having a specialist follow their progress via the teleconferencing network. More recently, TeleHealth expanded to include retinal screening for macular degeneration and diabetic retinopathy, common diseases that can lead to blindness if not treated early. Specially trained optical assistants visit remote areas with mobile units to examine patients and transmit photographs to Marshfield for diagnosis. When the American Telemedicine Association named Marshfield's TeleHealth one of the top three programs in the nation in 2002, Marshfield was offering the services of twenty-nine specialties and links to fifteen rural Wisconsin sites.

- Other clinic outreach activities for improving medical care in Wisconsin include overnight laboratory services and rapid-response electrocardiogram readings, videotaped lectures and conferences telecast to remote sites, and reference services from the clinic's library, home base of Northwoods HealthNet, a consortium serving small hospitals, clinics, county health departments, and educational institutions throughout northern Wisconsin.

Programs to Enhance Public Health Activities

- In the early 1990s Wisconsin had one of the worst Medicaid screening records in the nation for childhood immunizations. Tracking records is difficult because children need more than twenty immunizations by the age of two and often obtain them from a variety of sources. The staffs of the clinic and its Family Health Center (FHC) developed the Regional Early Childhood Immunization Network (RECIN), a computerized registry funded with mostly private donations that enables public and private immunization providers to record and coordinate children's immunizations on a common computer network. After three years in the RECIN program, Marshfield's home county increased its immunization compliance from 68 percent to 90 percent of all two-year-old children. In 2002, when the registry was deployed in twenty-two counties, the U.S. Centers for Disease Control and Prevention recognized it as one of the best in the nation.
- FHC sponsors many outreach services for all residents in its coverage area. These include elementary school dental screening, special programs for the elderly, annual health fairs for women and teens, pregnancy prevention services, and alcohol and other drug abuse programs.
- The Marshfield Clinic matched state and federal grants in 1999 to purchase and equip a forty-foot mobile unit that visits northern Wisconsin sites to screen low-income women aged eighteen and older for breast and cervical cancer, cardiovascular disease, diabetes, osteoporosis, depression, domestic violence, and other mental health problems. The unit is available to any rural community in the target area upon request. More recently, state and federal funding enabled FHC and the clinic to establish and staff a seventeen-chair dental clinic that serves residents in northern Wisconsin on a sliding fee scale.

- The clinic's regional centers sponsor support groups to help patients and their families deal with cancer, Alzheimer's disease, and other health and social problems.
- FHC received a grant of nearly $1 million from Wisconsin in 2000 for six community projects, including a registry to track, monitor, and educate individuals with diabetes so that patients can manage their condition and avoid long-term complications.

Programs to Provide Mental Health Services

In the late 1990s, 95 percent of the nation's most rural counties had no psychiatrists, 68 percent lacked psychologists, and 78 percent were without social workers. Failure to treat mental illness and addiction creates a serious burden for families, employers, and community law enforcement agencies. Security Health Plan has achieved considerable cost savings for itself, and for northern Wisconsin communities and families, by offering generous treatment benefits.

- The Marshfield Clinic and Saint Joseph's Hospital established new inpatient and outpatient alcohol and other drug treatment programs in 1995 that provide a wide range of health and social services for area patients and family members.

  After identifying alcohol and drug abuse as major public health problems in central Wisconsin in the early 1990s, FHC helped a community consortium obtain a $1.7 million strategic planning grant. That grant led to development of the Northwoods Coalition, coordinated since 1996 by the new clinic-supported Center for Community Outreach in Marshfield. Working with other programs, the center has obtained subsequent grants from a variety of funding sources, enabling communities, counties, and Native American nations throughout the state to develop grassroots programs for helping teens and young adults address a variety of behavioral and mental health issues, including pregnancy prevention; alcohol, tobacco, and other substance abuse; and depression and suicide. In 2004 clinic employees were serving residents in twenty-six communities.
- The clinic expanded its employee assistance program (EAP) in the late 1990s so that more central Wisconsin companies could help their

workers deal with stress, alcohol and drug abuse, family violence, depression, marriage problems, and difficulties with children. Evidence shows that employees and their families derive great benefit from such services. National reports show that every dollar that an employer spends on EAP services produces $14 in greater productivity because such services reduce absenteeism by an average of 21 percent and workplace accidents by 17 percent.

Programs That Put Research to Work

The Marshfield Medical Research and Education Foundation is the largest private medical research facility in Wisconsin and one of the largest in the nation. More than two hundred employees, a dozen basic scientists, and two hundred physician-researchers are involved in more than seven hundred active research projects. The foundation's major areas of emphasis are clinical research; genetics and biochemistry; rural health; epidemiology; and public and community health. Its extramural grants and contracts totaled $11.8 million in 1999, with 75 percent of the monies coming from the federal government, 13 percent from pharmaceutical companies, 5 percent from the state of Wisconsin, and 7 percent from other sources. Foundation scientists and statisticians work in conjunction with all the clinic's treatment centers to conduct epidemiological research that has widespread benefits.

- In 2000 foundation researchers who had participated in mapping the human genome were awarded a $22.6 million grant from the National Heart, Lung and Blood Institute to continue their search for genes that influence human health disorders. Another federal grant of $2.4 million enabled researchers to study whether education programs aimed at physicians and parents can reduce unnecessary antibiotic use.
- Nearly seventeen thousand patients in the clinic's system are participating in the National Cancer Institute's Prostate, Lung, Colorectal, and Ovarian Screening Trial to help evaluate a variety of cancer-screening methods. This study involves about 150,000 patients at ten centers nationwide.
- A five-year $3.2 million grant from the National Cancer Institute in 2003 enabled the Marshfield Clinic's Community Clinical Oncology Program to offer rural Wisconsin cancer patients state-of-the-art clinical trials

that help validate or improve cancer therapies. Marshfield's program was the only one in Wisconsin and one of only fifty in the country.

- In February 2001 a stem cell transplantation service at Marshfield Cancer Care and Saint Joseph's Hospital was the first in Wisconsin, and one of sixty-three out of 180 such centers in the United States, to be certified by the Foundation for the Accreditation of Hematopoietic Cell Therapy. Marshfield is affiliated with the Barbara Ann Karmanos Center Institute of Detroit, which is recognized by the National Marrow Donor Program as one of the largest and best bone marrow transplant centers in the nation. In its first affiliation outside Michigan, the Karmanos center agreed to work with Marshfield in developing a fully integrated bone marrow and stem cell transplant program that offers the latest experimental cancer treatments to Wisconsin residents.
- Atrial fibrillation is the most common heart abnormality that can cause clots to form inside the heart, which then travel to other parts of the body, resulting in stroke or other organ damage. The condition doubles the risk of death and increases the risk of stroke fivefold. In 2002 the Marshfield Clinic completed its participation in the six-year Atrial Fibrillation Follow-up Investigation of Rhythm Management (AFFIRM) Study sponsored by the National Institutes of Health. The study was designed to determine which of two therapies currently used to manage atrial fibrillation is better at prolonging life. Marshfield had the largest patient enrollment of 213 participating sites in the United States and Canada. (The investigators published their findings in the 5 December 2002 issue of the *New England Journal of Medicine*.)
- Research by the foundation has revealed many environmental hazards associated with farming and rural life. The results of such studies have had immediate applications for rural families everywhere. The foundation's work on farmers' lung disease and other respiratory ailments in the 1960s and 1970s attracted considerable national attention.
- The foundation organized the National Farm Medicine Center (NFMC) in 1981 to focus on the study, treatment, and prevention of diseases and injuries affecting farmers and their families. Studies include whether pesticide use is related to the high rates of prostate cancer among farmers; whether the physical and mental stress of farming is related to infertility; the causes of depression and high suicide rates among farmers; the prevention of farm accidents; and the risks that farmers face from sun exposure. NFMC sponsors many educational programs and

conferences. At the three-day Farm Progress Days held at different Wisconsin locations each year, squads of dermatologists screen farm families for skin cancer, and center staffers distribute hundreds of safety devices, including sun-safe hats, respirators for grain harvesting, sunglasses, and ear plugs.

- In an effort to curb the high rate of work-related injuries among farm children, NFMC convened the Child and Adolescent Injury Conference in March 1995; more than two hundred rural health and safety experts from the United States and Canada attended. Data presented at that conference revealed that rural children aged five to fourteen are twice as likely as their urban and suburban counterparts to die in accidents. The federally funded National Children's Center for Rural and Agricultural Health and Safety was created within NFMC in 1997 to focus more attention on environmental risks affecting rural children. Marshfield's center works closely with professionals engaged in improving the lives of rural children. In 2003 the center received a $3.3 million grant to work with agribusiness, media, insurers, major farm organizations, migrant farmworker groups, and national youth-serving groups to protect children at work and at play in agricultural settings.

- The research foundation's efforts to protect food supplies serve many industries and government agencies throughout the nation. Because of their unique combination of resources, Marshfield researchers have identified a number of disease-causing organisms that are transmitted from animals to humans and have developed the technology to implement wide use of the information. The foundation resources that make such discoveries possible include patient, veterinary, environmental health, food safety, and contaminant-isolation laboratories; the clinic's infectious disease department; an epidemiological research center; and records from the Marshfield Epidemiological Study Area, a stable population of patients who reside in zip code areas around Marshfield and who usually seek health care at the clinic.

- In 2002 the clinic started the Personalized Medicine Research Project, the largest study ever undertaken by the Marshfield Medical Research and Education Foundation. As of April 2004, more than eighteen thousand of forty thousand eligible central and northern Wisconsin residents had supplied samples of their genetic material so that researchers and physicians can learn more about how genetic alterations cause diseases that can be prevented or treated with early intervention. Researchers are already working to identify the 1 in 4 patients with a genetic variation that places them at risk of developing an adverse drug reaction, a problem that causes 100,000 people to die each year. Such information will help physicians determine the best drug and dosage for each patient. The clinic is well suited for this study because it has been following central Wisconsin's relatively stable population for many years. In addition, the foundation has an excellent record of genetic research, and the Marshfield Clinic Health Care System has a sophisticated electronic medical records system that captures and encodes very specific diagnostic data in a way that allows researchers to quickly retrieve significant sets and subsets of high-quality diagnostic data for both common and rare conditions. By linking population-based genetic data with environmental exposures and clinical data, this project will add a giant step to the scientific understanding of disease risk in populations. Area residents who participate in this project are protected by strict privacy rights regarding their genetic information.

Appendix 2

Acronym Definitions
and Descriptions

AAHP   American Association of Health Plans, formed when the Group Health Association of America merged with the American Managed Care Review Association in 1995.

AAPCC   Adjusted average per capita cost, a formula used to calculate Medicare reimbursement to HMOs based on the cost of serving all Medicare beneficiaries in a specified area.

AGPA   American Group Practice Association.

AHA   American Hospital Association, which represents the interests of member hospitals and the hospital industry.

AHIP   America's Health Insurance Plans, formed when the American Association of Health Plans merged with the Health Insurance Association of America in 2003.

AMA   American Medical Association, the dominant voice of organized medicine in the United States.

BCA   Blue Cross of America, the national association of Blue Cross plans.

BCS   Blue Cross Blue Shield Association, the national organization formed when the Blue Cross and Blue Shield plans merged in 1978.

BCBSU   Blue Cross Blue Shield United of Wisconsin, formed when the Blue Cross Associated Hospital Service and Blue Shield Surgical Care merged in 1980.

BCHS   Bureau of Community Health Services, administers community health and other federally funded health centers from within the U.S. Public Health Service.

BPHC   Bureau of Primary Health Care, formerly BCHS.

CAHPS   Consumer Assessment of Health Plan Study, used by
           Medicare to help beneficiaries select good health plans.
CMS   Center for Medicare and Medicaid Services, which re-
           placed HCFA, the Health Care Financing Administra-
           tion, in July 2001, is responsible for the administration of
           Medicare, Medicaid, and the State Children's Health In-
           surance Program (SCHIP).
DRG   Diagnostic-Related Group, a group of illnesses expected
           to require the same amount of hospital care, used by
           Medicare to reimburse hospitals on the basis of a patient's
           diagnosis rather than the services provided.
FHC   Family Health Center, a federally subsidized program for
           working poor established by the Marshfield Clinic Medical
           Research and Education Foundation in 1974.
FTC   Federal Trade Commission, provides consumer protection
           and antitrust enforcement.
GAO   General Accounting Office, the investigative arm of Con-
           gress, examines the use of public funds and evaluates
           public programs.
GHAA   Group Health Association of America, the leading voice
           of the prepaid health care industry (see AAHP and
           AHIP).
GMCHP   Greater Marshfield Community Health Plan, established
           in Marshfield, Wisconsin, by the Marshfield Clinic, Blue
           Cross Associated Hospital Service of Wisconsin, and Saint
           Joseph's Hospital in 1971.
HCFA   Health Care Financing Administration, created by the
           U.S. Department of Health, Education and Welfare in
           1977 to administer Medicare and Medicaid, was replaced
           by the Center for Medicare and Medicaid Services (CMS)
           in July 2001.
HEDIS   Health Plan Employer Data and Information Set, an as-
           sessment tool used by the National Committee for Quality
           Assurance to evaluate and accredit HMOs.
HEW   U.S. Department of Health, Education and Welfare.
HHS   U.S. Department of Health and Human Services, formerly
           HEW.
HIAA   Health Insurance Association of America.

HMO   Health maintenance organization, the term applied to pre-
            paid health plans in the 1970s.

HURA   Health to Underserved Rural Areas, federal program in
            effect from 1975 until 1981, when the Reagan administra-
            tion discontinued it as part its move to reduce federal in-
            volvement in health care.

IPA   Independent practice association, a prepaid health care
            plan that initially involved physicians in private practice
            who belonged to the same local medical society but now
            involves any group of physicians in private practice.

MCO   Managed care organization, a permutation of the health
            maintenance organization that relies on networks of physi-
            cians who are often fee-for-service providers.

MFN   Most favored nation, a clause commonly used by Blue
            Cross organizations to obtain the greatest possible dis-
            counts from health care providers.

NCHPP   North Central Health Protection Plan, an HMO in
            Wausau, Wisconsin, that participated in a "free-flow agree-
            ment" with the Greater Marshfield Community Health
            Plan for about a decade in the 1970s and 1980s, allowing
            enrollees of each plan to avail themselves of the services
            offered by both.

NCQA   National Committee for Quality Assurance, a private
            agency established by the HMO industry in 1979 to evalu-
            ate and accredit HMOs; which publishes annual reports
            on HMO performance using the Health Plan Data and In-
            formation Set.

NHC   Neighborhood Health Centers, federally subsidized health
            clinics serving low-income working families in inner-city
            neighborhoods.

NMC   National Medicare Competition, a Medicare risk-contract
            demonstration in the mid-1980s.

OBRA   Omnibus Budget Reconciliation Act, federal legislation
            enacted in 1981 and 1989.

OEO   Office of Economic Opportunity, established by President
            Lyndon B. Johnson as part of his 1960s "War on Poverty"
            to oversee the operation of several antipoverty programs.

PACE   Program of All-Inclusive Care for the Elderly, which enables low-income seniors to live at home instead of in nursing homes and is funded by Medicaid and Medicare.

PSRO   Professional standards review organization, one of a network of local physician organizations established by the Social Security Amendments of 1972 to monitor the cost and quality of hospital care provided to beneficiaries of federal programs.

RBRVS   Resource-based relative value scale, a measure that Medicare uses to compute physicians' fee-for-service reimbursements; it considers cognitive effort, training, time required to perform services, practice costs, malpractice premiums, and local circumstances.

SCHIP   State Children's Health Insurance Program, created by Congress in 1997 to provide health care coverage for children whose families earn too much to qualify for Medicaid but not enough to afford private insurance.

SHP   Security Health Plan, established by the Marshfield Clinic in September 1986 after dissolution of the Greater Marshfield Community Health Plan.

SMS   State Medical Society of Wisconsin.

TEFRA   Tax Equity and Fiscal Responsibility Act of 1982, federal initiatives to reduce hospital costs for Medicare beneficiaries and encourage their enrollment in HMOs.

USPHS   U.S. Public Health Service.

WIPRO   Wisconsin Peer Review Organization, one of several state and regional organizations created by the Tax Equity and Fiscal Responsibility Act of 1982 and authorized to apply sanctions and deny payments to physicians who order inappropriate hospital care for Medicare beneficiaries.

Notes

Introduction

1. Paul Starr, *The Social Transformation of American Medicine* (New York: Basis Books, 1982), 200–209; Jerome L. Schwartz, "Early History of Prepaid Medical Care Plans," *Bulletin of the History of Medicine* 39 (September–October 1965): 451–52.

2. C. R. Henderson, *Industrial Insurance in the United States* (Chicago: University of Chicago Press, 1909); *Experience with Mutual Benefit Associations in the United States* (New York: National Industrial Conference Board, 1923); C. W. Ferguson, *Fifty Million Brothers: A Panorama of American Lodges and Clubs* (New York: Farrar and Rinehart, 1937).

3. Donald Light and Sol Levine, "The Changing Character of the Medical Profession: A Theoretical Overview," *Milbank Quarterly* 66 (1988): 10–32 (supplement 2).

4. William A. MacColl, *Group Practice and Prepayment of Medical Care* (Washington, D.C.: Public Affairs Press, 1966), 11–12, 20–23.

5. For a philosophical discussion of the early grassroots movement that created managed care, see Laurie Zoloth, "The Best Laid Plans: Resistant Community and the Intrepid Vision in the History of Managed Care Medicine," *Journal of Medicine and Philosophy* 24 (1990): 461–91.

6. In 1850 the Franklin Health Assurance Company of Massachusetts was the first commercial company to offer coverage for nonfatal injuries. In 1860 the Travelers Insurance Company of Hartford, Connecticut, issued policies that became prototypes for hospital indemnity insurance. Six years later sixty companies were offering such coverage (*Source Book of Health Insurance Data, 1996* [Washington, D.C.: Health Insurance Association of America, 1996], 1).

7. Dorothy P. Rice and Barbara S. Cooper, "National Health Expenditures, 1929–1970," *Social Security Bulletin* 34 (January 1971): 15; Starr, *Social Transformation of American Medicine*, 258–60.

8. Odin W. Anderson, *Health Services in the United States: A Growth Industry Since 1875* (Ann Arbor, Mich.: Health Administration Press, 1985), 96–77;

Committee on the Cost of Medical Care, *Medical Care for the American People: The Final Report of the Committee on the Cost of Medical Care* (Chicago: University of Chicago Press, 1932), v–vi.

9. Committee on the Cost of Medical Care, *Medical Care for the American People,* 150.

10. Isidore S. Falk, *Security Against Sickness* (New York: Doubleday, Doran, 1936), 37.

11. Avedis Donabedian, S. J. Axelrod, and L. Wyszewianski, *Medical Care Chartbook,* 7th ed. (Ann Arbor, Mich.: Health Administration Press, 1980), 166; Kennett Lynn Simmons, "Managed Health Care: Right Idea—Wrong Rules" (Ph.D. diss., University of Texas at Austin, August 1992), 30; Pierce Williams, *The Purchase of Medical Care Through Fixed Periodic Payment* (New York: National Bureau of Economic Research, 1932), 220–26.

12. Committee on the Cost of Medical Care, *Medical Care for the American People,* 59–65.

13. Lawrence D. Brown, *Politics and Health Care Organization: HMOs as Federal Policy* (Washington, D.C.: Brookings Institution, 1983), 191.

14. Ibid., 159–66 and 193–94; Falk, *Security Against Sickness,* 279.

15. *Federal Emergency Relief Administration Rules and Regulations No. 7* (Washington, D.C.: Government Printing Office, 1933), 1.

16. Ibid., 2.

17. Edward D. Berkowitz, *America's Welfare State from Roosevelt to Reagan* (Baltimore, Md.: Johns Hopkins University Press, 1991), 155; Milton I. Roemer, *Ambulatory Health Services in America: Past, Present, and Future* (Rockville, Md.: Aspen Systems, 1981), 420; Odin W. Anderson, *The Uneasy Equilibrium: Private and Public Financing of Health Services in the United States, 1875–1965* (New Haven, Conn.: College and University Press, 1968), 104–9; Isidore S. Falk, "Some Lessons from the 50 Years Since the Committee on the Cost of Medical Care Final Report, 1932," *Journal of Public Health Policy* 4 (June 1983): 136–61; Social Security Online History, "Main Provisions of the 1935 [Social Security] Act," http://www.ssa.gov/history/law.html (accessed 2 May 2004).

18. Daniel M. Fox, *Health Policies, Health Politics: The British and American Experience, 1911–1965* (Princeton, N.J.: Princeton University Press, 1986), 149.

19. Starr, *Social Transformation of American Medicine,* 311–33.

20. Odin Anderson, *Blue Cross Since 1929: Accountability and the Public Trust* (Cambridge, Mass.: Ballinger, 1975), 42–87; Roemer, *Ambulatory Health Services,* 214–16 and 420; Louis Reed and Maureen Dwyer, *Health Insurance Plans Other Than Blue Cross or Blue Shield Plans or Insurance Companies; 1970 Survey,* Office of Research and Statistics, Social Security Administration, Research Report No. 35 (Washington, D.C.: Government Printing Office, 1971), 2; *Source Book of Health Insurance Data, 1996,* 2–3. According to Edwin J. Faulkner, *Health*

Insurance (New York: McGraw-Hill, 1960), 108, Liberty Mutual Insurance Company introduced the first major medical policy in 1949.

21. Light and Levine, "Changing Character of the Medical Profession," 25.

22. Alain C. Enthoven, "Consumer-Choice Health Plan (Part I), Inflation and Inequity in Health Care Today: Alternatives for Cost Control and an Analysis of National Health Insurance," *New England Journal of Medicine* 298 (March 1978): 651–52.

23. Ellis Cowling, *Cooperatives in America: Their Past, Present and Future*, rev. ed. (New York: Coward-McCann, 1943), 159; James P. Warbasse, *A Short History of the Cooperative League of the U.S.A.* (New York: Cooperative League, 1946), 22–23.

24. MacColl, *Group Practice and Prepayment*, 212–31.

25. John G. Smillie, *Can Physicians Manage the Quality and Costs of Health Care? The Story of the Permanente Medical Group* (New York: McGraw-Hill, 1991).

26. Ira G. Greenburg and Michael L. Rodburg, "The Role of Prepaid Group Practice in Relieving the Medical Care Crisis," *Harvard Law Review* 84 (1971): 887–1001.

27. Monte M. Poen, *Harry S. Truman Versus the Medical Lobby: The Genesis of Medicare* (Columbia: University of Missouri Press, 1979); Herman Somers and Anne Somers, *Medicare and the Hospitals* (Washington, D.C.: Brookings Institution, 1967); Berkowitz, *America's Welfare State;* Starr, *Social Transformation of American Medicine.*

28. Berkowitz, *America's Welfare State*, 175–76; Somers and Somers, *Medicare and Hospitals*, 12–16.

29. Rice and Cooper, "National Health Expenditures," 7; U.S. Public Health Service, National Center for Health Statistics, *U.S. Health and Prevention Profile* (Hyattsville, Md.: Government Printing Office, 1983), 177, 184–85; Berkowitz, *America's Welfare State*, 176–78.

30. Rice and Cooper, "National Health Expenditures," 7.

31. Charles Moritz, ed., *Current Biography* (New York: H. W. Wilson, 1964), 96.

32. Edward D. Berkowitz, *Mr. Social Security: The Life of Wilbur J. Cohen* (Lawrence: University Press of Kansas, 2000).

1. Dreams of a Medical Utopia

1. Lewis, notes, "Report on Planning Activities," undated, ca. February or March 1971, Lewis Papers, Wisconsin Historical Society Archives, Madison.

2. Lewis, interview by author, 17 February 1994.

3. Patrick Felker, interview by author, 9 January 1995.

4. John A. Nelson, "The History and Spirit of the HMO Movement: The Early Years," *HMO Practice* 1 (February 1987): 75. Almost every private medical group studied in a 1931 survey reported having at least one physician on its staff who had once been affiliated with the Mayo Clinic.

5. Reed Hall, Marshfield Clinic corporation counsel, interview by author, 28 February 1995.

6. Milton I. Roemer, *Ambulatory Health Services in America: Past, Present, and Future* (Rockville, Md.: Aspen Systems, 1981), 173–75, 187.

7. Ibid., 25; *Marshfield (Wis.) News-Herald,* 23 April 1966.

8. Hall interview.

9. According to Paul Starr, *The Social Transformation of American Medicine* (New York: Basic Books, 1982), 358, hospital-oriented specialties involving procedures such as surgery have consistently commanded higher salaries than specialties that are office based and provide consultative or cognitive services.

10. Lewis, interview by author, 7 April 1994. Clinic doctors abandoned their uniform salary system twenty-six years later, in 1980, when they needed to hire certain types of specialists who were in great demand and commanded high salaries.

11. Lewis, draft of "A History of the Greater Marshfield Health Plan," 30 September 1971, Lewis Papers.

12. Lewis, interview by author, 25 February 1994.

13. Lewis to Laird, 13 March 1968, Lewis Papers.

14. Lewis to Robert F. Froehlke, 28 February 1968, Lewis Papers.

15. Lewis, notes, "History of Recent Developments Involving the Federal Government and the Marshfield Clinic," undated (ca. July 1968), Lewis Papers.

16. Lewis, memorandum regarding telephone conversation with Carl Yordy, deputy director, Division of Regional Medical Programs, National Institutes of Health, 3 May 1968, Lewis Papers.

17. George Stevenson, Sentry Insurance, internal memorandum to Pat Clifford, 10 May 1968, Lewis Papers.

18. Lewis to Stevenson, 30 August 1968, Lewis Papers.

19. Dr. Gerald Porter to Lewis, 3 May 1968, Lewis Papers.

20. Miriam K. Clarke, "Five-County Health Survey, Wisconsin," National Opinion Research Center, University of Chicago, December 1969, Lewis Papers.

21. E. D. Rosenfeld Associates, "An Evaluation of Present Health Services and Long-Range Planning of Health Resources and Health Care Need for a Five-County Area in Rural Wisconsin," New York, 1968, pp. 136 and 145, Lewis Papers.

22. American Medical Association Council on Medical Services, *Voluntary Prepayment Medical Care Plans* (Chicago: American Medical Association, 1961), 21.

23. Employers Insurance of Wausau, internal memorandum, "Meeting with Mel Laird and members of his staff," 21 October 1968, Lewis Papers.

24. Lewis, notes of 5 November 1968 conversation with Laird, Lewis Papers.

25. Lewis, interview by author, 7 April 1994.

26. Lewis to Dr. Paul M. Ellwood Jr., 20 December 1968, Lewis Papers.

27. Lewis, notes for a talk, 17 April 1980, Lewis Papers.

28. Lewis, interview by author, 30 March 1994.

29. Position statements, State Medical Society of Wisconsin, mss #843, Wisconsin Historical Library, Madison; Earl Thayer, interviews by author, 21 November 1994 and 9 December 1994.

30. Thayer interview, 21 November 1994.

31. Lewis, notes, "History of Attempts to Get Comprehensive Health Insurance in Marshfield," December 1968; Lewis, report, "Insurance Meeting" of 28 May 1969, Lewis Papers.

32. Unsigned report of meeting in Marshfield on 31 June 1969 with visitors from the Chicago office of the U.S. Public Health Service and the Washington, D.C., office of the Group Practice Section of the Community Health Service, Lewis Papers.

33. Lewis to Dr. George H. Handy, assistant state health officer for Wisconsin, 12 December 1969, Lewis Papers.

34. Lewis interview, 17 February 1994.

35. Leo Suycott, testimony before the Subcommittee on Public Health and Welfare, House Interstate and Foreign Commerce Committee, *Hearings on Health Maintenance Organizations*, 92d Cong., 2d sess., May 1972, 985.

36. David Neugent, former vice president, Blue Cross Associated Hospital Service, interview by author, 30 November 1995; Leo Suycott, former president, Blue Cross Associated Hospital Service, interview by author, 1 December 1995; Joseph Voyer, former vice president, Blue Cross Associated Hospital Service, interview by author, 26 March 1996.

37. Suycott interview.

38. Neugent to Brad Larsen, clinic administrator, 12 July 1970, Lewis Papers.

39. Lewis, interview by author, 5 May 1994.

40. Suycott interview.

41. Rosemary Stevens, *In Sickness and in Wealth: American Hospitals in the Twentieth Century* (New York: Basic Books, 1989), 7–13.

42. Lewis interviews, 25 February 1994 and 5 May 1994; David Jaye, interview by author, 25 April 1995.

43. Floyd Detert, clinic administrator, memorandum to Lewis, Lawton, and Larson, 9 October 1970; Lewis, report of telephone conversation with Shearer, 3 November 1970, Lewis Papers.

44. Neugent interview.

45. Odin Anderson, *The Uneasy Equilibrium: Private and Public Financing of Health Services in the United States, 1875–1965* (New Haven, Conn.: College and University Press, 1968), 204.

46. Dustin L. Mackie, "Financial Planning," in Dustin L. Mackie and Douglas K. Decker, *Group and IPA HMOs* (Rockville, Md.: Aspen Systems, 1981), 127–29.

47. In 1971 eleven of the nation's well-established prepaid health care plans reported rates averaging $16.92 for single subscribers and $43.74 for families. See Senate Committee on Labor and Public Welfare, Subcommittee on Public Health and Environment, *Hearings on Physician Training Facilities and Health Maintenance Organizations,* 92d Cong., 2d sess., April–May 1972, table 4 following p. 1814.

48. Charles Gendron, clinic accountant, memorandum to Larson, 22 October 1970, Lewis Papers.

49. Suycott interview.

50. Lewis, draft, "History of Greater Marshfield Health Plan," Lewis Papers.

51. Lewis interview, 17 February 1994.

52. William B. Cherkasky to Lewis, 23 September 1970, Lewis Papers.

53. Neugent to John Allen, director, Medical Services, Wisconsin Department of Health and Social Services, 24 September 1970, Lewis Papers.

54. Lewis to Dr. E. M. Desslock, chair, State Medical Society of Wisconsin Commission on Medical Care Plans, 14 October 1970, Lewis Papers.

55. Thayer interview, 9 December 1994; Health Maintenance Plan (HMP) papers, Wisconsin Physicians Service summary history folder, personal files of Earl Thayer. Thayer said that Wisconsin Physicians Service started HMP in Wild Rose in response to prepaid plans that were forming elsewhere in central Wisconsin. Although HMP had a prepay element, Wisconsin Physicians Service was more concerned about the adequacy of the plan's reimbursement formula than with controlling or monitoring services to patients.

56. According to Gregory Nycz of the Marshfield Clinic Medical Research Foundation, Marshfield Clinic's leaders made the decision after GMCHP's first year to operate the plan at cost (85 percent of charges), with no profit (Gregory Nycz, interview by author, 19 May 1999).

57. The responsibilities of each of GMCHP's three partners were defined in "Prepaid Group Practice Plan Hospital Service Agreement with Saint Joseph's Hospital of Marshfield, Wisconsin, Inc.," "Medical Service Agreement with Marshfield Clinic," and "Prepaid Group Practice Group Master Contract," December 1970, all in Lewis Papers.

58. Helen E. Nelson, ed., *Consumers Organize for Health Care: Consumer-Sponsored Group Practice Health Care Plans* (Milwaukee: Center for Consumer Affairs, University of Wisconsin–Extension, 1970), 40.

59. Howard Eisenberg, "The New Boom in Prepaid Groups," *Medical Economics* 47 (28 September 1970): 272.

60. *Madison (Wis.) Capital Times,* 24 May 1972.

61. Neugent and Suycott interviews. (See note 80 for the definition of *tertiary care.*)

62. According to an anonymous, undated internal Blue Cross document in Lewis's papers, Blue Cross apportioned its expenses in three categories: management liaison, in-house task force, and special project task forces. The management category, including management salaries and fringe benefits for time spent on the Marshfield project, clerical support, travel, administrative services, and legal fees, cost approximately $164,000. The in-house task force, which included the services of seven managers and a vice president who held eighteen meetings and performed a variety of subcommittee assignments between November 1969 and May 1970, cost Blue Cross more than $16,000. Until the plan became operational, internal task forces for OEO development, marketing surveys, statistical and financial accounting, promotional literature, and sales contacts cost approximately $101,000.

63. The General Accounting Office (GAO) estimated in a 1 May 1979 report to Congress that sponsors would require $3 million to $5 million to develop and underwrite the initial operating deficits of an HMO. The costs would depend on whether the HMO involved an established group practice or a staff of independent physicians and what facilities they would need. The GAO predicted that an HMO's income and operating expenses would balance when enrollment reached thirty to forty thousand members.

64. *Madison (Wis.) Capital Times*, 24 May 1972.

65. Robert E. Schlenker et al., *HMOs in 1973: A National Survey* (Minneapolis, Minn.: Health Policy Division, InterStudy, February 1974), 4–5. According to a Blue Cross document that Voyer sent to me on 8 December 1995, Compcare was started by Milwaukee Blue Cross in May 1971 and had an enrollment of 15,452 twelve months later.

66. *Marshfield (Wis.) News-Herald*, 25 January 1972.

67. *Green Bay (Wis.) Press-Gazette*, 30 July 1972.

68. Russell F. Lewis, "The Greater Marshfield Community Health Plan—A Community Experiment," *Wisconsin Medical Journal* 72 (June 1973): 17–23.

69. Donald Nystrom, interview by author, 8 February 1995.

70. Lewis interview, 28 April 1994.

71. Independent Marshfield insurance agent quoted in a wire service story that ran in the *Des Moines (Iowa) Tribune*, 15 December 1972.

72. Joseph Voyer, personal communication, 8 December 1995.

73. The clinic's monthly capitation during GMCHP's first year of operation was $4.80, but the actual cost of medical services to subscribers averaged almost $8 per person per month. Clinic employees and their families cost $13, well above all other groups. Outpatient services to hospital employees and their families cost $7.80 and to employer group subscribers, $7.70. Nongroup subscribers, who tended to be sicker than group enrollees, cost the plan $9.60 per person per month. During rate negotiations for the plan's second year, clinic leaders accepted a capitation of $7.90 per month and wrote off additional expenses incurred by clinic

employees and their families (Lewis, memorandum to GMCHP's Community Committee, 4 April 1972, Lewis Papers).

74. GMCHP subscribers averaged 3.5 doctor visits per person per year. That rate was comparable to that of the Group Health Association in Washington, D.C., and only slightly higher than rates at Kaiser Permanente plans in Oregon and California. Marshfield's fee-for-service patients averaged only 2.8 doctor visits a year (Dr. John Mitchell, "Utilization and Cost of a Health Maintenance Organization: Initial Experience of the Greater Marshfield Community Health Plan," undated but about December 1972, Lewis Papers, hereafter cited as "Mitchell report").

75. Joel H. Broida and Monroe Lerner, "Knowledge of Patient's Method of Payment by Physicians in a Group Practice," *Public Health Reports* 90 (March–April 1975): 113–18.

76. According to the Mitchell report, the average clinic patient used less than half a day of hospital care per year before GMCHP started. Plan subscribers averaged 0.73 days during the first year. Fee-for-service hospital use increased by slightly more than 10 percent during that same period but remained less than half a day per year. The figure for the monetary loss of Saint Joseph's Hospital comes from a 1972 rate calculation document in the Lewis Papers.

77. According to the Mitchell report, some older HMOs, such as Kaiser Permanente, the Group Health Association in Washington, D.C., and the Community Health Association of Detroit, reported less than 0.6 hospital days per subscriber per year. However, these plans enrolled only workers and their families, who tended to be healthier than individual subscribers.

78. Joel H. Broida et al., "Impact of Membership in an Enrolled Prepaid Population on Utilization of Health Services in a Group Practice," *New England Journal of Medicine* 292 (10 April 1975): 780–83.

79. A good definition of tertiary care comes from the Johns Hopkins Medicine website (http://www.hopkinsmedicine.org/patients/insurance_footnotes.html): "Specialized consultative care, usually on referral from primary or secondary medical care personnel, by specialists working in a center that has personnel and facilities for special investigation and treatment. (Secondary medical care is the medical care provided by a physician who acts as a consultant at the request of the primary physician.)" (accessed April 27, 2004).

80. According to the Mitchell report, Wisconsin patients with standard Blue Cross health insurance policies averaged 1.18 hospital days per year in the early 1970s.

81. Dr. David Ottensmeyer, memorandum to clinic executive committee, 31 March 1972.

82. "Greater Marshfield Community Health Plan Calculation Rates, July 1, 1972 through June 30, 1973," Lewis Papers.

83. Lewis, personal communication, 21 February 1998; Ronald Pfannerstill, Marshfield Clinic fiscal affairs director, interview by author, 27 April 1995.

84. GMCHP's rates for 1972–1973 were $26.75 for single policyholders and $59.75 for families. The *Des Moines (Iowa) Tribune,* 14 December 1972, reported that rates for standard insurance policies in the Marshfield area ranged from $24 to $58 per month. Single premiums average $19.40, and family premiums averaged $55.05 at Kaiser Permanente in Oakland, California; Group Health Cooperative in Washington, D.C.; Columbia Medical Plan in Maryland; and Harvard Community Health Plan in Boston, according to an anonymous memo, 19 April 1972, Lewis Papers.

85. Detert, memorandum to Lawton, Lewis, and Larsen, 9 October 1970, Lewis Papers.

86. Lewis, memorandum to Lawton, 19 March 1971, Lewis Papers.

87. James Lube, memorandum to Larsen, 3 August 1970, Lewis Papers.

88. Gendron, memorandum to Detert, 21 April 1971, Lewis Papers.

89. Nystrom to Neugent, 6 August 1971, Lewis Papers.

90. Lewis to Neugent, 9 August 1971, Lewis Papers.

91. Neugent interview.

92. Nystrom, memorandum to Lewis and Detert, 16 August 1971, Lewis Papers.

93. Lewis, memorandum to Nystrom, 27 August 1971, Lewis Papers.

94. Nystrom interview.

95. Voyer to Gendron, 21 August 1972, Lewis Papers.

96. Lewis memorandum, 20 September 1972, Lewis Papers.

97. Nystrom to James Ensign, clinic executive director, 15 December 1972; Lewis to Ottensmeyer, 11 December 1973, both in Lewis Papers.

98. Lewis interview, 5 May 1994.

99. Marshfield Clinic memo, "Medical Staff," 6 October 1973, Lewis Papers.

100. "Greater Marshfield Community Health Plan Statement of Revenues and Expenses on an Incurred Basis for Nine Months Ended March 31, 1974," prepared 26 April 1974, Lewis Papers.

101. Marlyn Kefauver, "Avant Garde of County Medicine," *Health Services World,* April 1973, publication of the U.S. Health Services and Mental Health Administration, Rockville, Md.

102. Ingo Angermeier, "Impact of Community Rating and Open Enrollment on a Prepaid Group Practice," *Inquiry* 13 (March 1976): 48–53.

103. Lawrence D. Brown, *Politics and Health Care Organization: HMOs as Federal Policy* (Washington, D.C.: Brookings Institution, 1983), 212.

104. Schlenker et al., *HMOs in 1973,* 5–7; Richard McNeil Jr. and Robert E. Schlenker, "HMOs, Competition, and Government," *Milbank Memorial Fund Quarterly/Health and Society* 53 (1975): 197.

105. George B. Strumpf, "Health Maintenance Organizations, 1971–1976: Issues and Answers," draft of talk to be presented at the 104th meeting of the American Public Health Association, Medical Care Section, 19 October 1976, on file at

the office of American Association of Health Plans (formerly Group Health Association of America), Washington, D.C. Or see George B. Strumpf and Marie A. Garramone, "Why Some HMOs Develop Slowly," *Public Health Reports* 91 (November–December 1976): 496–503.

106. McNeil and Schlenker, "HMOs, Competition, and Government," 197–206. According to the authors, many states passed legislation after 1973 that was ostensibly designed to promote HMO formation. Many of these statutes imposed unfair burdens on prepaid plans and actually hindered their ability to compete with traditional insurance plans.

107. Sylvia A. Law, *Blue Cross: What Went Wrong?* (New Haven, Conn.: Yale University Press, 1974), 110; Eisenberg, "New Boom in Prepaid Groups," 31; Anne R. Somers, ed., *The Kaiser-Permanente Medical Care Program: A Symposium,* proceedings of a symposium sponsored by KPMCP, the Commonwealth Fund, and the Association of American Medical Colleges (New York: Commonwealth Fund, 1971), pp. 14–27, 36, and 223–32.

108. Lewis, notes on "Meeting of Medical Directors of Prepaid Health Programs, Denver Colorado, April 24 & 25, 1973," Lewis Papers.

109. Lewis to William H. Townsend, American Rehabilitation Foundation, 18 June 1971, Lewis Papers. HEW probably failed to respond when Lewis asked for help in starting GMCHP because agency staff members apparently knew no more about developing a prepaid health plan than he did.

110. Robert G. Shouldice and Katherine H. Shouldice, *Medical Group Practice and Health Maintenance Organizations* (Washington, D.C.: Information Resource Press, 1978), 103–4; Thomas F. Drury, "Access to Ambulatory Health Care, United States, 1974," *Advancedata,* no. 17, Public Health Service, National Center for Health Statistics, U.S. Department of Health, Education and Welfare, 1978, p. 4.

111. "Meet the HMO—A New Way to Buy Health Care," reprint from *Changing Times, The Kiplinger Magazine,* undated but about 1972, in Lewis's 1972–73 scrapbook, Marshfield Clinic archives; Joseph L. Dorsey, director of planning, Harvard Community Health Plan, testimony before the Senate Committee on Labor and Public Welfare, *Hearings on Physicians' Training Facilities,* 596–602; Irwin Miller, *American Health Care Blues: Blue Cross, HMOs and Pragmatic Reform Since 1960* (New Brunswick, N.J.: Transaction, 1996), 59.

112. Isidore S. Falk, "Community Group Health Plans: Response," *American Journal of Public Health* 59 (January 1969): 57–58.

113. E. Frank Harrelson and Kirk M. Donovan, "Consumer Responsibility in a Prepaid Group Health Plan," *American Journal of Public Health* 65 (October 1975): 1078.

114. Goldie Kranz, "San Joaquin Foundation for Medical Care," *American Journal of Public Health* 51 (January 1961): 23–27.

115. Richard H. Egdahl, "Foundations for Medical Care," *New England Journal of Medicine* 288 (8 March 1973): 491–98.

116. Richard Bohrer, Division of Community Health Centers, Bureau of Primary Health Care, U.S. Public Health Service, interview by author, 9 May 1995; Nycz interview.

117. Schlenker et al., *HMOs in 1973*, 5–7.

118. Miller, *American Health Care Blues*, 52–84.

119. Ibid.

120. Those forty HMOs included fourteen prepaid pioneers, such as the Group Health Cooperative in Washington, D.C.; Ross-Loos Clinic in Los Angeles; Health Insurance Plan of Greater New York in New York City; and Labor Health Institute in St. Louis.

121. David W. Stewart, Blue Cross, testimony before Subcommittee on Public Health and Welfare, *Hearings on Health Maintenance Organizations*, 946.

122. *New York Times*, 18 August 1973.

123. Blue Cross memorandum, "Problems with PGPs," undated, in my files; Suycott testimony, House Interstate and Foreign Commerce Committee, *Hearings on Health Maintenance Organizations*, 992.

124. McNeil and Schlenker, "HMOs, Competition, and Government," 197.

125. Schlenker et al., *HMOs in 1973*, 4–8 and 93–97.

2. The HMO Act and Its Aftermath

1. Robert G. Shouldice and Katherine H. Shouldice, *Medical Group Practice and Health Maintenance Organizations* (Washington, D.C.: Information Resource Press, 1978), 45.

2. See Patricia Bauman, "The Formulation and Evolution of the Health Maintenance Organization Policy, 1970–1973," *Social Science and Medicine* 10 (1976): 129–42, for many interesting details about the HMO legislative process.

3. Joseph L. Falkson, *HMOs and the Politics of Health System Reform* (Bowie, Md.: American Hospital Association and Robert J. Brady, 1980), 163.

4. Kennett Lynn Simmons, "Managed Health Care: Right Idea—Wrong Rules" (Ph.D. diss., University of Texas at Austin, August 1992), 288; Richard M. Nixon, *Nixon: The First Year of His Presidency* (Washington, D.C.: Congressional Quarterly, 1970).

5. "Health Care Warning," *Congressional Quarterly Weekly Report*, 18 July 1969, p. 1271.

6. James Singer, "Revised Medicare, Medicaid Programs Likely to Emerge from House Hearings," *National Journal*, November 1969, pp. 74–75.

7. Paul Starr, *The Social Transformation of American Medicine* (New York: Basic Books, 1982), 396.

8. James Singer, "Washington Pressures: The Committee of 100 for National Health Insurance," *National Journal,* December 1969, p. 458.

9. Falkson, *HMOs and the Politics of Health System Reform,* 10.

10. Richard M. Nixon, *Nixon: The Second Year of His Presidency* (Washington, D.C.: Congressional Quarterly, 1971), 1–4.

11. John K. Iglehart, "Health Report/Prepaid Group Medical Practice Emerges as Likely Federal Approach to Health Care," *National Journal,* 10 July 1971, pp. 1462–71.

12. Paul M. Ellwood Jr., et al, "Health Maintenance Strategy," *Medical Care* 10 (May–June 1971): 291–98.

13. Bauman, "Formulation and Evolution of HMO Policy," 130–31.

14. Iglehart, "Health Report/Prepaid Group," 1464; Rickey Hendricks, *A Model for National Health Care: The History of Kaiser Permanente* (New Brunswick, N.J.: Rutgers University Press, 1993), 3.

15. Lawrence D. Brown, *Politics and Health Care Organization: HMOs as Federal Policy* (Washington, D.C.: Brookings Institution, 1983), 210.

16. Ibid., 212.

17. Richard M. Nixon, "Message from the President of the United States Relative to Building a National Health Strategy," 18 February 1971, 92d Cong., 1st sess., H. Doc. 92–49; Brown, *Politics and Health Care,* 17–18.

18. Bauman, "Formulation and Evolution of HMO Policy," 133.

19. Elliot L. Richardson, "Toward a Comprehensive Health Policy for the 1970s: A White Paper," U.S. Department of Health, Education and Welfare, May 1971, pp. 31–37.

20. Brown, *Politics and Health Care,* 222.

21. Commission on Medical Care Plans, "Report on the Commission on Medical Care Plans: Findings, Conclusions and Recommendations," *Journal of the American Medical Association* (17 January 1959), 47–53, special edition.

22. House Committee on Ways and Means, Subcommittee on Health, *Hearings on National Health Insurance Proposals,* 92d Cong., 1st sess., 1971, 1967–74.

23. Edward M. Kennedy, "Introduction of the Health Security Act," *Congressional Record* 116 (1970): 30142–43.

24. Shouldice and Shouldice, *Medical Group Practice,* 109.

25. Jerome L. Schwartz, "Early History of Prepaid Medical Care Plans," *Bulletin of the History of Medicine* 39 (September–October 1965): 459–75.

26. American Medical Association Bureau of Medical Economics, *Organized Payments for Medical Services* (Chicago: American Medical Association, 1939), 132–35; Alma Howard, *We Knew We Could Do It: An Oral History of the Origins and Early Years of Group Health Cooperative of Puget Sound* (Seattle: n.p., 1983), 378; Schwartz, "Early History of Prepaid Medical Care," 468; John A. Nelson,

"The History and Spirit of the HMO Movement: The Early Years," *HMO Practice* 1 (February 1987): 83; Helen L. Johnston, "Rural Health Care Cooperatives," June 1950, Public Health Service bulletin no. 308, p. 55.

27. Robert W. Geist, "Sounding Board: Incentive Bonuses in Prepayment Plans," *New England Journal of Medicine* 291 (December 1974): 1306–8.

28. Iglehart, "Health Report/Prepaid Group," 1470.

29. Odin W. Anderson, *Health Services in the United States: A Growth Enterprise Since 1875* (Ann Arbor, Mich.: Health Administration Press, 1985), 205–6, 208, and 221.

30. Robert J. Samuelson, *The Good Life and Its Discontents: The American Dream in the Age of Entitlement, 1945–1995* (New York: Times Books, 1995), 96.

31. John K. Iglehart, "Washington Pressures/Skyrocketing Health-Care Costs Aggravate Mission of Hospital Lobby," *National Journal,* 22 April 1972, p. 680; Iglehart, "Economic Report/New Federal Health-Care Cost Controls Could Curtail Hospital Services," *National Journal,* 15 September 1973, pp. 1359–61; Iglehart, "Health Report/Explosive Rise in Medical Costs Puts Government in Quandary," *National Journal,* 20 September 1975, p. 1319.

32. Iglehart, "Health Report/Prepaid Group," 1467.

33. John K. Iglehart, "Health Report/Democrats Cool to Nixon's Health Proposal, Offer Own Alternatives," *National Journal,* 20 November 1971, pp. 1472–74; Iglehart, "Health Report/House Panel Moves Toward Compromise HMO Plan Despite Strong AMA Opposition," *National Journal,* 6 May 1972, p. 780.

34. House Committee on Ways and Means, *Hearings on National Health Insurance Proposals,* 139–49.

35. Ibid., 974–86.

36. John K. Iglehart, "Human Resources/Blue Cross 'Communications Network' Draws Critical Comment from Kennedy," *National Journal,* 13 November 1971, p. 2270.

37. Sylvia A. Law, *Blue Cross: What Went Wrong?* (New Haven, Conn.: Yale University Press, 1974), 19.

38. House Committee on Ways and Means, *Hearings on National Health Insurance Proposals,* 942–948.

39. Clark C. Havighurst, "Health Maintenance Organizations and the Market for Health Services," *Law and Contemporary Problems, Health Care Part II* 35 (August 1970): 748–50.

40. Count Gibson, M.D., testimony before Senate Committee on Labor and Public Welfare, Subcommittee on Public Health and Environment, *Hearings on Physicians' Training Facilities and Health Maintenance Organizations,* 92d Cong., 1st sess., 1971, 1527–45.

41. Shouldice and Shouldice, *Medical Group Practice,* 42–44.

42. Iglehart, "Health Report/House Panel," 777–80.

43. Brown, *Politics and Health Care,* 224.

44. Ernest W. Saward, "The Relevance of Group Practice to Effective Delivery of Health Services," testimony before House Committee on Ways and Means, *Hearings on National Health Insurance Proposals,* 2148–71.

45. Clark Havighurst, testimony before House Committee on Ways and Means, *Hearings on National Health Insurance Proposals,* 946.

46. Iglehart, "Health Report/House Panel, 778–79.

47. Ibid.

48. Ibid., 779–80.

49. Senate Committee on Labor and Public Welfare, *Hearings on Physicians' Training Facilities and Health Maintenance Organizations,* 92d Cong., 2d sess., 1972, 2612–23; House Committee on Ways and Means Committee Hearings, *Hearings on National Health Insurance Proposals,* 2175.

50. Richard V. Anderson and Nina Auger, "Community Rating in the Kaiser-Permanente Medical Care Program," *Topics in Health Care Financing* 8 (Winter 1981): 35–49.

51. Brown, *Politics and Health Care,* 418.

52. Senate Committee on Labor and Public Welfare, *Hearings on Physicians' Training Facilities,* 1972, 2611–12.

53. Iglehart, "Health Report/House Panel," 780. Legislation establishing the Professional Standards Review Organization, Public Law 92–603, 92d Cong., 2d sess., 30 October 1972, was supposed to prevent fraud and billing for unnecessary services by providers. HEW did not complete regulations to implement this legislation until 1975.

54. Joseph L. Dorsey, testimony before Senate Committee on Labor and Public Welfare, *Hearings on Physicians' Training Facilities,* 1971, 596–602.

55. Mark J. Mathiesen, "The Health Maintenance Organization Act of 1973—Federal Regulation and Support of Prepaid Group Health Care Plans—Preemption of Restrictive State Laws and Practices," *Vanderbilt Law Review* 27 (October 1974): 1043–56.

56. Paul Ellwood, testimony before House Committee on Interstate and Foreign Commerce, Subcommittee on Public Health and Environment, *Hearings on Health Maintenance Organizations,* 92d Cong., 2d sess., 1972, 403.

57. Iglehart, "Health Report/House Panel," 781.

58. Bauman, "Formulation and Evolution of HMO Policy," 134; Law, *Blue Cross: What Went Wrong?* 44 and 104–6.

59. John K. Iglehart, "Health Report/Intense Lobbying Drive by Medical Group Dims Prospects for HMO Legislation," *National Journal,* September 2, 1972, pp. 1404–5.

60. Shouldice and Shouldice, *Medical Group Practice,* 42–44.

61. Iglehart, "Health Report/Democrats Cool," 1476.

62. Iglehart, "Health Report/Intense Lobbying," 1404; Iglehart, "Congressional Actions," *National Journal,* 13 February 1973, p. 244.

63. Stuart Auerbach, "The Administration: Going Slow on Health Care," *Washington Post,* July 27, 1973.

64. Mathiesen, "The Health Maintenance Organization Act," 1054–55.

65. Cecil C. Cutting, "Group Practice Prepayment in the National Setting," *Group Practice* 20 (February 1971): 116–18.

66. Arnold J. Rosoff, "Phase Two of the Federal HMO Development Program: New Directions After a Shaky Start," *American Journal of Law and Medicine* 1 (Fall 1975): 225.

67. John K. Iglehart, "Health Report/Heralded HMO Programs Beset by Unexpected Problems," *National Journal,* 7 December 1974, pp. 1825–30; Iglehart, "The Federal Government as Venture Capitalist: How Does It Fare?" *Milbank Memorial Fund Quarterly/Health and Society* 58 (1980): 148–68; Brown, *Politics and Health Care,* 283, 340, 369, and 266.

68. National Academy of Sciences, Institute of Medicine, *Health Maintenance Organizations: Toward a Fair Market Test* (Washington, D.C.: National Academy of Sciences, May 1974).

69. Falkson, *HMOs and the Politics of Health System Reform,* 175–76.

70. Rosoff, "Phase Two of Federal HMO," 217—19.

71. Senate Committee on Labor and Public Welfare, Subcommittee on Health, *Hearings on Health Maintenance Organization Amendments,* 94th Cong., 1st and 2d sess., 21 November 1975–19 January 1976, 167–75, 350–53.

72. Ibid., 553–57 and 312–14.

73. Ibid., 414–29.

74. Ibid.

75. Brown, *Politics and Health Care,* 305 and 414.

76. Senate Committee on Labor and Public Welfare, Subcommittee on Health, *Hearings on Health Maintenance Organization Amendments,* 94th Cong., 1st and 2d sess., 21 November 1975–19 January 1976, 578–588.

77. Simmons, "Managed Health Care," 354.

78. Dustin L. Mackie, "An Overview of HMOs from the Federal Perspective," in Dustin L. Mackie and Douglas K. Decker, *Group and IPA HMOs* (Rockville, Md.: Aspen Systems, 1981), 45–46.

79. George B. Strumpf, "Health Maintenance Organizations, 1971–1976: Issues and Answers," draft of talk given at 104th American Public Health Association Meeting, Medical Care Section, 19 October 1976, on file at the office of American Association of Health Plans (formerly Group Health Association of America) Washington, D.C. Or see George B. Strumpf and Marie A. Garramone, "Why Some HMOs Develop Slowly," *Public Health Reports* 91 (November–December 1976): 496–503.

80. Paul S. Hughes et al., *Potential Impact of the Health Maintenance Organization Act of 1973 on the Development of Rural HMOs,* vol. 1: *Introduction, Analysis and Suggested Program Changes* (McLean, Va.: General Research, 21 April 1975).

81. Strumpf and Garramone, "Why Some HMOs Develop Slowly."

82. Andreas G. Schneider and Joanne B. Stern, "Health Maintenance Organizations and the Poor: Problems and Prospects, " *Northwestern University Law Review* 70 (1975): 101–3; Troyen A. Brennan and Donald M. Berwick, *New Rules: Regulations, Markets, and the Quality of American Health Care* (San Francisco: Jossey-Bass, 1996), 152–55; A. Taher Moustafa and David W. Sears, "Feasibility of Stimulation of HMOs," *Inquiry* 11 (July 1974): 145.

83. Cathy Tokarski and Janet Firshein, "Curbing Health Costs: Many Tried, None Succeeded," in *A New Deal for American Health Care: How Reform Will Reshape Health Care Delivery and Payment for a New Century,* ed. Richard M. Sorian et al. (Washington, D.C.: Healthcare Information Center, 1993), 70.

84. Richard McNeil Jr. and Robert E. Schlenker, "HMOs, Competition and Government," in *Politics in Health Care Milbank Reader,* ed. John B. McKinlay (Cambridge, Mass.: MIT Press, 1981), 6:169–82.

85. Brown, *Politics and Health Care,* 197.

86. Cutting, "Group Practice Prepayment," 116.

87. James A. Vohs, Richard V. Anderson, and Ruth Straus, "Critical Issues in HMO Strategy," *New England Journal of Medicine* 286 (May 1972): 1082–86.

3. Health Care in Rural America

1. Paul S. Hughes et al., *Potential Impact of the Health Maintenance Organization Act of 1973 on the Development of HMOs,* Vol. 1: *Introduction, Analysis and Suggested Program Changes* (McLean, Va.: General Research, 21 April 1975), 1.

2. Lawrence D. Brown, *Politics and Health Care Organizations: HMOs as Federal Policy* (Washington, D.C.: Brookings Institution, 1983), 503; Ira G. Greenberg and Michael L. Rodburg, "The Role of Prepaid Group Practice in Relieving the Medical Care Crisis," *Harvard Law Review* 84 (1971): 937.

3. GMCHP and the North Central Health Protection Plan, an independent practice association (IPA) in Wausau, Wisconsin, were the two largest rural prepaid health plans in the nation in the early 1970s. Two other medical group practice plans, the Geisinger Clinic in Danville, Pennsylvania, and the Shawnee Health Service in Carbondale, Illinois, each had fewer than two thousand subscribers. One hospital-sponsored and five consumer-sponsored plans also had very small enrollments. Three other rural IPAs, including one that was twenty-two years old and another that was thirty-six years old, had a combined enrollment of slightly more than twenty thousand (Jon B. Christianson et al., "The New Environment for Rural

HMOs," *Health Affairs* 5 [Spring 1986]: 105–6; Hughes et al., *Potential Impact of the HMO Act,* 17–42.

4. Hughes et al., *Potential Impact of the HMO Act,* 7–9, 49–50. Rural residents were still largely dependent on pediatricians and general internists for primary care in the early 2000s. The creation of family practice residencies in the 1970s halted the decline in the number of rural practitioners and gradually increased rural doctor-patient ratios. But recent declines in primary care residencies, in favor of more specialized training, may lead to fewer rural doctors after 2010. See Jack M. Colwill and James M. Cultice, "The Future Supply of Family Physicians: Implications for Rural America," *Health Affairs* 22 (January–February 2003): 190–98.

5. Daniel Richardson, member services and development representative, Wisconsin Farmers Union, Chippewa Falls, Wisconsin, interview by author, 4 June 1999; Robert Mimier, actuarial supervisor at Blue Cross from the early 1970s until he joined the Marshfield health plan in 1986, interview by author, 27 April 1995.

6. Milton I. Roemer, *Rural Health Care* (St. Louis: C. V. Mosby, 1976), 87.

7. Karen Davis, "Inequality and Access to Health Care," *Milbank Quarterly* 69 (1991): 262.

8. Roemer, *Rural Health Care,* 93; Marshfield Medical Research and Education Foundation's FHC grant application for July 1987 to June 1988, p. 56, personal files of Gregory Nycz.

9. Dick Clark, forward to *Proceedings of a National Conference on Rural HMOs, Louisville, Kentucky, July 8–10, 1974,* prepared for the Senate Committee on Agriculture and Forestry, Subcommittee on Rural Development (Washington, D.C.: Government Printing Office, 1974), iii; and Gregory Nycz, interview by author, 4 February 1995.

10. Hughes et al., *Potential Impact of the HMO Act,* 87–88.

11. Roemer, *Rural Health Care,* 73–74; Philip Cleveland, "Manpower: Summary of Overview Presentation," in *Delivery of Health Care in Rural America, an Invitational Conference in Washington, D.C., 1976* (Chicago: American Hospital Association, 1977), 11–13.

12. Roemer, *Rural Health Care,* 77; *Delivery of Health Care,* iv–v.

13. *Marshfield (Wis.) News-Herald,* 27 October 1969.

14. Natalie Holt, "'Confusion's Masterpiece': The Development of the Physician Assistant Profession," *Bulletin of the History of Medicine* 72 (Summer 1998): 2464–7.

15. Lewis to Neugent at Blue Cross, 17 August 1970, Lewis Papers.

16. *Marshfield (Wis.) News-Herald,* 28 September 1972, 22 January 1973, and 12 November 1973.

17. The American Medical Association, American Association of Family Physicians, American Academy of Pediatrics, American College of Physicians, and

Society of Internal Medicine were all involved in drafting the standards for physician's assistants. As late as 1981 the AMA opposed federal programs to train physician's assistants and supported certification of physician's assistants rather than licensure. Jarret Wise, "Prospectives of the Non-Physician Providers," in *Physician and Clinical Staffing in Prepaid Group Practices,* Proceedings of the Medical Directors Educational Conference, New Orleans, February 4–5, 1977, ed. Joseph L. Dorsey, Joseph Kane, and Sheila McCarthy (Washington, D.C.: Group Health Association of America, 1978), 92–111; Odin W. Anderson et al., *HMO Development: Patterns and Prospects: A Comparative Analysis of HMOs* (University of Chicago: Pluribus, 1985), 170.

18. Harold C. Sox Jr., "Quality of Patient Care by NPs and Physician Assistants: A Ten-Year Perspective," *Annals of Internal Medicine* 91 (September 1979), 461; American Medical Association Council on Medical Services, *Health Maintenance Organizations: Background Information Supplement to the Council on Medical Services Report A* (Chicago: American Medical Association, June 1980), 146–48.

19. "Health Opinions of the U.S. Population," Special Report—Robert Wood Johnson Foundation, no. 1 (1978), p. 14.

20. Lewis, draft report, "Meeting of Medical Directors of Prepaid Health Programs in Denver, Colorado, April 24 and 25, 1973," Lewis Papers; Donald Schaller, "Utilization of Physician Assistants in the Arizona Health Plan," in Dorsey, Kane, and McCarthy, *Physician and Clinical Staffing,* 73–79; Gordon Reid, "Use of Allied Health Professionals in the Primary health Care Team," in Dorsey, Kane, and McCarthy, *Physician and Clinical Staffing,* 80–85; Archie S. Golden and Henry Seidel, "Staffing Pattern of a Health Maintenance Organization," *Journal of the American Medical Association* 240 (27 October 1978): 1969–72.

21. F. N. Lohrenz et al., "Placement of Primary Care Physician's Assistants in Small Rural Communities," *Wisconsin Medical Journal* 75 (October 1975): 93–94.

22. Funding from the Comprehensive Health Manpower Training Act of 1971 enabled medical schools to increase their physician training capacity substantially. Although the number of medical school graduates and new doctors enrolled in postgraduate residency programs doubled between 1965 and 1980, from seventy-four hundred to fifteen thousand, relatively few graduates became general practitioners. House Committee on Ways and Means. *Committee on Ways and Means Green Book,* 104th Cong., 2d sess., 4 November 1996, Committee Print 104–14, 1025.

23. Lewis, interview by author, 28 April 1994.

24. David L. Draves, "Marshfield Medical Foundation, Rural Health Initiative Evaluation Report, July 1, 1976–Sept. 30, 1979, on the Northcentral Wisconsin Rural Health Network," Grant No. 05 H 000525 01 0/CS H27, pp. 10–11, Nycz files.

25. Ibid., 8–9.

26. Ibid., 20–21.

27. Ibid., 21–26 and 13–16.

28. Nycz, interview by author, 10 February 1995.

29. "The Marshfield Clinic . . . for the one in four," Marshfield Clinic recruitment brochure, undated but ca. 1975, Marshfield Clinic archives, Marshfield Clinic Library, Marshfield, Wisconsin.

30. Lewis interview, 28 April 1994.

31. *Marshfield (Wis.) News-Herald,* 18 May 1971.

32. Gregory Nycz, "Health Care Manpower Survey, 1972–78," Marshfield Medical Research and Education Foundation, Nycz files.

33. David Zaresky, *President Johnson's War on Poverty: Rhetoric and History* (Tuscaloosa: University of Alabama Press, 1986); H. Jack Geiger, "Community Health Centers: Health Care as an Instrument of Social Change," in *Reforming Medicine: Lessons of the Last Quarter Century,* ed. Victor W. Sidel and Ruth Sidel (New York: Pantheon, 1984), 12.

34. Geiger, "Community Health Centers," 13.

35. Alice Sardell, "The Neighborhood Health Center: Model and Federal Policy," *Health PAC Bulletin* 12 (1980): 1–21 27; Jude T. May and Peter K. New, "Neighborhood Health Center Directors: Perceptions of Community and Organizational Restraint," unpublished draft for presentation at meetings of the American Anthropological Association, Mexico City, 20 November 1974, pp. 15–18, from the files of the American Association of Medical Plans (formerly Group Health Association of America), Washington, D.C.

36. Richard Bohrer, Division of Community Health Centers, Bureau of Primary Health Care, U.S. Public Health Service, interview by author, 9 May 1995.

37. Frederick Wenzel, testimony before Senate Committee on Labor and Public Welfare, Subcommittee on Public Health and Environment, *Hearings on Physicians' Training Facilities and Health Maintenance Organizations,* 92d Cong., 2d sess., November–December 1972, 830–35.

38. Lawton to Lewis, 15 December 1971; Lewis to David Ottensmeyer, Marshfield Clinic president, 3 February 1972; Lewis to Jeanette Treat, Office of Health Affairs at OEO, 5 April 1972; Richard J. Green, M.D., at OEO to Lewis, undated but received 22 May 1972; Lewis to Carl Wallace, Laird's special assistant, 2 June 1972; and Lewis to Charles Goulet, grant consultant, 29 June 1972, all in Lewis Papers.

39. *Marshfield (Wis.) News-Herald,* 23 June 1972.

40. Lewis to Dr. Hazel Swann, Division of Health Care Services, Health Services and Mental Health Administration, 2 September 1972, Lewis Papers.

41. *Milwaukee Sentinel,* 19 September 1972.

42. *Health Services Information,* a publication of the U.S. Public Health Service, 22 April 1974, p. 2, Nycz files. Nycz told me that HEW allowed all its

health centers to offer inpatient hospital services based on Marshfield's experience; when the agency withdrew all such waivers in 1982, Marshfield's FHC was the last federally subsidized health center in the nation to terminate inpatient benefits (Nycz interview, 8 February 1995).

43. The Blue Cross marketing staff arranged for GMCHP farmers to have their premiums deducted from their dairy milk checks shortly after the health plan started. In the 1980s, when economic circumstances forced GMCHP to charge direct-pay subscribers higher premiums than group subscribers, arrangements were made for farmers to join or remain in the plan by paying group premiums through their dairy cooperatives.

44. FHC families averaged 5.64 members, compared to 4.2 members in GMCHP families. The average age of FHC members was nineteen and of GMCHP members, twenty-six (Nycz, "Family Health Center Enrollment," 4 October 1974, and "Family Health Center Profile," 12 November 1974, both in Lewis Papers).

45. The Health Revenue Sharing and Health Services Act of 1975 (Public Law 94-63) combined all the health centers and placed them under the Office of Community Health Centers, Bureau of Community Health Services in the Health Services Administration. In 2004 health centers were administered by the Division of Community and Migrant Health, Bureau of Primary Health Care, in the Health Resources and Services Administration.

46. Frederick J. Wenzel, director, Marshfield Medical Research and Education Foundation, to Cayetano Santiago, Region V Community Health Services, 5 February 1974, Lewis Papers.

47. Wenzel, memorandum to Ottensmeyer, 9 April 1974; Family Health Center notice, 26 December 1974, all in Lewis Papers.

48. Wenzel proposal to Region V, HEW, 11 November 1974; Norbert M. Sabin, D.D.S., to members of the Second Councilor District, Wisconsin Dental Association, 30 January 1975, both in Lewis Papers. The American Dental Association declared in 1973 that HMOs ought to provide dental care as an essential service, but they "should provide beneficiaries with an individual choice between prepaid group practice and care by other practitioners" (photocopy of appendix A-93 from a report of the American Dental Association Conference on HMOs and Dentistry in Chicago, 14–15 February 1973, Lewis Papers.

49. Family Health Center notice, 20 February 1975, Lewis Papers; Marshfield Medical Research and Education Foundation, FHC grant application, March 1976, pp. 4–6.

50. In 1983 the Marshfield FHC established a program to provide dental screening for all elementary school children in GMCHP's service area, aided by voluntary participation of area dentists and dental hygienists. FHC money paid for promotion, education, direct materials costs, and restorative care for children in low-income families. More than thirteen hundred children from sixty-one

schools were seen during the program's first year. Because private well water was not fluoridated, students from communities of fewer than twenty-five hundred residents had nearly 85 percent more cavities than students from larger communities with centralized water supplies. The Wisconsin Division of Health nominated the Marshfield FHC dental program for national recognition by the Center for Disease Control's Bureau of Health Promotion in 1985 (Nycz interview, 8 February 1995; Nycz memos, 20 February and 24 May 1976, Lewis Papers).

51. Marshfield Medical Research and Education Foundation's FHC grant application, March 1979, pp. 1–7, 15–16. A University of Wisconsin study found that low-income people used preventive health services when they had financial coverage and when services were accessible and responsive to their needs (Nycz interview, 8 February 1995; Doris P. Slesinger, Richard C. Tessler, and David Mechanic, "The Effect of Social Characteristics on the Utilization of Preventive Medical Services in Contrasting Programs," *Medical Care* 14 (May 1976): 392–404).

52. Nycz interview, 19 May 1999.

53. Marshfield Medical Research and Education Foundation, FHC grant application, March 1976, p. 6.

54. Bohrer interview.

55. Ibid.; Merwyn R. Greenlick et al., "Comparing the Use of Medical Care Services by a Medically Indigent and a General Membership Population in a Comprehensive Prepaid Group Practice Program," *Medical Care* 10 (May–June 1972): 187. When Kaiser-Permanente compared use experiences of 346 previously uninsured people with a demographically similar control group enrolled in commercial insurance in the early 1990s, the previously uninsured had 30 percent more ambulatory visits, but the cost of serving them from the outset was not substantially higher than for the control group members. Kaiser offered its subsidized enrollees medical benefits that were comparable to Marshfield's but apparently did not have to use outreach services to improve utilization patterns among those who were previously uninsured. (See H. Bograd et al., "Extending HMOs to the Uninsured: A Controlled Measure of Health Care Utilization," *Journal of the American Medical Association* 277 [1997]: 167–72.)

56. Bohrer interview.

57. Chris Bale, "Neighborhood Health Centers: Group Practices of the Future?" *Group Practice* 26 (January–February 1977): 18–20.

58. Marshfield Medical Research and Education Foundation, FHC grant application, March 1981, appendix 1.

59. Ibid.

60. Community Committee, minutes, 1 April 1971; Lewis memorandum to Lawton, 16 April 1971, Lewis Papers.

61. Community Committee, minutes, 7 May and 18 October 1971, 28 February 1972; committee chair to William Enright, Blue Cross, 2 March 1972, Lewis Papers.

62. Lewis to Community Committee chair, 3 and 5 April 1972, Lewis Papers.

63. Staff, confidential memorandum to Lewis, 17 April 1972, Lewis Papers.

64. Lewis to Community Committee chair, 29 April 1972, Lewis Papers.

65. Community Committee, minutes, 4 May 1972, Lewis Papers.

66. GMCHP newsletter, August 1972, Lewis Papers.

67. Community Committee chair to Jaye, 22 September 1972, Nycz files.

68. "Statement of Purpose and Guidelines for the Operation of the Community Committee of the Greater Marshfield Community Health Plan," 22 January 1973, Lewis Papers.

69. Family Health Center Governing Board, minutes, 15 November 1978, Lewis Papers.

70. Nycz interview.

71. E. Frank Harrelson and Kirk M. Donovan, "Consumer Responsibility in a Prepaid Group Health Plan," *American Journal of Public Health* 65 (October 1975): 1077–86.

72. Robert G. Shouldice and Katherine H. Shouldice, *Medical Group Practice and Health Maintenance Organizations* (Washington, D.C.: Information Resource Press, 1978), 156.

73. U.S. Department of Health, Education and Welfare, Health Maintenance Organization Service, Office of Consumer Education and Information, *Selected Papers* (Washington, D.C.: Government Printing Office, 1973), 14–17, 26.

74. The reference is to Jerome L. Schwartz, *Medical Plans and Health Care* (Springfield, Ill.: Charles C. Thomas, 1968), cited in Shouldice and Shouldice, *Medical Group Practice,* 140–49.

75. Ewell Paul Roy, *Cooperatives: Today and Tomorrow* (Danville, Ill.: Interstate Printers, 1964), 150–52.

76. *Marshfield Clinic Pulse,* 1 March 1999.

4. Affiliated Providers and Necessary Compromises

1. Lewis interview, 24 March 1994.

2. Confidential letter from the State Medical Society of Wisconsin (hereafter, SMS) to Lewis, 3 August 1973; Henry Ashe, M.D., chair, Grievance Committee, SMS, to three doctors, 13 August 1973; and SMS Office Memorandum, No. 74-43, 16 October 1974, Lewis Papers.

3. "Fee Comparisons," 5 May 1975, Lewis Papers.

4. "GMCHP Affiliated Physician Medical Service Sub-Contract," attached to memo from David Gruel, prepaid health plan coordinator, to GMCHP administrators, 22 May 1978, Lewis Papers.

5. "Hospital Data—All Prepaid Programs," undated but after September 1975, Lewis Papers.

6. U.S. Bureau of HMOs and Resource Development, *Considerations in Developing a Rural HMO* (Washington, D.C.: U.S. Department of Health and Human Services, 1985), 39–40.

7. Dr. Nelson Moffat, interview by author, 27 April 1995.

8. Dr. Dean Emanuel, interview by author, 26 April 1995.

9. Report of 1 October 1974 meeting with area optometrists; Lewis memorandum to Nystrom, 25 February 1975; reports of meetings with affiliated optometrists, 5 April 1976, 6 June 1978, and 9 July 1979; report by Lewis of meeting with clinic ophthalmologists, 23 January 1986, Lewis Papers.

10. Lewis memorandum to Dr. David Ottensmeyer, clinic president, 8 February 1972, Lewis Papers.

11. Internal Blue Cross memoranda and W. O. Vogel to R. C. Haskins, 11 April 1972; Vogel to A. Schumacher et al., 14 April 1972; Neugent to Vogel and Nitschke, 10 May 1972; Nitschke to Neugent, 5 June 1972; J. B. Guenther, chief pharmacist, Saint Joseph's Hospital, to Neugent, undated; Neugent to Guenther, 19 April 1972, all attached to memo from Nitschke to Neugent, 5 June 1972, Lewis Papers.

12. Lewis memorandum to Lawton, 11 June 1971, Lewis Papers.

13. Fritz Wenzel, "Report of Discussion of Dental Prepayment Plan Meeting, July 14, 1971," Lewis Papers.

14. Lewis report of meeting with Marshfield Dental Clinic, 18 October 1972, Lewis Papers.

15. Roy A. Menzel, executive director, Wisconsin Dental Service, to Lewis, 20 April 1973; report of 18 June 1973 dental insurance meeting, presumably by Lewis; Richard Peters, clinic oral surgeon, memorandum to Lewis, 6 July 1973; Lewis memorandum to Ottensmeyer, 9 July 1973; "The Marshfield Incentive Dental Plan," attached to Peters memorandum to Lewis, 12 July 1973; report by Lewis of a dental insurance meeting, 8 October 1973; Peters to Lewis, 19 October 1973, all in Lewis Papers.

16. Robert P. Coopmans, a Marshfield dentist, to area dentists, 22 September 1975; report from Peters of dental peer review meeting, 23 January 1978, Lewis Papers.

17. David Gruel, memorandum to Lewis and Wenzel, 21 April 1980; Lewis to Wausau dentist, 16 May 1980, Lewis Papers.

18. Lewis memorandum to clinic and affiliated oral surgeons, 26 November 1985, Lewis Papers.

19. Minutes of psychiatry department meetings, 30 January and 20 March 1978, Lewis Papers.

20. "Memorandum of Understanding," attached to letter from Lewis to Bruce Willett, director, Taylor County Department of Social Services, 31 October 1978, Lewis Papers.

21. Warren W. Garitano, clinic psychiatrist, to Lewis, 27 March 1979, Lewis Papers.

22. Lewis memorandum to Reed Hall, 22 August 1979, attached to draft of "Memorandum of Understanding"; Hall to Lewis, 17 July and 24 July 1979 and 20 August 1979, all in Lewis Papers.

23. Lewis, notes, "Mental Health Provider Problem," 7 January 1980; revised "Memorandum of Understanding," approved 5 August 1980, Lewis Papers.

24. Nycz memorandum regarding GMCHP outpatient mental health expenses, 9 April 1986, Lewis Papers.

25. "Site Visit Report on the GHAA Health Plan Membership Application of Greater Marshfield Community Health Plan, Marshfield, Wisconsin, Sept. 20–21, 1976," Lewis Papers. The inspection team consisted of John G. Smillie, M.D., assistant to executive director, Permanente Medical Group; H. Frank Newman, M.D., Group Health Cooperative of Puget Sound; and Joseph Kane, Medical Directors Division, GHAA.

26. Ibid.

27. Ibid.

28. Ibid.

29. George B. Strumpf, deputy director, "Health Maintenance Organizations, 1971–1976: Issues and Answers," p. 10, draft of talk given at the 104th American Public Health Association Meeting, Medical Care Section, 19 October 1976, on file at the office of American Association of Health Plans (formerly Group Health Association of America), Washington, D.C.; U.S. Public Health Service, Division of Program Promotion, "National HMO Census of Prepaid Plans" (U.S. Department of Health, Education and Welfare, Rockville, Md., July 1976).

30. Emanuel interview.

5. Emerging Problems with Medicare and Medicaid

1. John K. Iglehart, "Explosive Rise in Medical Costs Puts Government in Quandary," *National Journal,* 20 September 1975, pp. 1319–28.

2. Debra A. Freund and Robert E. Hurley, "Managed Care in Medicaid: Selected Issues in Program Origins, Design and Research," *Annual Review of Public Health* 8 (1987): 137–38; Steven Jonas, *An Introduction to the U.S. Health Care System,* 3d ed. (New York: Springer, 1992), 132–33; Kennett Lynn Simmons, "Managed Health Care: Right Idea—Wrong Rules" (Ph.D. diss., University of Texas at Austin, August 1992), 261.

3. Andreas G. Schneider and Joanne B. Stern, "Health Maintenance Organizations and the Poor: Problems and Prospects," *Northwestern University Law Review* 70 (1975): 101–37, esp. 127–30; Sidney Trieger, Trudi W. Galblum, and Gerald Riley, *HMOs: Issues and Alternatives for Medicare and Medicaid* (Washington, D.C.: Department of Health and Human Services, April 1981), 3.

4. *Hearing on Medi-Cal Fraud and Abuse, Findings and Recommendations,* S. Rep., 95th Cong., 2d sess., 47–57; Simmons, "Managed Health Care," 390–91, 418–19; Tom Lovett et al., "Report of HURA Project: A Case Study of a Medical Assistance/HMO Contract in Wisconsin," Marshfield Medical Research and Education Foundation, 1 February 1981, p. 6, personal files of Gregory Nycz.

5. Unless otherwise noted, information about the Marshfield HURA project in this and subsequent paragraphs is from Lovett et al., "Report of HURA Project," 11–31.

6. H. Ross Perot, the founder of Electronic Data Systems, became, without competitive bidding, the Texas Blue Cross claims subcontractor in 1965. Perot then arranged for an $8 million loan from the Republic National Bank of Dallas, whose chief operating officer was also the chair of Texas Blue Cross, to develop the capacity to handle the new account. By 1970 Perot's firm had nine Medicaid and Medicare contracts. The Texas contract, which established a precedent for noninsurers' administering health insurance programs, led to the rise of "third-party" health care administration in the 1980s (Robert Claiborne, "The Great Health Care Rip-off," *Saturday Review,* 1 January 1978, p. 16; Simmons, "Managed Health Care," 255).

7. Karen Davis, "Inequality and Access to Health Care," *Milbank Quarterly* 69 (1991): 262; Marshfield Medical Research and Education Foundation's FHC grant application for 1979–1980, p. 20, Nycz files.

8. Lovett et al., "Report of HURA Project"; Lewis interview, 18 July 1994.

9. HURA was in effect from 1975 until 1981, when discontinued by the Reagan administration as part of a move to reduce federal involvement in health care. See Larry T. Patton, "Developing Rural Health Care Agenda for the Future," in *Financing Rural Health Care,* ed. LaVonne A. Straub and Norman Walzer (New York: Praeger, 1988), 165.

10. Lewis to Donald E. Percy, secretary, Wisconsin Department of Health and Social Services, 17 September 1981, Lewis Papers.

11. Lovett et al., "Report of HURA Project," 67.

12. The Joint HCFA/USPHS Task Force Report's findings and recommendations appear in Lovett et al., "Report of HURA Project," 6–10.

13. Economically depressed areas had few HMOs, and most of their potential subscribers were Medicaid recipients. (Harold S. Luft, "Assessing the Evidence on HMO Performance, "*Milbank Memorial Fund Quarterly* 58 [1980]: 530.)

14. Clifton Gaus, Barbara Cooper, and Constance Hirshman, "Contrasts in HMO and Fee-for-Service Performance," *Social Security Bulletin,* May 1976, pp. 3–14.

15. Norman A. Fuller and Margaret W. Patera, *Study of Medicaid Utilization of Services in a Prepaid Group Practice Health Plan* (West Hyattsville, Md.: Department of Health, Education, and Welfare, 1976).

16. L. J. Kinbell and D. E. Yett, "An Evaluation of Policy Related Research on

the Effects of Alternative Health Care Reimbursement Systems," Human Research Center, University of California–Los Angeles, 1975, p. 453, table IV-19.

17. Freund and Hurley, "Managed Care in Medicaid," 140; Ellen M. Morrison and Harold S. Luft, "Health Maintenance Organization Environments in the 1980s and Beyond," *Health Care Financing Review* 12 (Fall 1990): 86.

18. Milton I. Roemer, Carl E Hopkins, Lockwood Carr, and Foline Gartside, "Copayments for Ambulatory Care: Penny-Wise and Pound-Foolish," *Medical Care* 13 (June 1975): 456–66; Gerald E. Porter, Marshfield Clinic pediatrician, to Lewis, 20 September 1982, Lewis Papers.

19. Michael McDonald, associate director of prepaid plans, GMCHP, to Martin A. Preizler, director, Bureau of Health Care Financing, Wisconsin Department of Health and Social Services, 19 January 1983, Lewis Papers.

20. Lewis, memorandum to clinic physicians, 1 March 1983; Lewis to affiliated physicians, 23 September 1983; undated Wisconsin Department of Health and Social Services announcement to central Wisconsin Medicaid recipients regarding enrollment in GMCHP, Lewis Papers.

21. According to an undated Wisconsin Department of Health and Social Services document titled "HMO Preferred Enrollment Initiative in Dane and Milwaukee County" in the Lewis Papers, estimated monthly fee-for-service costs for Medicaid recipients during the 1984 state fiscal year were $46.48 in the Marshfield area and $55.11 in Dane County. Estimated monthly costs for the 1985 fiscal year were $48.80 for the Marshfield area, $57.87 for Dane County, and $75.83 for Milwaukee County.

22. Gregory Nycz, interview by author, 9 February 1995.

23. Nycz to Katie Morrison, Wisconsin Department of Health and Social Services, 7 February 1984; minutes of Greater Marshfield partnership meeting, 28 June 1984; Lewis to Morrison, 16 July 1984; Frederick Wenzel, clinic executive director, to Morrison, 16 July 1984; Morrison to Wenzel, 7 August 1984; Lewis's draft of a Medicaid termination notice for GMCHP's newsletter, 25 September 1988, all in Lewis Papers.

24. Freund and Hurley, "Managed Care in Medicaid," 141–63.

25. Nicole Lurie, N. B. Ward, M. F. Shapiro, and R. H. Brook, "Termination from Medi-Cal: Does it Affect Health?" *New England Journal of Medicine* 311 (1984): 480–84; J. E. Ware Jr. et al., "Comparison of Health Outcomes at a Health Maintenance Organization with Those of Fee-for-Service Care," *Lancet* 1 (1986): 1017–22.

26. Simmons, "Managed Health Care," 422.

27. Louis Reed and Maureen Dwyer, *Health Insurance Plans Other Than Blue Cross or Blue Shield or Insurance Companies: 1970 Survey*, Office of Research and Statistics, Social Security Administration, Research Report No. 35 (Washington, D.C.: U.S. Government Printing Office, 1971), 52.

28. James B. Bonanno and Terrie Wetle, "HMO Enrollment of Medicare Recipients: An Analysis of Incentives and Barriers," *Journal of Health Politics, Policy, and Law* 9 (Spring 1984) : 41–62, esp. 43; Dustin L. Mackie and Robert L. Biblo, "Marketing Analysis and Implementation," in Dustin L. Mackie and Douglas K. Decker, *Group and IPA HMOs* (Rockville, Md.: Aspen Systems, 1981), 85–107; Richard McNeil Jr. and Robert E. Schlenker, "HMOs, Competition, and Government," *Milbank Memorial Fund Quarterly/Health and Society* 53 (1975): 211–13.

29. Marshfield Medical Research and Education Foundation, "Draft Final Report, September 30, 1982: Alternative Models for Prepaid Capitations Financing of Health Care Services for Medicare/Medicaid Recipients," 19 March 1983, p. 5, files of Gregory Nycz, Marshfield Medical Research and Education Foundation.

30. Trieger, Galblum, and Riley, *HMOs: Issues and Alternatives,* 4; Eugenia Warhol, ed., *Proceedings of the 29th Annual Group Health Institute: 1979 Management and Policy Issues in HMO Development* (Washington, D.C.: Group Health Association of America, 1979), 146–55.

31. Gail Lee Cafferata, *Private Health Insurance Coverage of the Medicare Population* (Rockville, Md.: U.S. Department of Health and Human Services, 1983).

32. Bonanno and Wetle, "HMO Enrollment," 42; Trieger, Galblum, and Riley, *HMOs: Issues and Alternatives,* 2.

33. "Health Insurance for Older People: Filling the Gaps in Medicare," *Consumer Reports,* January 1976, pp. 27–34.

34. Marshfield Medical Research and Education Foundation, "Draft Final Report," 4–5.

35. Lewis interview, 8 September 1998.

36. Thor E. Anderson, "An HMO Experiment in Medicare Prepayment," *Medical Group Management* 27 (September–October 1980): 40–41.

37. Morrison and Luft, "Health Maintenance Organization Environments," 85.

38. Greg R. Nycz and Frederick J. Wenzel, "A View from Under the Microscope: Medicare Prospective Risk Contracting," *Medical Group Management* 30 (May–June 1983): 20–21.

39. Marshfield's cost for treating people with end-stage renal disease was well below the statewide average. As a result Medicare reimbursements for GMCHP patients with renal disease were nearly 63 percent greater than expenses (more than $360,000) during the demonstration project (G. R. Nycz, F. J. Wenzel, R. J. Greisinger, and R. F. Lewis, "Medicare Risk Contracting: Lessons from an Unsuccessful Demonstration," *Journal of the American Medical Association* 257 [6 February 1987]: 658).

40. Cafferata, *Private Health Insurance Coverage,* 3–4.

41. Anderson, "HMO Experiment," 41–43; Louis Rossiter, Alan Friedlob,

and Kathryn Langwell, "Exploring Benefits of Risk-Based Contracting Under Medicare," *Healthcare Financial Management* 39 (May 1985): 24.

42. Nycz interview, 10 February 1995; Marshfield Medical Research and Education Foundation, "Draft Final Report," 23.

43. Marshfield Medical Research and Education Foundation, "Draft Final Report," 62–63.

44. Marshfield Medical Research and Education Foundation, "Alternative Models for Prepaid Capitation Financing of Health Care Services for Medicare/Medicaid Recipients," annual report, 19 April 1980–28 July 1981, dated 30 November 1981, p. 55.

45. Marshfield Medical Research and Education Foundation, "Draft Final Report," 43, 50, 54, and 60; Lewis interview, 5 May 1994.

46. Testimony of Russell F. Lewis and Gregory Nycz before the Special Senate Committee on Aging, *Medicare Reimbursement to Competitive Medical Plans*, hearings, 97th Cong., 1st sess., 20 July 1981, 86; testimony of John P. O'Connell, executive director, Fallon Community Health Plan in Worcester, Massachusetts, before the Special Senate Committee on Aging, *Medicare Reimbursement to Competitive Medical Plans*, 92–99; testimony of Merwyn R. Greenlick, vice president of research, Kaiser Foundation Hospital, Portland, Oregon, before the Senate Subcommittee on Health of the Committee on Finance, *Medicare Reimbursement of HMOs*, 97th Cong., 1st sess., 30 July 1981, 15, and before the Special Senate Committee on Aging, *Medicare Reimbursement to Competitive Medical Plans*, 77–84.

47. Lewis testimony, *Medicare Reimbursement to Competitive Medical Plans*, 106; testimony of James Reynolds, M.D., MedCenters Health Plan, St. Louis Park, Minnesota, *Medicare Reimbursement of HMOs*, 12–13, 27; testimony of Richard E. YaDeau, M.D., president, Bethesda Health Care Organization, St. Paul, Minnesota, *Medicare Reimbursement of HMOs*, 166.

48. Paul R. Ginsburn and Glenn M. Hackbarth, "Alternative Delivery Systems and Medicare," *Health Affairs* 5 (Spring 1986): 20; Nycz interview, 10 February 1995. When Congress incorporated HCFA's Medicare risk contracting into the Tax Equity and Fiscal Responsibility Act of 1982, the legislation did not permit not permit HMOs to adjust their rates or determine enrollment eligibility based on health status.

49. Lewis and Nycz testimony, *Medicare Reimbursement to Competitive Medical Plans*, 85–106, and *Medicare Reimbursement of HMOs*, 133–37.

50. According to testimony by J. P. O'Connell, *Medicare Reimbursement of HMOs*, 43; Greenlick testimony, *Medicare Reimbursement of HMOs*, 15; Nycz and Wenzel, "View from Under the Microscope," 26–27, GMCHP's hospital utilization dropped from a high annualized rate of 2.89 days per member to 2.35 days. Fallon's rates were 2.70 days per member and Portland's 1.70.

51. Nycz and Wenzel, "View from Under the Microscope," 26; internal HCFA memorandum from acting director, Office of Research, Demonstrations and Statistics, to HCFA administrator, 23 September 1981, Lewis Papers.

52. In 1982 HCFA's capitation was $88 for GMCHP, $153 for Fallon, $140 for Kaiser, $138 for Health Central in Michigan, and $180 the four Twin Cities HMOs (Frederick J. Wenzel, "Medical Perspective," and Jan Malcolm, "HMO Perspective," in "Medicare Rick Contracts: Success or Failure?" *Medical Group Management* 33 [May–June 1986]: 30–33). Fallon's capitation of $195 in 1984 was so generous that the health plan eliminated copayments for prescription drugs; nevertheless, in four years the program enrolled only 15 percent of its resident Medicare population (D. B. Wolfson, C. W. Bell, and D. A. Newbery, "Fallon's Senior Plan: A Summary of the Three-Year Marketing Experience," *Group Health Journal* 5 [Spring 1984]: 4–7).

53. Nycz interview, 9 February 1995.

54. Internal HCFA document from Nancy Row, Office of Demonstrations and Evaluation, to director, Office of Research and Demonstrations, 27 August 1982, p. 7, Lewis Papers.

55. Congressional Budget Office, *Containing Medical Care Cost Through Market Forces* (Washington, D.C.: Government Printing Office, 1982), 27.

56. Internal HCFA memorandum, "Continuation of Marshfield HMO Demonstration—DECISION," from acting director, Office of Research, to administrator, Health Care Financing Administration, 23 September 1981, Lewis Papers.

57. Nycz memorandum to GMCHP executive committee, 4 January 1983, Lewis Papers.

58. Nycz, memorandum to Lewis, 9 January 1984, Lewis Papers.

59. Typescript of a talk by Lewis, 9 January 1983, Washington, D.C., where he chaired a panel discussion on Medicare demonstration projects, Lewis Papers.

60. House Committee on Ways and Means, *Green Book*, 104th Cong., 2d sess., 1996, 1126.

61. J. S. McCombs, J. D. Kasper, and G. F. Riley, "Do HMOs Reduce Health Care Costs? A Multivariate Analysis of Two Medicare HMO Demonstration Projects," *Health Services Research* 25 (October 1990): 593–613.

62. Nycz, Wenzel, Greisinger, and Lewis, "Medicare Risk Contracting," 656–59; John K. Iglehart, "Health Policy Report: The Future of HMOs," *New England Journal of Medicine* 307 (12 August 1982): 455.

63. Internal HCFA memo, acting director, 23 September 1981; Trieger, Galblum, and Riley, *HMOs: Issues and Alternatives*, 13–14.

64. Walter McClure, "On the Research Status of Risk-Adjusted Capitation," *Inquiry* 21 (Fall 1984): 261.

65. Ibid.

66. Ginsburn and Hackbarth, "Alternative Delivery Systems," 7.

67. Judith B. Collins and JoElyn McDonald, "Health Care for Medicare Beneficiaries: The HMO Option," *Nursing Economics* 2 (July–August1984): 260.

68. Bonanno and Wetle, "HMO Enrollment," 49–56.

69. Paul L. Grimaldi, "Relying on HMOs to Trim Medicare and Medicaid Spending," *Nursing Management* 12 (April 1984): 75–76.

70. Collins and McDonald, "Health Care for Medicare Beneficiaries," 261.

71. Morrison and Luft, "Health Maintenance Organization Environments," 85.

72. Katherine M. Langwell et al., "Early Experience of Health Maintenance Organizations Under Medicare Competition Demonstrations," *Health Care Financing Review* 8 (April 1987), HCFA Pub. No. 03237, Office of Research and Demonstrations, Washington, D.C.

73. Rossiter, Friedlob, and Langwell, "Exploring Benefits," 49–50; Wolfson, Bell, and Newbery, "Fallon's Senior Plan," 4–7.

74. Michael Zimmerman, "Testimony Before the House Aging Committee," *Caring* (May 1986), 63–67.

75. Cafferata, *Private Health Insurance Coverage*, 251 and 161.

76. Rossiter, Friedlob, and Langwell, "Exploring Benefits," 56; Warhol, *Proceedings of the 29th Annual Group Health Institute*, 146–55.

77. Nycz interview, 9 February 1995; Nycz, Wenzel, Greisinger, and Lewis, "Medicare Risk Contracting," 656–59.

6. Entering a Management Revolution

1. Elements of a successful a HMO are discussed in Paul S. Hughes et al., *Potential Impact of the Health Maintenance Organization Act of 1973 on the Development of Rural HMOs*, Vol. 1: *Introduction, Analysis and Suggested Program Changes* (McLean, Va.: General Research, 21 April 1975); Milton I. Roemer, *Rural Health Care* (St. Louis: C. V. Mosby, 1976); Jon B. Christianson et al., "The New Environment for Rural HMOs," *Health Affairs* 5 (Spring 1985): 105–21; U.S. Congress, Office of Technology Assessment, *Health Care in Rural America* (Washington, D.C.: Government Printing Office, September 1990). Most works cited take note of GMCHP's successes.

2. Lewis to Dr. George H. Handy, assistant Wisconsin state health officer, 12 December 1969, Lewis Papers.

3. Don Nystrom, interview by author, 8 February 1995.

4. Lewis thought there was "no need to worry about spending in-house to meet the needs of the health plan" (Lewis, report of his talk with Ron Pfannerstill, clinic fiscal affairs director, 26 April 1978, Lewis Papers).

5. Dr. Frederic P. Westbrook and Joseph W. Mitlyng, memorandum to Marshfield Clinic executive committee regarding Corporate Strategy-Health Plan, 29

January 1980; executive committee report, 29 January 1981; GMCHP executive committee minutes, 17 February 1981, Lewis Papers.

6. Lewis, report of a meeting in Wausau, 20 April 1972, Lewis Papers; Jacob Spies of Employers to James Ensign, clinic executive director, 20 September 1973, Lewis Papers; Lewis interview, 12 May 1994.

7. Lewis, minutes of meeting with the Wausau Medical Center, 18 January 1977, Lewis Papers.

8. The Robert Wood Johnson Foundation approved a grant to Wausau Hospitals in 1976 to build a clinic in the neighboring community of Weston but withdrew its offer when the Wausau Medical Center objected that the proposed clinic would duplicate and pose a threat to its own nearby business. Because of considerable criticism from Wausau business leaders and residents, doctors at the Wausau Medical Center believed that they needed a presence in Mosinee to deflect the criticism and demonstrate their desire to improve access to medical care in the area. Wausau Hospitals and Wausau Medical Center subsequently drafted a grant application to build and operate a clinic in the nearby town of Kronenwetter (Dr. Gerald Porter, summary of meeting with Wausau physicians, 18 January 1977, Lewis Papers; draft of "Goals and Objectives of Wausau Hospitals, Its Medical Staff and the Wausau Medical Center in the Establishment of a Group Practice Through a Grant from the Robert Wood Johnson Foundation," undated but about 16 March 1977, Lewis Papers).

9. G. Michael Hammes, Employers Insurance, report of a joint meeting on 5 December 1977; two reports of a meeting in Wausau on 30 January 1978, one by Lewis and the other anonymous, all in Lewis Papers.

10. Lewis to Leo Suycott at Blue Cross, 20 April 1978, with 13 April 1978 draft of "Agreement for Joint Affiliation Between North Central Health Protection Plan and Greater Marshfield Community Health Plan" attached; Suycott to Lewis, 8 May 1978; Steven E. Keane at Foley & Lardner in Milwaukee to Blue Cross of Wisconsin, 8 May 1978; Lewis to Lloyd Mathwick at Employers, 10 May 1978; minutes of the Prepaid Policy Group, 18 May 1978; Mathwick to Lewis, 23 May 1978; Roger Drayna, public relations director at Employers, to Frederick Wenzel, 11 May 1978, all in Lewis Papers.

11. According to minutes of meetings at Sentry Insurance in Stevens Point, 16 February 1978, Lewis Papers, Sentry and Portage County Healthguard considered participating in the agreement as well. The free-flow affiliation arrangement between GMCHP and NCHPP was unique until similar agreements were reached in the early 1990s between Group Health Cooperative and Health Partners in Minneapolis, and Group Health Cooperative and Virginia Mason in Seattle (James Coleman, interview by author, 25 April 1995). Coleman worked for Employers at NCHPP in the late 1970s and early 1980s before accepting a position with GMCHP in 1985.

12. Lewis, notes of conversation with Leo Suycott on 25 May 1978, transcribed 31 May 1978, Lewis Papers.

13. Lewis to resident, 24 May 1978, Lewis Papers.

14. David R. Jaye Jr., president, Saint Joseph's Hospital, to Lewis, 13 June 1978, Lewis Papers.

15. Lewis, memorandum to Dr. Nelson Moffat, 30 January 1980; Lewis, memorandum to Dr. William Maurer, 17 January 1983, with 25 July 1978 GMCHP Memorandum of Understanding attached, Lewis Papers; Lewis interview, 24 March 1994.

16. Lewis interview, 24 March 1994.

17. Minutes of the partnership meeting, 17 January 1978; Lewis, memorandum to Lawton, 28 September 1979; GMCHP executive committee minutes, 17 May 1981, all in Lewis Papers.

18. Sheila L. Simler, "Orange's Hospital Center Sponsors the Struggling Central Essex Health Plan," *Modern Healthcare* 7 (December 1977): 32–35.

19. Harold S. Luft, "Assessing the Evidence on HMO Performance," *Milbank Memorial Fund Quarterly* 58 (1980): 501–36.

20. Comptroller General, General Accounting Office, "Health Maintenance Organizations: Federal Financing Is Adequate but HEW Must Continue Improving Program Management," report to Congress, 1 May 1979, 7–21; U.S. Public Health Service, Division of Program Promotion, "National HMO Census of Prepaid Plans, June 30, 1980," USPHS 80–50159, U.S. Department of Health and Human Services, Rockville, Md., 1981, p. 5; John K. Iglehart, "The Federal Government as Venture Capitalist: How Does It Fare?" *Milbank Memorial Fund Quarterly/Health and Society* 58 (1980): 546–666.

21. Except for losses during its first year and a slight deficit at the end of its fourth year, GMCHP remained solvent throughout most of the 1970s. In 1979, after eight years of operation, Greater Marshfield was using cash reserves of more than $1 million to stabilize premiums and provide protection against unexpected usage (Marshfield Medical Research Foundation's FHC grant application for 1979–1980, p. 9, from the personal files of Gregory Nycz).

22. Lewis, notes, "Consideration of Insurance Program," undated but about October 1971, Lewis Papers.

23. Lewis interview, 12 May 1994.

24. Lewis interview, 5 May 1994.

25. David Gruel, interview by author, 17 April 1995.

26. Lewis, memorandum to Lawton, 18 May 1977, Lewis Papers.

27. Lewis, memorandum to Lawton, 28 June 1977; draft job description by Lewis, 17 August 1977, Lewis Papers; Lewis interview, 24 May 1994.

28. Lewis interview, 7 April 1994. In the 1990s the clinic started to allow presidents to serve six consecutive years but continued to limit the terms of members

of the executive committee to three consecutive years. Most clinic physicians favored annual elections and limited terms for the president because they felt that presidents would be better attuned to the needs and views of their peers if they remained in active practice.

29. Lewis, memorandum to members of the new policy group, 20 March 1978, Lewis Papers.

30. Moffat, memorandum announcing appointments on 19 May 1980, and Lewis, memorandum to Maurer, 17 January 1983, both in Lewis Papers; Dr. Nelson Moffat, interview by author, 27 April 1995.

31. Lewis and Wenzel, memorandum to Moffat and the executive committee, 19 May 1980, Lewis Papers.

32. Lewis, memoranda to Moffat, 25 March and 4 April 1980, Lewis Papers.

33. Lewis to Dean Arnold Brown, 14 July 1981, Lewis Papers.

34. Suycott to Lewis, 30 April 1980; GMCHP executive committee minutes, 2 December 1980; job description for associate director, prepaid plans, GMCHP executive committee minutes, 1 July 1980; job description for medical director, prepaid plans, GMCHP executive committee minutes, 13 January 1981, all in Lewis Papers.

35. Draft of newsletter to GMCHP's affiliated providers, 15 May 1981, and Moffat, memorandum to Lewis, 8 February 1982, both in Lewis Papers; Lewis interview, 6 April 1994.

36. Lewis, notes about an HMO conference in Washington, D.C., 10 March 1978, and Dr. John Smillie, Kaiser Permanente Medical Group, to Lewis, 28 July 1980, both in Lewis Papers; Lawrence D. Brown, *Politics and Health Care Organization: HMOs as Federal Policy* (Washington, D.C.: Brookings Institution, 1983), 100; Robert Rosenberg and Dustin L. Mackie, "Physicians and Prepaid Group Practices," in Dustin L. Mackie and Douglas K. Decker, *Group and IPA HMOs* (Rockville, Md.: Aspen Systems, 1981), 111–12.

37. Lewis interview, 6 August 1994.

38. Lewis interview, 7 April 1994.

39. Lewis interview, 24 May 1994; Lewis to Edward Edwards of Blue Cross, 1 August 1984; Lewis to Robert J. DeVita, 11 September 1984, all in Lewis Papers.

40. Alain C. Enthoven, "Consumer-Choice Health Plan (Part 1), Inflation and Inequity in Health Care Today: Alternatives for Cost Control and an Analysis of National Health Insurance," *New England Journal of Medicine* 298 (March 1978): 650–58.

41. "Utilization Review in the U.S.: Results from a 1976–77 Survey of Hospitals," *Medical Care* 17 (August 1979): 1.

42. American Medical Association Council on Medical Services, *Health Maintenance Organizations: Background Information Supplement to the Council on Medical Services Report A* (Chicago: American Medical Association, June 1980),

138; *Information Needs, Information Systems: Some Concerns for Developing HMOs Reflecting the Experiences of Eight Operation Plans* (Boston: Harvard Center for Community Health and Medical Care, July 1975).

43. John Mitchell, draft of "Utilization and Cost of a Health Maintenance Organization: Initial Experience of the Great Marshfield Community Health Plan," undated but about 1 December 1972, Lewis Papers.

44. Minutes of Task Force on Cutting Cost for the Insurance Program, 1 September 1972; John Mitchell, memorandum to clinic administrators, "Proposed Activities," 1 December 1972, both in Lewis Papers.

45. Frank N. Lohrenz, memorandum to clinic physicians, 19 June 1973; Lewis to Dr. Paul Gottschalk and Don Nystrom re cost control measures, 20 June 1972; utilization report by Nycz, undated but after 26 October 1973, Lewis Papers.

46. Joseph Voyer of Blue Cross, memorandum to Lewis and Lawton, 12 November 1975, Lewis Papers; Milton I. Roemer, "Bed Supply and Hospital Utilization: A Natural Experiment" *Hospitals* 35 (November 1961): 36–42.

47. Voyer to Ensign and Jaye, 17 January 1973, Lewis Papers.

48. Lewis, notes on causes of rising costs, November 1975, Lewis Papers.

49. In 1976, when GMCHP's enrollment increased by 16 percent to almost 33,000 members, hospital utilization also rose 16 percent, to 777.5 days per 1,000 members. The national average for HMO hospital utilization that year was only 449 days per 1,000 members. See Nycz, memorandum to members of the Community Committee, "Population and Utilization Data for Fiscal 1975–1976," 19 October 1976, and attached "Summary of National HMO Census of Prepaid Plans, June 1976," a mid-1976 census of HMOs conducted by the Blue Cross Association, the National Association of Blue Shield Plans, InterStudy, and the Division of Health Maintenance Organizations, Lewis Papers.

50. Nycz memo on prepaid statistics for November 1976, tables 1 and 3, 2 January 1977, Lewis Papers.

51. Henry L. Sutton Jr., George V. Stennes and Associates, to Wenzel, 3 April 1975, Lewis Papers.

52. Memorandum regarding protocol for three-day procedures, 31 March 1981; "Greater Marshfield Protocol for Same-Day Surgery," 10 February 1982, both in Lewis Papers.

53. "Outpatient/Same-Day Surgery Summary," 1 January 1982, Lewis Papers.

54. Greg Nycz, interview by author, 18 April 2000.

55. "Summary of National HMO Census"; M. I. Roemer et al., *Health Insurance Effects: Services, Expenditures and Attitudes Under Three Types of Plans* (Ann Arbor: School of Public Health, University of Michigan, 1972), 33; Gloria J. Gardocki, *Utilization of Outpatient Care Resources, 1982* (Hyattsville, Md.: U.S. Department of Health and Human Services, 1985), 4; Harold S. Luft, *Health*

Maintenance Organizations: Dimensions of Performance (New York: John Wiley, 1981), 137–38.

56. Robert L. Harrington, "Characteristics of High Outpatient Users," in *Finance and Marketing in the Nation's Group Practice HMOs: Proceedings of the 31st Annual Group Practice Health Institute,* ed. Eugenia Warhol (Washington, D.C.: Group Health Association of America, 1981), 37–41; Sidney Garfield, "The New Primary Care Delivery Systems," *Medical Informatics* 7 (July–September 1982): 165–68.

57. F. N. Lohrenz, G. R. Nycz, F. J. Wenzel, and C. L. Jacoby, "The Evaluation of Medical Care in Patients with 25 or More Office Visits per Annum in a Prepaid Plan," *Wisconsin Medical Journal* 75 (February 1977): S31–32.

58. Lewis to Moffat, 30 January 1980 and 22 December 1981; Lewis to Maurer, 17 January 1983, all in Lewis Papers.

59. Wenzel, memorandum dated 10 February 1981, re February 6 meeting at Employers; Lewis, notes dated 24 June 1981, of conversation with former president of Employers Insurance, Lewis Papers.

60. "North Central Health Protection Plan (A Cooperative Plan) and Marshfield Clinic Enrollee Free-Flow Agreement," attached to letter from NCHPP executive director William Mineau to Wenzel, 10 February 1982, Lewis Papers.

61. Jeffrey Zriny, NCHPP, to Wenzel, 15 February 1983, with sample copy of letter to affiliated physician dated 11 February 1983 attached, Lewis Papers.

62. James Coleman, NCHPP administrator, to Wenzel and Dr. Boyd Groth, Mosinee, 3 March 1983, Lewis Papers.

63. Wenzel, memorandum dated 30 March 1983, re capitation proposal; "Capitation Reimbursement Agreement Between North Central Health Protection Plan (A Cooperative Plan) and Marshfield Clinic," 25 October 1983; NCHPP, "Participating Physician Newsletter," 12 December 1983 and 2 May 1984; minutes of joint utilization review committee meetings, 10 September and 24 October 1984, all in Lewis Papers. During the 1983–84 fiscal year the Marshfield Clinic received nearly $902,000 in capitation and provided NCHPP subscribers with services valued at nearly $930,000. That same year the clinic paid NCHPP $1,073,683 for treating GMCHP subscribers. NCHPP routinely provided more care to GMCHP members than GMCHP doctors furnished to NCHPP members because the Marshfield plan had a much larger enrollment (Nycz, "Joint Affiliation Financial Statistics Comparative Analyses for FY 1980–1981 and FY 1981–1982," Lewis Papers).

64. Coleman interview.

65. Gerald B. Meier and John K. Tillotson, *Physician Reimbursement and Hospital Use in HMOs* (Minneapolis: InterStudy, September 1978), 69–78.

66. Richard McNeil Jr. and Robert E. Schlenker, "HMOs, Competition, and

Government," *Milbank Memorial Fund Quarterly/Health and Society* 53 (1975): 195–224, esp. 220–21. Two decades later L. C. Baker, in "Association of Managed Care Market Share and Health Expenditures for Fee-for-Service Medicare Patients," *Journal of the American Medical Association* 281 (1999): 432–37, reported that high managed care market penetration influences the practice patterns of all physicians, reducing utilization rates among prepaid as well as fee-for-service patients.

7. Assessing HMO Quality and Consumer Satisfaction in the 1980s

1. Clark C. Havighurst and James F. Blumstein, "Coping with Quality/Cost Trade-Offs in Medical Care: The Role of PSROs," *Northwestern University Law Review* 70 (1975): 15–21.

2. Ronald Anderson, R. McL. Greeley, Joanna Kravits, and Odin W. Anderson, *Health Service Use: National Trends and Variations* (Washington, D.C.: Center for Health Administration Studies, University of Chicago, 1972).

3. Avedis Donabedian, "Evaluating the Quality of Medical Care," *Milbank Memorial Fund Quarterly/Health and Society* 44 (1966): 166–206.

4. For example, see John Newport and Milton I. Roemer, "Comparative Perinatal Mortality Under Medical Care Foundations and Other Delivery Models," *Inquiry* 12 (March 1975): 10–17; S. I. Wilner, S. C. Schoenbaum, R. C. Monson, and R. N. Winickoff, "A Multiple-Indicator Comparison of the Quality of Maternity Care Between a Health Maintenance Organization and Patients of Fee-for-Service Practices," in *Proceedings of the 30th Annual Group Health Institute: Skills Development for the HMO Managers of the 1980s,* ed. Eugenia Warhol, (Washington, D.C.: Group Health Association of America, 1980), 247–57.

5. John W. Williamson, Frances C. Cunningham, and David L. Ward, "Quality of Health Care in HMOs as Compared to Other Settings: A Literature Review and Policy Analysis, Executive Summary," Office of Health Maintenance Organizations, Department of Health, Education and Welfare, Rockville, Maryland, April 1979, pp. 1–2.

6. Troyen A. Brennan and Donald M. Berwick, *New Rules: Regulations, Markets, and the Quality of American Health Care* (San Francisco: Jossey-Bass, 1996), 94–114; R. H. Brook et al., *Quality of Medical Care Assessment Using Outcome Measures,* Vol. 1: *An Overview of the Method* (Santa Monica, Calif.: Rand Corporation, August 1976), v–vii.

7. Avedis Donabedian, "An Evaluation of Prepaid Group Practice," *Inquiry* 6 (September 1969): 3–27; Milton I. Roemer, "Evaluation of Health Service Programs and Levels of Measurement," *Health Services and Mental Health Administration Reports* 86 (September 1971): 840–48; Michael A. Newman, ed., *The Medical Director in Prepaid Group Practice HMOs: Proceedings of a Conference*

in Denver, CO, 1973 (Rockville, Md.: U.S. Department of Health Education and Welfare), 133–34; Milton I. Roemer and William Shonick, "HMO Performance: The Recent Evidence," *Milbank Memorial Fund Quarterly—Health and Society* 51 (Summer 1973): 271–317; American Medical Association Council on Medical Services, *Health Maintenance Organizations: Background Information Supplement to the Council on Medical Services Report A* (Chicago: American Medical Association, June 1980), 149–59; Harold S. Luft, *Health Maintenance Organizations: Dimensions of Performance* (New York: John Wiley, 1981), 210–12.

8. Claudia B. Galiher and Marjorie A. Costa, "Consumer Acceptance of HMOs," *Public Health Reports* 90 (March–April 1975): 106–112.

9. Daniel M. Barr and Clifton R. Gaus, "A Population-Based Approach to Quality Assessment in Health Maintenance Organizations," *Medical Care* 11 (November–December 1973): 523–28.

10. Henry L. Sutton Jr., George V. Stennes and Associates, to Wenzel, 3 April 1975, Lewis Papers.

11. Lawrence D. Brown, *Politics and Health Care Organization: HMOs as Federal Policy* (Washington, D.C.: Brookings Institution, 1983), 415.

12. U.S. Department of Commerce, Economics and Statistics Administration, *Statistical Abstract of the United States* (Washington, D.C.: Bureau of the Census, 1998), 472; AMA Council on Medical Services, *HMOs: Background Information*, 110.

13. Only 1.5 percent of Medicare recipients and less than 1 percent of the nation's Medicaid population belonged to HMOs in 1981. See Tom Lovett et al., "Report of HURA Project: A Case Study of a Medical Assistance/HMO Contract in Wisconsin," Marshfield Medical Research and Education Foundation, 1 February 1981, p. 6, personal files of Gregory Nycz; James B. Bonanno and Terrie Wetle, "HMO Enrollment of Medicare Recipients: An Analysis of Incentives and Barriers," *Journal of Health Politics, Policy and Law* 9 (Spring 1984): 42.

14. David Mechanic and Richard C. Tessler, "An Inquiry into the Dynamics of Patient Behavior and the Organization of Medical Care," in *Growth of Bureaucratic Medicine: An Inquiry into the Dynamics of Patient Behavior and the Organization of Medical Care,* ed. David Mechanic (New York: John Wiley, 1976); Seth B. Goldsmith, "Choosing an HMO: A Review of Consumer Behavior Research," *Journal of Ambulatory Care Management* 2 (August 1979): 41–48; Ernest W. Saward and Scott Fleming, "Health Maintenance Organizations," *Scientific American,* October 1980, pp. 47–53.

15. S. E. Berki and Marie L. F. Ashcraft, "HMO Enrollment: Who Joins What and Why, a Review of the Literature," *Milbank Memorial Fund Quarterly* 58 (1980): 588–632; Mark S. Blumberg, "Health Status and Health Care Use in Type of Private Health Coverage," *Milbank Memorial Fund Quarterly* 58 (1980): 633–55; H. S. Luft, J. B. Trauner, and S. C. Maerki, "Adverse Selection in a Large

Multiple-Operation Health Benefits Program: A Case Study of the California Public Employees Retirement System," in *Advances in Economic and Health Service Research,* ed. R. M. Scheffler and L. F. Rossiter (Greenwich, Conn.: JAI Press, 1985); Luft, *HMOs: Dimensions of Performance,* 40–51; Gail R. Wilensky and Louis F. Rossiter, "Patient Self-Selection in HMOs," *Health Affairs* 5 (Spring 1986): 68–70.

16. As late as 1980, federal agencies did not refer to direct-pay enrollees in reports about the nation's health plans (U.S. Public Health Service, Division of Program Promotion, "National HMO Census of Prepaid Plans, June 30, 1980," USPHS 80–50159, U.S. Department of Health and Human Services, Rockville, Md., 1981.

17. Lewis, memorandum regarding telephone call from Lloyd Mathwick, Employers, 2 June 1978, Lewis Papers.

18. Narrative about the GMCHP-NCHPP agreement in Marshfield Medical Research and Education Foundation's FHC grant application for 1979–80, p. 23, Nycz files; Lewis interview, 13 October 1994.

19. Nycz, memoranda regarding GMCHP enrollment characteristics, un-dated but about January 1973; 5 March 1975, and 19 February 1980, all in Lewis Papers.

20. John K. Iglehart, "HMOs Are Alive and Well in the Twin Cities Region," *National Journal,* 22 July 1978, pp. 1160–65.

21. AMA Council on Medical Services, *HMOs: Background Information,* 155–56.

22. Ibid., 156–57.

23. Sidney R. Garfield, "The Delivery of Medical Care," *Scientific American,* April 1970, pp. 15–23, Garfield, "Prevention of Dissipation of Health Services Resources," *Journal of the Indiana State Medical Association,* October 1972.

24. AMA Council on Medical Services, *HMOs: Background Information,* 157–59.

25. Frederick J. Wenzel, "Assessing Health Care Needs in a Prepaid Group Practice and an Independent Practice Association by Using Consumer Response," in *Proceedings of the 29th Annual Group Health Institute: Management and Policy Issues in HMO Development,* ed. Eugenia Warhol (Washington, D.C.: Group Health Association of America, 1979), 202–7.

26. Ronald Anderson, "Policy Implications of a National Survey of Access to Medical Care," in Lu Ann Aday, Ronald Anderson, and Gretchen V. Flemming, *Health Care in the United States: Equitable for Whom?* (Beverly Hills, Calif.: Sage, 1980), 285–86.

27. Wenzel, "Assessing Health Care Needs," 202–7.

28. Lewis, notes for talk, 21 October 1984, Lewis Papers.

29. GMCHP memorandum, "Decisions Regarding Procedures and Other Services," 24 February 1986, Lewis Papers.

30. HMOs faced a number of problems when hiring or contracting for dental services, including restrictive state laws governing dental care (Brown, *Politics and Health Care Organization,* 294–96 and 411–12).

31. According to Klaus A. Hieber, "Pharmacy Benefit Administration Options," *Journal of Managed Care Pharmacy* 2 (May–June 1996): 272–73, the United Auto Workers was the first union to negotiate pharmacy benefits into its contracts with the "Big Three" automobile makers in the 1960s. The union's model, which usually required a $2 copayment for each prescription purchase, quickly spread to other industries.

32. Merian Kirchner, "A Brake on Costs," *Medical Economics* 55 (29 May 1978): 125.

33. Bruce L. Levin, "State Mandates for Mental Health, Alcohol, and Substance Abuse Benefits: Implications for HMOs," *GHAA Journal* (Winter 1998): 48–69.

34. C. P. Hall, "Financing Mental Health Services Through Insurance," *American Journal of Psychiatry* 131 (1974): 1079–87; Odin W. Anderson et al., *HMO Development: Patterns and Prospects: A Comparative Analysis of HMOs* (Chicago: Pluribus, 1985), 198; Lewis interview, 14 August 1994.

35. Levin, "State Mandates," 48–69; and Brown, *Politics and Health Care Organization,* 411.

36. Bruce L. Levin and J. H. Glasser, "A Survey of Mental Health Service Coverage Within Health Maintenance Organizations," *American Journal of Public Health* 69 (1979): 1120–25.

37. Jan Stein, "Does Psychotherapy Really Work? The Government Tries to Find Out," *National Journal,* 23 December 1980, pp.: 2113–15.

38. Marion Becker, R.N., "Mental Health Services," in Warhol, *Proceedings of 30th Annual Group Health Institute,* 60–63; E. W. Hoeper et al., "Diagnosis of Mental Disorder in Adults and Increased Use of Health Services in Four Outpatient Settings," *American Journal of Psychiatry* 175 (1980): 207–10; Stein, "Does Psychotherapy Really Work?" 2113–15; Darrl E. Regier et al., "Specialist/Generalist Division of Responsibility for Patients with Mental Disorders," *Archives of General Psychiatry* 39 (February 1982): 219–24.

The Health Insurance Plan of Greater New York spent $7.50 per member per year for mental health services, according to Raymond Kink, "Financing Outpatient Mental Health Care Through Psychiatric Insurance," *Mental Hygiene* 55 (April 1971): 148; the Harvard Community Health Plan spent $10.44 per year, according to "A Study of Integrated Comprehensive Mental Health Services in Health Maintenance Organizations," Health Services Mental Health Agency

Contract HSM-42–72–201, February 1973, p. 46; and an Arizona HMO spent $9.72 per year for broad mental health benefits in 1974, according to Thomas E. Bittaker and Scott Idzorek, "The Evolution of Psychiatric Services in a Health Maintenance Organization," *American Journal of Psychiatry* 135 (March 1978): 339–42.

39. Sandra L. Putnam, "A Comparison of HMO Services Used by Alcoholics and Matched Controls," in Warhol, *Proceedings of the 30th Annual Group Health Institute*, 212–29.

40. Kenneth A. Kessler, "Benefit Design, Utilization Review, Case Management, PPOs Contain Cost," *Benefits Today*, 9 May 1986.

41. In a letter to Bruce Willet, Human Services Center of Taylor County, Wisconsin, 31 October 1978, Lewis said it was his belief that "alcoholics deserve treatment" and his "policy was to give blanket approval for that disease entity," Lewis Papers.

42. Lewis, memorandum to Dr. Richard Dart, 16 January 1984; Lewis, memorandum to Marshfield Clinic physicians and GMCHP's affiliates, announcing the opening of Saint Joseph's alcohol unit on 19 July 1984, Lewis Papers; Lewis interview, 14 August 1994.

43. Lewis to Dr. Warwick Dean, 11 March 1981; Lewis, memoranda to GMCHP staff, 8 September 1981; Dr. William Maurer, memorandum to Dean, 31 August 1982; Dean, memorandum to Maurer, 10 September 1982; Lewis to all clinic doctors and GMCHP affiliates, 5 October 1983; Lewis to Guerdon Coombs, 28 August and 23 September 1986, all in Lewis Papers.

44. Luft, *HMOs: Dimensions of Performance*, 393 and 205; and Luft, "Why Do HMOs Seem to Provide More Health Maintenance Services?" *Milbank Memorial Fund Quarterly/ Health and Society* 56 (1978): 163–65.

45. Debra Cascardo, "Factors Affecting Cost Containment in an HMO: A Review of the Literature," *Ambulatory Care Management* 5 (August 1982): 58; Ernest W. Saward, testimony before the House Committee on Interstate and Foreign Commerce, Subcommittee on Public Health and Environment, *Health Maintenance Organizations*, 92d Cong., 2d sess., 12 April 1972, 181; Paul Ellwood Jr., testimony before House Committee on Interstate and Foreign Commerce, *Hearings on Health Maintenance Organizations*, 2–5 May 1972, 388.

46. Harold S. Luft, "Assessing the Evidence on HMO Performance," *Milbank Memorial Fund Quarterly* 58 (1980): 516; Lewis, notes for talk, 21 October 1984; Lewis interview, 5 May 1994.

47. Sarah J. Nasser, "Health Education," in Warhol, *Proceedings of the 29th Annual Group Health Institute*, 97–101.

48. Odin W. Anderson, *Health Services in the United States: A Growth Enterprise Since 1875* (Ann Arbor, Mich.: Health Administration Press, 1985), 314.

49. Roger W. Birnbaum, "Review of a Variety of Studies Regarding What At-

tracts People, Who Enrolls and Why They Stay or Leave," in Warhol, *Proceedings of the 31st Annual Group Health Institute*, 59–69; Milton I. Roemer, *Ambulatory Health Care in America: Past, Present and Future* (Rockville, Md.: Aspen Systems, 1981), 251–83.

50. Robert G. Shouldice and Katherine H. Shouldice, *Medical Group Practice and Health Maintenance Organizations* (Washington, D.C.: Information Resource Press, 1978), 147; Richard Tessler and David Mechanic, *Consumer Satisfaction with Prepaid Group Practice: A Comparative Study* (Madison: Research and Analytic Report Services, University of Wisconsin, 1974), 21–23; Avedis Donabedian, *Explorations in Quality Assessment and Monitoring*, Vol. 1:, *The Definition of Quality and Approaches to Its Assessment* (Ann Arbor, Mich.: Health Administration Press, 1980), 4–5; Donald K. Freeborn, "Physician Satisfaction in a Prepaid Group Practice HMO," *Group Health Journal* 6 (Spring 1985): 10; Leon Weszewianski, John R.C. Wheeler, and Avedis Donabedian, "Market-Oriented Cost-Containment Strategies and Quality of Care," *Milbank Memorial Fund Quarterly/Health and Society* 60 (Fall 1982): 535–36; David Mechanic et al., "A Model of Rural Health Care: Consumer Response Among Users of the Marshfield Clinic," *Medical Care* 18 (June 1980): 597–608; Edwin W. Hoeper, *Proceedings of the Fourth Annual Family Health Center Conference at Grand Portage, MN* (Rockville, Md.: U.S. Department of Health, Education and Welfare, 1976), 731.

51. Hoeper, *Proceedings of the Fourth Annual FHC Conference*, 938; Ernest W. Saward and E. K. Gallagher, "Reflections on Change in Medical Practice: The Current Trend to Large-scale Medical Organizations," *Journal of the American Medical Association* 250 (1983): 2820–25.

52. Carolyn Dana Andre and Harry Sharp, "An Analysis of Greater Marshfield Community Health Plan Terminations," a report from the University of Wisconsin Survey Research Laboratory, Madison, December 1973.

53. National Industry Council for HMO Development, *The Health Maintenance Organization Industry: Ten Year Report, 1973–1983* (Washington, D.C.: National Industry Council for HMO Development, 1984), 9.

54. U.S. Department of Health and Human Services, National Center for Health Services Research, "Who Are the Uninsured?" *Data Preview* 1 (1980).

55. R. H. Egdahl, C. H. Taft, J. Friedland, and K. Linde, "The Potential of Organizations of Fee-for-Service Physicians for Achieving Significant Decreases in Hospitalization," *Annals of Surgery* 186 (September 1977): 388–99.

56. Report on survey of physicians' attitudes about HMOs, *Medical World News* 19 (March 6, 1978): 89–92.

57. Reginald W. Rhein Jr., "HMOs: Feds Vow to Make Them Grow," *Medical World News* 19 (March 6, 1978): 89.

58. *Alternative Health Care Delivery Systems: "The HMO Concept"* (Chicago: American Medical Association, December 1978).

59. AMA Council on Medical Services, *HMOs: Background Information.*

60. Randall Bovbjerg, "The Medical Malpractice Standard of Care: HMOs and Customary Practice," *Duke Law Journal* (1975): 1375–1414; Randall R. Bovbjerg and Clark C. Havighurst, "Medical Malpractice: An Update for Noncombatants," *Business and Health* 2 (September 1965): 38–42.

61. William J. Curran and George B. Moseley III, "The Malpractice Experience of HMOs," *Northwestern University Law Review* 70 (1975): 70–71; Stuart S. Burstein, "Prepaid Health Care in the United States," *Illinois Medical Journal* 160 (August 1981): 83–85.

62. Ira G. Greenburg and Michael E. Rodburg, "Role of Prepaid Group Practice in Relieving the Medical Care Crisis," *Harvard Law Review* 84 (1971): 887–1001; David Mechanic, *The Organization of Medical Practice and Practice Orientations Among Physicians in Prepaid and Non-Prepaid Primary Care Settings,* Research and Analytic Report Series (Madison: Center for Medical Sociology and Health Services Research, University of Wisconsin, 1974), 21–25; Uwe E. Reinhardt, "A Framework for Deliberations on the Compensation of Physicians," *Journal of Medical Practice Management* 3 (Fall 1987) : 85–95; Saward and Gallagher, "Reflections on Change in Medical Practice," 2820–25; Luft, *HMOs: Dimensions of Performance,* 99; Freeborn, "Physician Satisfaction," 3–12.

63. Freeborn, "Physician Satisfaction," 3; Luft, "Assessing the Evidence," 520–21.

64. Louis Harris and Associates, *Summary Report—A Report Card on HMOs, 1980–1984,* prepared for the Henry J. Kaiser Family Foundation (New York: Gannett, 1984); D. L. Dolan, ed., "Blue Cross and Blue Shield's Personal Care Plan—Physician Forum," *North Carolina Medical Journal* 49 (1985): 451–54.

65. Judith B. Collins and JoElyn McDonald, "Health Care for Medicare Beneficiaries: The HMO Option," *Nursing Economics* 2 (July–August 1984): 264; Beth C. Weitzman, "The Quality of Care: Assessment and Assurance," in *Health Care Delivery in the United States,* ed. Anthony R. Kovner, 4th ed. (New York: Springer, 1990), 358.

8. Idealism Confronts Realities

1. For example, see Edward D. Berkowitz and Wendy Wolff, *Group Health Association: A Portrait of a Health Maintenance Organization* (Philadelphia: Temple University Press, 1988); Walt Crowley, *To Serve the Greatest Number: A History of Group Health Cooperative of Puget Sound* (Seattle: University of Washington Press, 1996).

2. Karen Davic, F. G. Anderson, D. Rowland, and E. P. Steinberg, *Health Care Cost Containment* (Baltimore: Johns Hopkins University Press, 1990), 104–5.

3. Linda E. Demkovich, "Business, as a Health Care Consumer, Is Paying Heed to the Bottom Line," *National Journal,* 24 May 1980, pp. 851–54; *Control-*

ling Health Care Costs: Crisis in Employee Benefits (Washington, D.C.: Bureau of National Affairs, 1983), 106; Kennett Lynn Simmons, "Managed Health Care: Right Idea—Wrong Rules" (Ph.D. diss., University of Texas at Austin, August 1992), 444.

4. Gail A. Jensen and Jon R. Gabel, "The Erosion of Purchased Health Insurance," *Inquiry* 25 (Fall 1988): 328–43.

5. Ibid.; Health Insurance Association of America, *Source Book of Health Insurance Data* (Washington, D.C.: Health Insurance Association of America, 1996), 4; H. E. Frech III and Paul B. Ginsburg, "Competition Among Health Insurers, Revisited," *Journal of Health Politics, Policy and Law* 13 (Summer 1988): 279–91.

6. *Controlling Health Care Costs*, 11; Frech and Ginsburg, "Competition Among Health Insurers," 282.

7. Lewis to Everett Edwards, 3 March 1981, Lewis Papers.

8. Nycz, memorandum, "Health Plan Demographic and Rate Considerations for GMCHP Executive Committee," 19 April 1984, Lewis Papers; Nycz interview, 9 February 1995.

9. GMCHP Executive Committee meetings minutes 24 May and 20 July 1982, Lewis Papers.

10. Prepaid Partnership executive committee minutes, 22 July 1982; GMCHP executive committee minutes, 3 August 1982; notes by Lewis, "GMCHP Controversy over the Deductible Plan," undated but about 1985, all in Lewis Papers; Lewis interview, 24 March 1994. According to Lewis, that year's negotiations were the most controversial of his fifteen-year tenure as medical director.

11. Lewis to Robert Pollock, executive director, Sentry Insurance, 31 August 1982; Nycz, "Statistics on GMCHP Enrollment, Demographics and Ambulatory Utilizations," 25 January 1984, Lewis Papers.

12. GMCHP executive committee minutes, 20 July 1982, Lewis Papers.

13. Nycz, memorandum, "Components of the Program to Collaborate with the Clinic in Support of High Risk Greater Marshfield Participants," undated but early 1988, Lewis Papers; Nycz, memorandum to clinic president William Maurer, "GMCHP Enrollment History," 11 October 1983, all in Lewis Papers; GMCHP executive committee minutes, 18 October 1983, Lewis Papers.

14. John W. Hutter, Region IV director, International Woodworkers of America, AFL-CIO, to Lewis, 1 September 1983, Lewis Papers.

15. Daniel J. McCarty et al., "Equity in Physician Compensation: The Marshfield Experiment," *Perspectives in Biology and Medicine* 35 (Winter 1992): 261–70.

16. Compared with national figures, the Marshfield Clinic's fees for procedures were about average, but its fees for the types of nonprocedural services performed by internists and pediatricians were somewhat higher than average (Merian Kirchner, "Are Fees Breaking All Restraints?" *Medical Economics* 63 [6 October 1986]: 122–55).

17. Dr. Stanley Custer, interview by author, 9 January 1995; Lewis interview,

17 February 1994. Blue Cross reported that GMCHP's costs for medical services were too high because they accounted for 51 percent of its premiums, while medical services costs at Kaiser Permanente plans averaged only 48 percent to 49 percent of their premiums (Blue Cross interoffice memo, undated but after 30 January 1984, Lewis Papers). Nycz reported that GMCHP's costs for medical services fell within the average range when the costs of items not usually considered in that category were removed (Nycz, "FY83 Health Plan Clinic Disbursements as a Percent of FY Health Plan Expenses," 8 February 1984, Lewis Papers).

18. Peter Mick, Blue Cross sales manager for GMCHP in Marshfield, memorandum, 20 April 1983, Lewis Papers.

19. Letter attached to lengthy response by Lewis, 3 August 1982, Lewis Papers.

20. Nycz, "Statistics on GMCHP Enrollment, Demographics and Ambulatory Utilizations," 25 January 1984, and Nycz, "Health Plan Demographic and Rate Considerations for GMCHP Executive Committee," 19 April 1984, both in Lewis Papers.

21. "Direct-Pay Rating/Underwriting," undated but after August 1985; "Underwriting Report," prepared for 11 November 1986 for clinic board of directors meeting; Lewis to affiliated physician, 1 December 1986; Nycz, "Components," all in Lewis Papers.

22. Lewis to Pollock, 31 August 1982, Lewis Papers.

23. Porter to Lewis, 28 July 1982; Porter and Sautter to Lewis, two letters dated 12 August 1982, Lewis Papers.

24. Reed Hall, Marshfield Clinic corporation counsel, interview by author, 10 February 1995.

25. Nycz interview, 10 February 1995.

26. Family Health Center governing board and community committee minutes, 25 August 1980, 23 February 1981, and 30 March 1981, Lewis Papers; Nycz interviews, 17 February 1995 and 19 May 1999.

27. In 1982 two-thirds of FHC enrollees had an income that was less than 75 percent of the poverty line, and more than two-fifths had an income equal to less than half of the poverty line (Nycz interview, 17 February 1995). A family of five with an income of less than $11,684 was considered to be living below the poverty line in 1982 (U.S. Census Bureau, "Historic Poverty Thresholds for Families of Specified Size, 1955–2000," 6 October 2003, http://www.census.gov/hhes/poverty/histpov/hstpov1.html (accessed 14 May 2004).

28. Marshfield Medical Research and Education Foundation's FHC grant application for July 1982 to June 1983, pp. 19 and 24, files of Gregory Nycz.

29. Ibid.

30. FHC was operating in all or parts of nine counties by 1986. Its governance had been transferred from the Medical Research Foundation's board of directors to a newly created eleven-member FHC council consisting of seven FHC en-

rollees and four individuals representing the clinic, Saint Joseph's Hospital, and the foundation board. The council was responsible for all aspects of FHC's operations, but the foundation board retained authority for overall program management (Marshfield Medical Research and Education Foundation's FHC grant applications for 1984 to 1985 and 1986 to 1987; the foundation's 1986 annual report, Nycz files).

31. Nycz interview, 8 February 1995.

32. David Jaye, interview by author, 25 April 1995.

33. Porter, interview by author, 9 January 1995.

34. GMCHP's reimbursement to Saint Joseph's Hospital came to more than 100 percent of its charges in FY1979–80 and 93 percent of its charges in FY1980–81 (Minutes of rate-setting staff meeting, 12 May 1982, Lewis Papers).

35. Lewis interview, 14 August 1994; Jaye interview.

36. Thomas Hoyer, "Hospice and Future of End-of-Life Care: Approaches and Funding Ideas," *Journal of Palliative Medicine* 5 (2002): 259–262, esp. 260.

37. Paul R. Ginsburn and Glenn M. Hackbarth, "Alternative Delivery Systems and Medicare," *Health Affairs* 5 (Spring 1986): 6–22; U.S. Bureau of HMOs and Resource Development, *Considerations in Studying the Feasibility of Rural HMOs* (Washington, D.C.: Department of Health and Human Services, 1985), 183; Rosemary Stevens, *In Sickness and in Wealth: American Hospitals in the Twentieth Century* (New York: Basic Books, 1989), 325; Cathy Tokarski and Janet Firshein, "Curbing Health Costs: Many Tried, None Succeeded," in A *New Deal for American Health Care: How Reform Will Reshape Health Care Delivery and Payment for a New Century,* ed. Richard M. Sorian et al. (Washington, D.C.: Healthcare Information Center, 1993), 76.

38. Simmons, "Managed Health Care," 400; Beth C. Weitzman, "The Quality of Care: Assessment and Assurance," in *Health Care Delivery in the United States,* ed. Anthony R. Kovner, 4th ed. (New York: Springer, 1990), 374.

39. Paul L. Grimaldi and Julie A. Micheletti, *Prospective Payment: The Definitive Guide to Reimbursement* (Chicago: Pluribus, 1985), 1; Bernard R. Tresnowski, "HMOs Are Rolling—and We Can All Benefit," *Inquiry* 21 (Fall 1984): 205–13.

40. Minutes of GMCHP rate-setting meeting, 12 July 1983, Lewis Papers.

41. Lewis interview, 14 August 1994.

42. John K. Iglehart, "Government Searching for Most Cost-Efficient Way to Pay Hospitals," *National Journal,* 25 December 1976, pp. 1822–29; Clark C. Havighurst, "The Changing Locus of Decision Making in the Health Care Sector," *Journal of Health Politics, Policy and Law* 11, no. 4 (1986): 697–735, esp. 710–24.

43. Richard Carlson, Saint Joseph's Hospital vice president, to Richard Smith, Blue Cross manager of sales, 5 October 1983; Thomas Gazzana, Blue Cross vice president, memorandum to Smith, 13 October 1983; Lewis to Harlan J. Failor, CEO, Carle Clinic Association, 14 February 1983, Lewis Papers.

44. Peter Mick, memorandum, "State of Wisconsin HMO Rates for 1983," 13 June 1983, Lewis Papers. Another report prepared for a state employee enrollment period later that year revealed that GMCHP's monthly premiums were $20 higher than those of any other HMO or insurance plan listed. While other plans used experience to rate groups and generally gave state employees more favorable rates, Marshfield charged all groups the same premium ("It's Your Choice," information for Wisconsin state employee's dual choice enrollment period, 3–28 October 1983, Lewis Papers).

45. Dr. Richard Leer, president, Marshfield Clinic, interview by author, 22 April 1996; Porter interview.

46. Lewis, notes, "GMCHP Reimbursement," undated but shortly after 30 January 1984, Lewis Papers.

47. Leon Weszewianski, John R. C. Wheeler, and Avedis Donabedian, "Market-Oriented Cost-Containment Strategies and Quality of Care," *Milbank Memorial Fund Quarterly/Health and Society* 60 (Fall 1982): 518–50.

48. Lewis to a GMCHP utilization review nurse, 18 April 1984, Lewis Papers.

49. Report on Marshfield Clinic Ambulatory Surgery Center, 27 March 1985, Lewis Papers.

50. *Marshfield Clinic Pulse,* 21 October 2004.

51. Nycz, "Length of Stay for Selected Diagnoses at Hospitals in Greater Marshfield's Core Area," 18 January 1985, Lewis Papers.

52. "Out-of-Area Services and Out-of-Area Referrals," undated but after 30 September 1983, Lewis Papers.

53. Lewis to affiliated providers, 14 August 1986; out-of-area referral report, May 1987, both in Lewis Papers.

54. "Inpatient Care Costs for AODA Programs," 4 January 1985; "Out of Area Drug/Alcohol Outpatient Referrals," September 1984; Lewis to Carlson at Saint Joseph's Hospital, 3 October 1984, Lewis Papers.

55. Lewis interview, 12 May 1994.

56. Michael McDonald, GMCHP manager, to health plan affiliates, 22 April 1981, Lewis Papers.

57. Confidential letter from an affiliated physician to Lewis, 15 July 1983; letter from Lewis to affiliated physician, 26 July 1983, Lewis Papers.

58. Sam Main, Alexander Grant and Co., to Wenzel, 17 April 1984, Lewis Papers.

59. Lewis to WIPRO Director Donald J. McIntyre, 11 June 1984; report by Lewis of a meeting with McIntyre and WIPRO's Don Schlais regarding arrangements for review, 20 June 1984; Lewis to Schlais, 21 September 1984, all in Lewis Papers.

60. WIPRO report to Lewis, 14 November 1984, Lewis Papers.

61. Lewis to Everett Edwards, president of Wisconsin Blue Cross–Blue

Shield, 27 November 1984; "Minutes of the Meeting with Blue Cross," 19 December 1984, both in Lewis Papers.

62. Lewis to affiliated hospital director, 5 March 1985; Lewis to Jaye, 6 March 1985, both in Lewis Papers.

63. Lewis, report of a meeting with affiliates and GMCHP representatives, 7 March 1985; Lewis to WIPRO, 15 March 1985; Lewis to affiliates, 19 March 1985, all in Lewis Papers.

64. Lewis, report of a telephone conversation with director of affiliated hospital, 3 April 1985, Lewis Papers.

65. Lewis memorandum to GMCHP staff, 23 September 1985, Lewis Papers.

66. Ibid.; Lewis to affiliated doctor, 2 October 1985; affiliated hospital director to Lewis, 15 October 1985, both in Lewis Papers.

67. For example, a utilization review nurse reported eleven questionable cases at one affiliated site, four at another, and two at the Marshfield Clinic, 28 April 1986, Lewis Papers.

68. Lewis to affiliated doctor, re delivery rates, 15 January 1986; Lewis to clinic oncologist, 25 March 1986; clinic oncologist to Lewis, 23 April 1986 and 31 May 1986, all in Lewis Papers.

69. Lewis to affiliated doctor, 20 February 1986.

70. Lewis to clinic physician, confidential, 26 March 1986 and 29 April 1986; clinic physician to Lewis, confidential, 30 April 1986, all in Lewis Papers.

71. Lewis to Gazzana at Blue Cross, 1 May 1986, with WIPRO agreement attached; Jaye to Lewis, 6 May 1986, all in Lewis papers.

72. WIPRO to Lewis with WIPRO report attached, 7 November 1987, Lewis Papers.

73. Dr. Sidney Johnson to Lewis, 9 December 1986; "Summary of GM Audit Regarding WIPRO Review," prepared by GMCHP utilization review nurses, 20 January 1987, Lewis Papers.

74. "Summary of GM Audit Regarding WIPRO Review."

75. Director of an affiliated hospital to Lewis, 16 February 1987, Lewis Papers.

76. By 1985 the Office of HMOs had assumed oversight responsibility for experiments using HMOs to control expenses in federal health insurance programs. It was subsequently renamed Office of Prepaid Health Care (OPHC) and transferred to HCFA; Ed Moy, the director of OPHC, advocated repeal of the HMO Act at the end of the decade (Simmons, "Managed Health Care," 394).

77. Howard R. Veit, "Future of the Federal Government Role in Development of HMOs," in *Skills Development for HMO Managers in the 1980s, Proceedings of the 30th Annual Group Health Institute,* ed. Eugenia Warhol (Washington, D.C.: Group Health Association of America, 1980), 3–8.

78. Lawrence D. Brown, *Politics and Health Care Organization: HMOs as Federal Policy* (Washington, D.C.: Brookings Institution, 1983), 496–97.

79. Anthony J. Mahler and John Friedland, "Identifying Available Options," in *Industry and HMOs: A Natural Alliance, Industry and Healthcare, No. 5*, ed. Richard H. Egdahl and Diana Chapman Walsh (New York: Springer-Verlag, 1978), 45–46; Louis J. Segadelli, "Management Perspectives on Independent Practice Associations," in Dustin L. Mackie and Douglas K. Decker, *Group and IPA HMOs* (Rockville, Md.: Aspen Systems, 1981), 173–91; "Preferred Provider Organizations and Direct Provider Contracting: Analysis of DRG Prospective Payment," *Wisconsin Medical Journal* 82 (May 1983): 20–26; Martha Kendrick, "PPOs: A Challenge to HMOs?" *Group Health Journal* 6 (Fall 1985): 22–27; Gordon K. MacLeod, "An Overview of Managed Health Care," in *The Managed Health Care Handbook*, ed. Peter R. Dongstvedt (Gaithersburg, Md.: Aspen, 1993), 7.

80. Some of the largest multistate HMO plans included Kaiser Permanente Medical Care; Blue Cross and Blue Shield plans; HealthAmerica; PruCare, operated by Prudential Health Care Plans; INA Health Plans, operated by CIGNA and Connecticut General; Maxicare and CNA Health Plans; Health Insurance Plans of Greater New York and Greater New Jersey (*The HMO Industry: Ten Year Report, 1973–1983* [Washington, D.C.: National Industry Council for HMO Development, 1984], 6 and 21–23).

81. Irwin Miller, *American Health Care Blues: Blue Cross, HMOs and Pragmatic Reform Since 1960* (New Brunswick, N.J.: Transaction, 1996), 108.

82. J. A. Hale and M. M. Hunter, *From HMO Movement to Managed Care Industry: The Future of HMOs in a Volatile Health Care Market* (Excelsior, Minn.: InterStudy, June 1988); U.S. Bureau of HMOs and Research Development, *Contraction Activities of HMOs and State Medicaid Agencies* (Rockville, Md.: U.S. Department of Health and Human Services, 30 August 1985), 3–4.

83. Frech and Ginsburg, "Competition Among Health Insurers," 279; Odin W. Anderson et al., *HMO Development, Patterns and Prospects: A Comparative Analysis of HMOs* (Chicago: Pluribus, 1985), 298.

84. U.S. Bureau of HMOs, *Considerations in Studying the Feasibility of Rural HMOs*, 6; U.S. Congress, Office of Technology Assessment, *Health Care in Rural America* (Washington, D.C.: Government Printing Office, September 1990), 101–2 and 315.

85. MacLeod, "An Overview of Managed Health Care," 9.

86. Anderson et al., *HMO Development*, 301.

87. Hale and Hunter, *From HMO Movement to Managed Care Industry*.

88. Marsha Gold, *HMO Industry Profiles*, Vol. 1: *Benefits, Premiums and Market Structure* (Washington, D.C.: Group Health Association of America, June 1988), x.

89. Ibid., 48; U.S. Bureau of HMOs, *Considerations in Studying the Feasibility of Rural HMOs*, 43–44.

90. Anderson et al., *HMO Development*, 209.

91. Simmons, "Managed Health Care," 12.

92. Anderson et al., *HMO Development*, , 208.

93. Miller, *American Health Care Blues*, 104.

94. In 1994, well after many plans had converted all or part of their operations to for-profit, the Blue Cross Blue Shield Association officially allowed its license holders to drop their nonprofit status. See Jack Needleman, "Nonprofit to For-profit Conversions by Hospitals, Health Insurers and Health Plans," *Public Health Reports* 114 (March–April 1999): 108–19.

95. Warren Greenberg, *Competition, Regulation and Rationing in Health Care* (Ann Arbor, Mich.: Health Administration Press, 1991), 49–50.

96. Milton I. Roemer, "Bed Supply and Hospital Utilization: A Natural Experiment," *Hospitals* 35 (November 1961): 36–42.

97. Steven Jonas, *An Introduction to the U.S. Health Care System*, 3d ed. (New York: Springer, 1992), 25. (Earlier editions were by Milton I. Roemer.)

98. Donald Light and Sol Levine, "The Changing Character of the Medical Profession: A Theoretical Overview," *Milbank Quarterly* 66 (1988): 10–32 (supplement 2).

99. Kathy Shannon, "Special Edition: Ambulatory Surgery," *Hospitals* 59 (16 May 1985): 54–62, esp. 61. The number of inpatient surgical procedures decreased in the 1980s, but the growing acceptance of highly technical operations such as coronary bypasses and joint replacements increased total surgical costs dramatically. See Institute of Medicine, Committee on Utilization Management by Third Parties, *Controlling Costs and Changing Patient Care? The Role of Utilization Management* (Washington, D.C.: National Academy Press, 1989), 43.

100. Karen Davis, "Inequality and Access to Health Care," *Milbank Quarterly* 69 (1991): 253–73.

101. William A. Rothman Sr., "The Impact of an HMO on Hospital Operations," in Warhol, *Skills Development for HMO Managers in the 1980s*, 125–30.

102. William R. Fifer, "Prospective Payment Strategy—Is It Working?" *Pennsylvania Medicine* 87 (December 1984): 38–42; Frech and Ginsburg, "Competition Among Health Insurers," 287; "DRGs' First Six Months: Many Hospitals Are Doing Better Than They'd Expected," *Modern Healthcare*, June 1984, p. 42.

103. James B. Bonanno and Terrie Wetle, "HMO Enrollment of Medicare Recipients: An Analysis of Incentives and Barriers," *Journal of Health Politics, Policy, and Law* 9 (Spring 1984): 41–62; Needleman, "Nonprofit to For-profit Conversions," 111.

104. Institute of Medicine, Committee on Implications of For-Profit Enterprise in Health Care, *For-Profit Enterprise in Health Care*, ed. Bradford H. Gray (Washington, D.C.: National Academy Press, 1986), 182–204.

105. Ibid., 205.

106. Greenberg, *Competition, Regulation and Rationing*, 30–41.

107. Clark Havighurst, *Deregulating the Health Care Industry: Planning for Competition* (Cambridge, Mass.: Ballinger, 1982), 77–106; *Goldfarb v. Virginia State Bar,* 421 U.S. 773 (1975).

108. Warren Greenberg, "HMOs Stimulate Competition, FTC Concludes," *Hospital Care* 9 (May–June 1971): 291–98.

109. Light and Levine, "Changing Character of the Medical Profession," 24.

110. Greenberg, *Competition, Regulation and Rationing,* 15–23; Kenneth M. Ludmerer, *Time to Heal: American Medical Education from the Turn of the Century to the Era of Managed Care* (New York: Oxford University Press, 1999).

111. Edmund D. Pellegrino, "Health and the Spirit of Man," in *Financing and Marketing in the Nation's Group Practice HMOs: Proceedings of the 31st Annual Group Health Institute,* ed. Eugenia Warhol (Washington, D.C.: Group Health Association of America, 1981), 47–52.

112. Arnold S. Relman and Uwe E. Reinhardt, "Debating For-Profit Health Care and the Ethics of Physicians," *Health Affairs* 5 (Summer 1986): 5–31, especially 13–14.

113. Dr. John L. Cory Jr., interview by Dennis L. Breo, *American Medical News,* 16 May 1986, pp. 1, 33.

114. Simmons, "Managed Health Care," 397.

115. Lewis, notes for talk, "How Does Competition Affect Access?" 7 May 1984, Lewis Papers.

116. Frech and Ginsburg, "Competition Among Health Insurers," 290.

117. Hale and Hunter, *From HMO Movement to Managed Care Industry.*

118. Patricia McDonnell, Abbie Guttenberg, Leonard Greenberg, and Ross H. Arnett III, "Self-Insured Plans," *Health Care Financing Review* 8 (Winter 1986): 1; Frech and Ginsburg, "Competition Among Health Insurers," 281–82.

119. *Controlling Health Care Costs,* 105–6.

120. Joseph P. Newhouse et al., "Some Interim Results from a Controlled Trial of Cost Sharing in Health Insurance," *New England Journal of Medicine* 305 (17 December 1981): 1503.

121. *The HMO Industry: Ten Year Report,* 13; *Controlling Health Care Costs,* 31.

122. Congressional Budget Office, *Containing Medical Care Cost Through Market Forces* (Washington, D.C.: Government Printing Office, 1982), x and 14.

123. Newhouse et al., "Some Interim Results," 1501–7.

124. National Center for Health Statistics, *Advanced Data,* no. 201 (18 January 1991): 1–2.

125. C. C. Havighurst, J. Blumstein, and R. Bovbjerg, "Strategies in Underwriting the Costs of Catastrophic Disease," *Law Contemporary Problems* 40 (1976): 122–95; Havighurst, "The Changing Locus of Decision Making," 713.

126. Bradford H. Gray and Walter J. McNerney, "Special Report: For-Profit

Enterprise in Health Care, The Institute of Medicine Study," *New England Journal of Medicine* 314 (5 June 1986): 1523–28, especially 1527.

127. Alain Enthoven, "Managed Competition of Alternative Delivery Systems," *Journal of Health Politics, Policy and Law* 13 (Summer 1988): 305–21.

9. Competing Values Doom a Partnership

1. Leo Suycott, interview by author, 1 December 1995.

2. Irwin Miller, *American Health Care Blues: Blue Cross, HMOs and Pragmatic Reform Since 1960* (New Brunswick, N.J.: Transaction, 1996), 99–106.

3. H. E. Frech III and Paul B. Ginsburg, "Competition Among Health Insurers, Revisited," *Journal of Health Politics, Policy and Law* 13 (Summer 1988): 279–91. According to Emily Friedman in "What Price Survival? The Future of Blue Cross and Blue Shield," *Journal of the American Medical Association* 270 (17 June 1998): 1963–69, by the late 1990s the Blues had little in common but their logo, which was "pure gold and ranked only second to Coca-Cola in terms of public recognition."

4. *Eau Claire (Wis.) Leader Telegram,* 5 June 1982, Lewis Papers.

5. Prepaid Plans Policy Group minutes, 20 December 1979, Lewis Papers.

6. Ibid., 22 June 1981, Lewis Papers.

7. Charles Paine, SHP administrator, interview by author, 26 April 1995.

8. Frederick Wenzel to E. Everett Edwards, 1 February 1984; Prepaid Plans Policy Group minutes, 9 February 1984, both in Lewis Papers. Wenzel set clinic losses at $989,000 and estimated Blue Cross losses at $1.8 million.

9. David Gruel, GMCHP coordinator, memoranda regarding data-processing problems, 14, 21, and 28 October and 12 November 1986, Lewis Papers.

10. Lewis to Thomas Gazzana, Blue Cross vice president, 30 April and 16 May 1986, Lewis Papers.

11. Tina Daniell and Neil D. Rosenberg, "Insurance Ills: Complaints About Blue Cross Continue at a High Level," *Milwaukee Journal,* 25 January 1987, Lewis Papers.

12. Suycott to Lewis, 21 February 1986, Lewis Papers; Lewis interview, 6 August 1994.

13. James Coleman, SHP manager, interview by author, 25 April 1995.

14. Dr. Richard Sautter to Lewis, reporting conversation with Edwards of Blue Cross, 14 February 1985, Lewis Papers.

15. Lewis to Sautter, 23 October 1985; draft of letter from Lewis to unknown recipient(s), 10 January 1986, Lewis Papers.

16. Lewis, draft report of Group Health Association of America meeting in Dallas, in which he described formation of the Clinic Club, 12–16 June 1983, Lewis Papers.

17. Lewis interview, 6 August 1994.

18. The Dean Clinic in Madison, Wisconsin; the Geisinger Clinic in Danville, Pennsylvania; the Carle Clinic in Urbana, Illinois; and the Scott & White Clinic in Temple, Texas, all owned their own prepaid health plans and encouraged the Marshfield Clinic to acquire its plan (Lewis interview, 6 August 1994).

19. Lewis, notes, "Thoughts About Blue Cross Relationship," 29 October 1985, and "Relationship with Blue Cross," 5 February 1986, Lewis Papers; Lewis interview, 14 August 1994.

20. Sautter to Lewis, 14 February 1985 and 25 September 1985, Lewis Papers.

21. Blue Cross memorandum, "Greater Marshfield Intermediate and Long-Range Organizational Proposals," 9 July 1985, Lewis Papers.

22. Edwards to Dr. William F. Maurer, 3 December 1985, Lewis Papers.

23. Maurer to GMCHP executive committee, 5 December 1985, Lewis Papers.

24. Lewis interview, 6 August 1994; Lewis, notes, "Blue Cross Relations and Negotiations," 17 December 1985; Maurer to Edwards, 10 January 1986; Edwards to Maurer, 21 January 1986, all in Lewis Papers.

25. Lewis, memorandum, "Relationship with Blue Cross," 5 February 1986; Sidney Johnson, memorandum to clinic physicians, 7 February 1986; Hall, notes of 24 February partnership meeting, 25 February 1986, all in Lewis Papers.

26. Dr. Norman Desbiens to other clinic physicians, 11 February 1986, Lewis Papers.

27. Lewis draft, " Blue Cross Relationship—Next Phase," 13 February 1986, and second draft to clinic physicians, 17 February 1986, Lewis Papers.

28. Wenzel, report of joint conference committee meeting, 19 February 1986, Lewis Papers.

29. Edwards to Lewis, 17 March 1986; Lewis to Edwards, 18 March 1986, both in Lewis Papers.

30. Fritz Wenzel, "Greater Marshfield Community Health Plan," 26 Feb. 1986, prepared for clinic board of directors meetings of 4 and 11 March 1986; information packets distributed to clinic board of directors, 27 February 1986 and about 4 March 1986, all in Lewis Papers.

31. Marshfield Clinic interoffice communication, "Summary of GMCHP Partnership Meeting, 12 September 1986," Lewis Papers.

32. Gazzana to Johnson and David Jaye, 26 September 1986, Lewis Papers.

33. Summary of GMCHP Partnership meeting, 6 October 1986, Lewis Papers.

34. Hall and Coleman, notes of a meeting with the Office of the Commissioner of Insurance, 24 February 1986; Security Health Plan certificate of authority, 3 September 1986, under Chapter 613 of Wisconsin statutes as a service corporation, both in Lewis Papers.

35. Gazzana to Johnson and Jaye, 9 December 1986, Lewis Papers.

36. Gregory Nycz to Wenzel, 9 December 1986, Lewis Papers.

37. Robert DeVita, notes of a 15 January meeting with Blue Cross staff, 19 January 1987; Ronald F. Pfannerstil memo to Wenzel and Hall, 31 May 1989, both in Nycz files.

38. Lewis, notes, "Thoughts on the Ministry Corporation," 13 March 1987.

39. Dr. William Maurer, SHP medical director, interview by author, 8 February 1995; Jaye to Wenzel, 5 November 1986; Sister Lois Bush, president, Sisters of the Sorrowful Mother Ministry Corporation, to Johnson, 4 December 1986, all in Lewis Papers.

40. David Jaye, interview by author, 25 April 1995.

41. Nycz, memorandum, "Importance of Greater Marshfield Health Plan to the Marshfield Clinic," 8 November 1983, Lewis Papers.

42. Joseph Voyer, interview by author, 26 March 1996.

43. Suycott, interview by author, 1 December 1995.

44. Beverly Zupanc, Marshfield Clinic memorandum, "HMO Participants as of 10 April 1987," 15 April 1987, Lewis Papers.

45. Robert Mimier, interview by author, 27 April 1995.

46. DeVita, memorandum, "Rate Group Ideas," 6 May 1986; GMCHP Rate Calculations, 1 October 1986 to 1 October 1987, both in Lewis Papers.

47. Marshfield Clinic Prepaid Plans Committee, minutes, 28 July 1987, Lewis Papers.

48. Paine interview.

49. Security Health Plan executive committee minutes for January 1988, corporate files of the Marshfield Clinic.

50. Maurer interview in *Marshfield Clinic Pulse*, 20 August 1987, files of the Marshfield Clinic.

51. Security Health Plan executive committee minutes, 16 February 1988 and 22 March 1988, clinic files.

52. Security Health Plan executive committee minutes, 19 May 1988 and 16 May 1989, clinic files.

53. Nycz, memorandum, "Components of the Program to Collaborate with the Clinic in Support of High Risk Greater Marshfield Health Plan Participants," undated but after FY 1987; Mimier, memorandum to Nycz, "Healthshare Direct Experience," 7 April 1988; Nycz to Nicholas F. Desien, vice president, Sisters of the Sorrowful Mother Ministry Corporation, 1 May 1988, all in Lewis Papers; Coleman interview.

54. Wisconsin Office of the Commission of Insurance, "Health Insurance Risk-Sharing Plan: Background and Policy Considerations," Wisconsin Office of the Commissioner of Insurance, Madison, January 1996. According to "Insurance Program on the Mend," *Wisconsin State Journal*, 14 May 2000, the annual pre-

mium for a man in his sixties was then $5,400 with a $1,000 deductible, or $4,656 with a $2,500 deductible.

55. Robert Kuttner, "Must Good HMOs Go Bad? Part II: The Search for Checks and Balances," *New England Journal of Medicine* 338 (28 May 1998): 1635–39.

56. Nycz interview, 18 April 2000.

57. Mimier interview, 22 May 2000.

58. Maurer interview.

59. Ibid.

60. SHP executive committee minutes, 15 September 1987, and 22 March and 27 June 1989, clinic files; Coleman interview.

61. Maurer report to SHP board, "An All Clinic Out of Area Referral Control System," 1 August 1991, and cost of referrals report, 20 August 1991, SHP files at SHP office in Marshfield.

62. Pfannerstil, interview by author, 27 April 1995..

63. Gruel, interview by author, 27 April 1995.

64. Mimier interview, 27 April 1995.

65. Maurer interview.

66. Gerald Porter to Johnson, 1 June 1989, Lewis Papers.

67. The IRS extended tax exemption to the clinic's satellite clinics in 1993. Although not required to do so, the clinic donated more than $1 million in lieu of taxes to communities in which it operated in 1996 (Reed Hall, interview by author, 10 February 1995; *Marshfield Clinic Pulse,* 13 November 1997).

68. Hall, memorandum to Lewis, 16 September 1988, Lewis Papers. After a protracted legal battle the Geisinger Clinic failed to achieve tax-exempt status for its HMO. See Thomas L. Driscoll, "Special Report on Taxation and Health Care Delivery Systems," *Healthcare Law Newsletter* 7 (December 1992): 1616–22; Driscoll, "Tax Court Overruled in Geisinger Case" *Healthcare Law Newsletter* 8 (May 1993): 19–21; Driscoll, "No Tax Exemption for Geisinger Health Plan," *Healthcare Law Newsletter* 8 (August 1993): 20–22; Driscoll, "Geisinger Loses Appeal of Its HMO's Tax Status," *Modern Healthcare,* 22 February 1993, p. 13; Phillip G. Royalty, "IRS Toughens Its Guidelines on Tax Exemption for HMOs," *Healthcare Financial Management* 45 (January 1991): 58–60.

69. Lewis to Dr. Richard Leer, Marshfield Clinic president, 5 April 1990. Lewis Papers.

70. Nancy Kraus, Michelle Porter, and Patricia Ball, "Managed Care: A Decade in Review 1980–1990," *InterStudy Edge,* special edition, newsletter published by Ellwood's HMO study group in Minnesota, 1991, pp. 17–45.

71. Wenzel, report of a 27 June 1989 meeting with Thomas Hefty, BCBSU president and CEO, Lewis Papers.

10. The Perils of Antitrust in the Health Care Marketplace

1. Robert DeVita, interview by author, 22 April 1996; Robert Mimier, interview by author, 7 April 1995; Frederick Wenzel, memorandum, 27 June 1989, Lewis Papers.

2. *Blue Cross & Blue Shield United of Wisconsin and Compcare Health Services Insurance Corporation v. the Marshfield Clinic and Security Health Plan of Wisconsin, Inc.* (hereafter, *Blue Cross v. Marshfield Clinic*), summary of actions prepared by Reed Hall, Marshfield Clinic corporation counsel, 22 September 1999, and hereafter called "Hall summary," in Lewis Papers.

3. Dean M. Harris, "Legal Issues," in *Creating Community Care Networks: Issues and Opportunities, Report of the 1993 National Forum on Hospital and Health Affairs, Durham, N.C., May 19–21, 1994*, ed. J. Alexander McMahon (Durham, N.C.: Fuqua School of Business, Duke University, 1994), 54.

4. Troyen A. Brennan and Donald M. Berwick, *New Rules: Regulations, Markets, and the Quality of American Health Care* (San Francisco: Jossey-Bass, 1996), 229.

5. See, for example, *AMA v. U.S.*, 317 U.S. 519 (1943), in which the Court upheld an AMA conviction under the Sherman Antitrust Act for conspiracy to restrain trade; and *Group Health Cooperative of Puget Sound v. King County Medical Society*, 237 P.2d (Wash. 1951), *rehearing denied* (1952), in which the Washington Supreme Court found that the King County Medical Society was illegally trying to prevent competition from physicians engaged in prepaid health care. Others cases include *United States v. Oregon State Medical Society*, 343 U.S. 346 (1952), and *Complete Service Bureau v. San Diego County Medical Society*, 43 Cal. 2d 201, 272 P.2d 497 (1954).

6. *Goldfarb v. Virginia State Bar*, 421 U.S. 773 (1975).

7. Congressional Budget Office, *Containing Medical Care Cost Through Market Forces* (Washington, D.C.: Government Printing Office, 1982), 8–9; Clark C. Havighurst, "Antitrust Enforcement in the Medical Services Industry: What Does It All Mean?" *Milbank Memorial Fund Quarterly/Health & Society* 58 (Winter 1980): 89–124; Robert Kuttner, "Physician-Operated Networks and the New Antitrust Guidelines," *New England Journal of Medicine* 336 (30 January 1997): 386–91.

8. Havighurst, "Antitrust Enforcement"; Kennett Lynn Simmons, "Managed Health Care: Right Idea—Wrong Rules" (Ph.D. diss., University of Texas at Austin, August 1992), 363 and 395.

9. Bernard T. Ferrari and Thomas H. Sponsler, "Health Maintenance Organizations and the Specter of Antitrust Law," *Specialty Law Digest—Health Care* 9 (January 1988): 7–34.

10. Lawrence G. Goldberg and Warren Greenberg, "The Health Maintenance Organization and Its Effects on Competition," *Economic Report* (publication of the Federal Trade Commission), July 1977.

11. *Arizona v. Maricopa County Medical Society,* 457 U.S. 332 (1982); Sammis B. White, *Innovative Approaches to Health Care in Wisconsin: A Review of Three Business-Initiated Alternative Health Care Plans* (Milwaukee: Wisconsin Policy Research Institute, about 1993).

12. Kuttner, "Physician-Operated Networks," 386.

13. Ferrari and Sponsler, "HMOs and Specter of Antitrust Law," 17–19.

14. Warren Greenberg, *Competition, Regulation and Rationing in Health Care* (Ann Arbor, Mich.: Health Administration Press, 1991), 126; Barry F. Rosen and Bradford W. Warbasse, "Physician Relationships with Health Maintenance Organizations Cause Antitrust Problems," *HealthSpan* 10 (May 1993): 7–8; Joel L. Michails, *Legal Issues in the Fee-for-Service/Prepaid Medical Group* (Denver: Center for Research in Ambulatory Health Care Administration, Medical Group Management Association, 1990), 48–51.

15. Marilyn Weber Serafini, "Not So Fast," *National Journal,* 17 December 1994, pp. 2967–70; "U.S. Issues Guidelines to Help Doctors Form Health Networks," *New York Times,* 29 August 1996, p. A1; Michael Werner, "New Guidelines Give Physicians Greater Flexibility in Integration," *Annals of Internal Medicine* 126 (1 February 1997): 253.

16. *Blue Cross v. Marshfield Clinic,* trial transcript, 13 December 1994, sec. 16, line 20, to sec. 33, line 22; Anita J. Slomski, "Is This Group an Illegal Doctor Monopoly?" *Medical Economics* 71 (26 September 1994): 64–76.

17. Slomski, "Is This Group an Illegal Doctor Monopoly?" 64.

18. Jeff Miles, "Antitrust Suit Could Bode Ill for Integrated Systems," *American Medical News* 37 (14 March 1994): 14.

19. *Blue Cross v. Marshfield Clinic,* defendant's motion for summary judgment, 5 July 1994.

20. *Blue Cross v. Marshfield Clinic,* 881 F. Supp. 1309 (W.D. Wis. 1994).

21. Slomski, "Is This Group an Illegal Doctor Monopoly?" 65.

22. Richard Eggleston, "Medical Monopoly: Clinic Loses Case," *Madison (Wis.) Capital Times,* 30 December 1994. One week after the jury award in *Blue Cross v. Marshfield Clinic,* consumers in western Wisconsin filed a class action lawsuit charging that Blue Cross had negotiated secret discounts with providers but had not shared them with consumers. A BCBSU spokesperson responded that the discounts that it obtained were "well publicized." Blue Cross–Blue Shield of Tennessee settled a similar suit out of court for $8.4 million in 1991, and at least six similar suits were pending in other states in 1995 (*Milwaukee Journal* and *Milwaukee Sentinel,* 13 January 1995).

23. *Marshfield Clinic Pulse,* 12 January 1995.

24. Brennan and Berwick, *New Rules,* 246.

25. Robert Imre, "Healthy Precedent? Clinic Case May Alter Care Industry's Path," *Milwaukee Journal,* 11 January 1995.

26. Ibid.

27. Jim Montague, "Playing by the Rules: MD Groups and Antitrust," *Hospitals and Health Networks,* 20 March 1995, pp. 56–58.

28. Letters from two jurors to Shabaz, 13 January 1995, Marshfield Clinic corporate files.

29. *Marshfield Clinic Pulse,* 5 January 1995; Reed Hall, interview by author, 10 February 1995.

30. *Blue Cross v. Marshfield Clinic,* 883 F. Supp. 1247 (W.D. Wis. 1995).

31. Geeta Sharma-Jensen, "Blues' Ads Rip Marshfield Clinic Adding Insult to Injury," *Milwaukee Journal Sentinel,* 14 April 1995.

32. *Marshfield (Wis.) News-Herald,* 14 April and 19 April 1995.

33. *Blue Cross v. Marshfield Clinic,* 65 F.3d 1406 (7th Cir. 1995).

34. *Marshfield Clinic Pulse,* 29 June 1995.

35. Lewis interview, 14 August 1995.

36. *Blue Cross v. Marshfield Clinic,* 65 F.3d 1406, 1409 (7th Cir. 1995).

37. Ibid., 1413.

38. Ibid., 1416.

39. Ibid.

40. Ibid., 1408, 1416–17.

41. James A. Carlson, Associated Press, "Monopoly Suit Against the Clinic Rejected," *Stevens Point (Wis.) Journal,* 19 September 1995.

42. James Mara, *Marshfield (Wis.) News-Herald,* 19 September 1995.

43. James R. Troupis and William E. Snyder, "Analysis of Seventh Circuit's Decision in *Blue Cross & Blue Shield United of Wisconsin and Compcare Health Services Insurance Corp. v. Marshfield Clinic and Security Health Plan of Wisconsin, Inc.,*" *Digest Analysis* 23 (October 1997): 3–10.

44. Robert E. Bloch and Scott P. Perlman, "Most Favored Nation Clauses in Contracts between Healthcare Networks and Providers: The Search for Practical Antitrust Guidance," *Digest Analysis* 23 (May 1997): 3–11.

45. Brian McCormick, "Justice, FTC Seek Rehearing of Marshfield Antitrust Case," *American Medical News* 38 (23 October 1995): 3.

46. BCBSU press release, 3 October 1995, Lewis papers.

47. Marshfield Clinic press release, 3 October 1995; Reed Hall, memorandum to clinic executive committee, 3 October 1995, both in Lewis Papers.

48. *Blue Cross v. Marshfield Clinic,* 65 F.3d 1406 (7th Cir. 1995); Jodie De-Jonge, "Blue Cross Seeks Retrial Delay to Take Suit to Supreme Court," *Wisconsin State Journal,* 20 October 1995.

49. Jamie Mara, "High Court May Get Clinic Case: Blue Cross Files Petition

to Appeal Lower Court Ruling Favoring Clinic," *Marshfield (Wis.) News-Herald,* 12 January 1996.

50. Richard Eggleston, "State Asks U.S. Supreme Court to Take Clinic Case," *Wisconsin State Journal,* 16 February 1996.

51. *Marshfield Clinic Pulse,* 15 February 1996.

52. *Blue Cross v. Marshfield Clinic,* 65 F.3d 1406 (7th Cir. 1995), *cert. denied,* 116 S. Ct. 1288 (1996).

53. "High Court Won't Review Clinic Monopoly Case," *Wisconsin State Journal,* 20 March 1996.

54. Julie Johnsson, "Boost for Antitrust Relief: Marshfield Case Pushes Fed to Reconcile Guidelines, Rulings," *American Medical News* 39 (15 April 1996): 1, 28.

55. Art Grillo, "Blue Cross Case Prompts Questions About Health Care Competition," *(Milwaukee) Business Journal,* 30 March 1996, p. 22.

56. Jamie Mara, "Clinic Legal Tab $4.5 Million in Blue's Suit," *Marshfield (Wis.) News-Herald,* 30 March 1996.

57. Warren Greenberg, "Private Antitrust as a Public Good," *Loyola Consumer Law Reporter* 8 (1996): 118–23.

58. *Blue Cross v. Marshfield Clinic,* U.S. District Court for the Western District of Wisconsin, opinion and order, 10 September 1996.

59. *Blue Cross v. Marshfield Clinic,* U.S. District Court for the Western District of Wisconsin, opinion and order, 1 April 1997, pp. 5 and 19.

60. *Blue Cross v. Marshfield Clinic,* U.S. District Court for the Western District of Wisconsin, opinion and order, 7 April 1997, pp. 2 and 4.

61. *Blue Cross v. Marshfield Clinic,* 980 F. Supp. 1298, 1302 (W.D. Wis. 1997).

62. *Blue Cross v. Marshfield Clinic,* 152 F.3d 588 (7th Cir. 1998).

63. "Merrill Joins Clinic Practice," *Marshfield (Wis.) News-Herald,* 20 November 1995.

64. *Marshfield Clinic Pulse,* 15 February 1996.

65. "Clinics Here, Wausau OK Merger," *Marshfield (Wis.) News-Herald,* 12 December 1996. Marshfield Clinic press release, "Marshfield Clinic and Wausau Medical Center Reach Agreement with State Attorney General: Proceed with Plans to Merge," 18 June 1987; "FTC Allows Wausau Medical Center, Marshfield Clinic Merger to Proceed," *Marshfield Clinic Pulse,* 24 July 1997; "It's Official: Wausau Medical Center Joins the Marshfield Clinic System," *Pulse,* 2 October, 1997.

66. *Marshfield Clinic Pulse,* 1 October 1997.

67. Ibid., 9 October 1997 and 8 January 1998.

68. Ibid., 17 June 1999.

69. *Rozema v. Marshfield Clinic/Security Health Plan (Class Action),* U.S. District Court, Western District of Wisconsin, No. 96-C-592-C, 24 July 1996.

70. *Halida v. Marshfield Clinic/Security Health Plan, Rhinelander Medical Center, North Central Health Protection Plan (Class Action),* U.S. District Court, Western District of Wisconsin, 96 C 730 C, 23 August 1996.

71. *Rozema v. Marshfield Clinic/Security Health Plan,* 977 F. Supp. 1362 (W.D. Wis. 1997).

72. *Malek v. Marshfield Clinic/Security Health Plan, Rhinelander Medical Center, North Central Health Protection Plan (Class Action),* U.S. District Court, Western District of Wisconsin, 96-C-916-C, 14 November 1996.

73. "Third Suit Against Clinic 'Unusual,'" *Marshfield (Wis.) News-Herald,* 14 November 1996.

74. *Rozema v. Marshfield Clinic/Security Health Plan,* 977 F. Supp. 1362 (W.D. Wis. 1997).

75. Ibid.

76. Preliminary settlement approved by Judge Barbara Crabb on 24 October 1997, and fairness hearing held on 8 December 1997.

77. Mary Lawson and Sarah Fuelleman, "Clinic, Blue Cross, Former Enemies, Sign Preferred Provider Agreement," *Marshfield (Wis.) News-Herald,* 22 January 1999.

78. Hall summary, 22–23.

79. Mark L. Glassman, "Can HMO Markets Wield Market Power? Assessing Antitrust Liability in the Imperfect Market for Health Care Financing," *American University Law Review* 46 (October 1996): 91–147. David Bruda, in "Lax Enforcement Paints Favorable Legal Outlook," *Modern Healthcare,* 1 January 1996, pp. 49–50, suggested further litigation was likely to be brought by private parties, such as insurers who were "locked out of markets by dominant provider groups" or by provider groups that are denied markets by dominant insurers. State enforcers, such as the attorneys general who sought reconsideration of Posner's decision, were also likely "to bring antitrust actions similar to those in Marshfield."

80. William M. Sage, "Judge Posner's RFP: Antitrust Law and Managed Care," *Health Affairs* 16 (November–December1997): 44–61.

81. Clark C. Havighurst, testimony before the House Committee on Judiciary, *Antitrust Health Care Advancement Act of 1996: Hearings on H.R. 2925,* 104th Cong., 2d sess., 28 February 1996, 390–556, including insertion of documents by Havighurst on 428–52, 468–87.

82. "U.S. Issues Guidelines"; Werner, "New Guidelines," 253.

83. Federal Trade Commission/Department of Justice Policy Statement, 28 August 1996, Federal Trade Commission website, http://www.ftc.gov/opa/1996/08/hlth3.htm (accessed 8 June 2000).

84. Warren Greenberg, "Marshfield Clinic, Physician Networks, and the Exercise of Monopoly Power," *Health Services Research* 33 (December 1998): 1461–76.

85. Kuttner, "Physician-Operated Networks," 386–91.

86. Ibid.

87. Sara Rosenbaum, "The Application of Antitrust Law," in Rand E. Rosenblatt, Sylvia A. Law, and Sara Rosenbaum, *Law and the American Health Care System* (Westbury, N.Y.: Foundation Press, 1997), 689–700.

11. HMOs and Public Programs in the 1990s and Early 2000s

1. Kennett Lynn Simmons, "Managed Health Care: Right Idea—Wrong Rules" (Ph.D. diss., University of Texas at Austin, August 1992), 422.

2. House Committee on Ways and Means, "Beneficiaries Enrolled in Medicare Risk HMOs, 1990–2000," p. 165, fig. 4.2, *Medicare and Health Care Chartbook, May 17, 1999*, Committee Print, 106th Cong., 1st sess., 6 January 1999, http://www.access.gpo.gov/congress/house/ways-and-means/sec4.pdf (accessed 1 May 2004).

3. Previous presidential efforts included proposals by Franklin D. Roosevelt and Harry Truman for comprehensive prepaid national health insurance financed through Social Security; Lyndon Johnson's attempts to insure all Americans before he settled on Medicare and Medicaid for the elderly and poor; and Nixon's Comprehensive Health Insurance Program, which would have provided extensive coverage to both employed and unemployed Americans. See Robert J. Blendon, introduction to *A New Deal for American Health Care: How Reform Will Reshape Health Care Delivery and Payment for a New Century*, ed. Richard M. Sorian et al. (Washington, D.C.: Health Care Information Center, 1993), 1–3.

4. Julie Kosterlitz, "Looking for Explanations," *National Journal*, 24 September 1994, p. 2250.

5. Hilary Stout, "Doctors' and Insurers' Groups Step up Ads Lambasting Health Care Overhaul," *Wall Street Journal*, 25 January 1994.

6. Julie Kosterlitz, "From the K Street Corridor," *National Journal*, 14 May 1994, p. 1143; Julie Kosterlitz and James A. Barnes, "From the K Street Corridor," *National Journal*, 28 May 1998, p. 1245.

7. Blendon, introduction, 1–3.

8. "The Uninsured," *Kaiser Public Opinion Update*, publication of the Kaiser Family Foundation, Menlo Park, California, April 2000.

9. Robert J. Bendon and John M. Benson, "Americans' Views on Health Policy: A Fifty-Year Historical Perspective, "*Health Affairs* 20 (March–April 2001): 33–45.

10. Lauran Neergaard, "U.S. Ranked Low for Health Care," *Wisconsin State Journal*, 21 June 2000.

11. Thomas M. Kickham and William D. Clark, "Cost Containment and Access in the United States: The Challenge to Control Costs While Expanding

Access," in *Cost Control for Quality Care: Meeting the Challenge of Health System Financing,* Studies and Research No. 32 (Geneva: International Social Security Association, 1992), 69; Ellen Morrison et al., "Global Budgets in the United States: Feasibility and Implications," in *Transforming the System: Building a New Structure for a New Century: The Future of Health Care,* vol. 4, ed. Robert J. Blendon and Mollyann Brodie (Washington, D.C.: Healthcare Information Center, 1994), 27–28.

12. Gerard F. Anderson and Peter S. Hussey, "Questioning the Need to Ration," *Lancet* 358 (7 July 2001): 81.

13. Janet Hook, Los Angeles Times Wire Service, "Number Lacking Health Insurance Rises to 44.3 M," *Madison (Wis.) Capital Times,* 4 October 1999; "Bush, Gore Wrong on Health Care," *Wisconsin State Journal,* 15 October 2000.

14. Dennis P. Andrulis, "Access to Care Is the Centerpiece in the Elimination of Socioeconomic Disparities in Health," *Annals of Internal Medicine* 129 (1 September 1998): 412–16; Joseph P. Shapiro, "No Time for the Poor," *U.S. News and World Report,* 5 April 1999, p. 57; John Holahan and Johnny Kim, "Why Does the Number of Uninsured Americans Continue to Grow?" *Health Affairs* 19 (July–August 2000): 188–94; Steven A. Schroeder, "Health Policy 2001: Prospects for Expanding Health Insurance Coverage," *New England Journal of Medicine* 344 (15 March 2001): 847–52.

15. David Mechanic, "The Changing Elderly Population and Future Health Care Needs," *Journal of Urban Health: Bulletin of the New York Academy of Medicine* 76 (March 1999): 24–38; Sara Rosenbaum, "Health Policy Report: Medicaid," *New England Journal of Medicine* 346 (21 February 2002): 636–37.

16. Rosenbaum, "Health Policy Report,": 635–40.

17. Bruce C. Vladeck, "Where the Action Is: Medicaid and the Disabled," *Health Affairs* 22 (January–February 2003): 90–100.

18. David Mechanic, "Managing Behavioral Health in Medicaid," *New England Journal of Medicine* 348 (8 May 2003): 1914–16.

19. Rosenbaum, "Health Policy Report."

20. Thomas Rice and Kathleen R. Morrison, "Patient Cost Sharing for Medical Services: A Review of the Literature and Implications for Health Care Reform," *Medical Care Review* 51 (Fall 1994): 235–87.

21. John Holahan and Shinobu Suzuki, "Medicaid Managed Care Payment Methods and Capitation Rates in 2001," *Health Affairs* 22 (January–February 2003): 204–218.

22. Marilyn Werber Serafini, "Another Looming Crisis," *National Journal,* 2 and 9 January 1999, pp. 32–36.

23. John Holahan, Stephen Zuckerman, Alison Evans, and Suresh Rangarajan, "Medicaid Managed Care in Thirteen States," *Health Affairs* 17 (May–June 1998): 43–63; John Holahan, Suresh Rangarajan, and Matthew Schirmer,

"Medicaid Managed Care Payment Methods and Capitation Rates: Results of a National Survey," Urban Institute, 1 May 1999, http://newfederalism.urban.org/html/occa26.html (accessed 20 April 2004).

24. Paul L. Grimaldi, "Navigating the Waters of Medicaid Managed Care Contracting," *Healthcare Financial Management* 49 (June 1995): 72–80; J. E. Bailey et al., "Academic Managed Care Organizations and Adverse Selection Under Medicaid Managed Care in Tennessee," *Journal of the American Medical Association* 282 (15 September 1999) 282: 1067–72.

25. Nancy Taplin McCall, "Monitoring Access Following Medicare Price Changes: Physician Perspective," *Health Care Financing Review* 14 (Spring 1993): 97–117; Uwe E. Reinhardt, "Wanted: A Clearly Articulated Social Ethic for American Health Care," *Journal of the American Medical Association* 278 (5 November 1997): 1446–47; Patricia Simms, "Dentists Needed to Treat the Poor," *Wisconsin State Journal,* 19 July 2000.

26. Kaiser Family Foundation, "Health Insurance Enrollment," *Trends and Indicators in the Changing Health Care Marketplace,* exhibit 2.16: Medicaid Managed Care and Traditional Enrollment, 1990–2002, http://www.kff.org/insurance/7031/ti2004-2-16.cfm (accessed 5 May 2004).

27. Suzanne Felt-Lisk, Pam Silberman, Sheila Hoag, and Rebecca Slifkin, "Medicaid Managed Care in Rural Areas: A Ten-State Follow-Up Study," *Health Affairs* 18 (March–April 1999): 238–45.

28. LaVonne A. Straub and Norman Walzer, "Financing Demand for Rural Health Care," in *Rural Health Care: Innovation in a Changing Environment,* ed. LaVonne A. Straub and Norman Walzer (Westport, Conn.: Praeger, 1992), 3–19; David Hartley, Lois Quam, and Nicole Lurie, "Urban and Rural Differences in Health Insurance and Access to Care," *Journal of Rural Health* 10 (Spring 1994): 98–108.

29. Debra Freund, L. Rossiter, and P. Fox, "Evaluation of Medicaid Competition Demonstrations," *Health Care Financing Review* 11 (Fall 1989): 81–97; J. W. Krieger, F. A. Connell, and J. P. LoGerfo, "Medicaid Prenatal Care: A Comparison of Use and Outcomes in Fee-for-Service and Managed Care," *American Journal of Public Health* 82 (February 1992): 183–190.

30. Janet Currie and John Fahr, "Medicaid Managed Care: Effects on Children's Medicaid Coverage and Utilization," *JCPR (Joint Center for Poverty Research) Policy Briefs* 2 (8 February 2000), http://www.jcpr.org/policybriefs/vol2_num5.html (accessed 1 May 2004).

31. Robert E. Hurley and Stephen A. Sommers, "Medicaid and Managed Care: A Lasting Relationship?" *Health Affairs* 22 (January–February 2003): 77–88.

32. Congress's welfare reform efforts were contained in the Personal Responsibility and Work Opportunity Reconciliation Act of 1996.

33. Bowen Garrett and John Holahan, "Health Insurance Coverage After Welfare," *Health Affairs* 19 (January–February 2000): 175–84; Robert Pear, *New York Times* News Service, "States Aren't Taking Advantage of Post-Welfare Funds," *Wisconsin State Journal*, 21 May 2000.

34. Jenny Price, "Anti-Smoking Effort Boosted," *Wisconsin State Journal*, 19 May 1999.

35. Sarah Wyatt, "BadgerCare for Poor Families Set to Start," *Wisconsin State Journal*, 28 June 1999; U.S. Department of Health and Human Services, "The 1999 HHS Poverty Guidelines," http://aspe.os.dhhs.gov/poverty/99poverty.htm (accessed 2 May 2004).

36. "Setbacks Fail to Slow Down BadgerCare," *Wisconsin State Journal*, 4 April 2000.

37. *Marshfield Clinic Pulse*, 27 April 2000.

38. Robert Pear, "Forty States Forfeit Health Care Funds for Poor Children," *New York Times*, 24 September 2000.

39. Charles Ornstein, "Federal Deadline to Spend Millions Missed by Texas: Congress Could Give Back Some Money for Kids' Health Insurance," *Dallas Morning News*, 5 October 2000; "Talk of Health-Care Reform Is Just Talk," editorial, *Wisconsin State Journal*, 25 October 2000.

40. Marsha Gold, Jessica Mittler, Debra Draper, and David Rousseau, "Participation of Plans and Providers in Medicaid and SCHIP Managed Care," *Health Affairs* 22 (January–February 2003): 230–40.

41. Kristen Harknett et al., "Do Public Expenditures Improve Child Outcomes in the U.S.? A Comparison Across Fifty States," Center for Research on Child Wellbeing, working paper no. 03-02, http://crcw.princeton.edu/working papers/WP03–02-Harknett.pdf (accessed 20 April 2004).

42. Jeff Mayers, "GOP Seeks Short-Term Fix for BadgerCare," *Wisconsin State Journal*, 22 March 2000.

43. Gold, Mittler, Draper, and Rousseau, "Participation of Plans and Providers"; Debra A. Draper and Marsha R. Gold, "Provider Risk Sharing in Medicaid Managed Care," *Health Affairs* 22 (May–June 2003): 159–67.

44. Rosenbaum, "Health Policy Report"; "Approved HIFA Demonstrations" are listed at Centers for Medicare and Medicaid Services, http://www.cms.hhs .gov/hifa/hifaadem.asp (accessed 1 May 2004).

45. John K. Iglehart, "Health Policy Report: The Dilemma of Medicaid," *New England Journal of Medicine* 348 (22 May 2003): 2140–47; Diane Rowland and James R. Tallon Jr., "Medicaid: Lessons from a Decade," *Health Affairs* 22 (January–February 2003): 138–44.

46. "Badger-Style Welfare Can Work Nationwide," editorial, *Wisconsin State Journal*, 29 May 2002.

47. Iglehart, "Health Policy Report: The Dilemma of Medicaid"; Laura Meckler, Associated Press, "Bush Plan Would Give States Power to Remake Medicaid, *Wisconsin State Journal,* 1 February, 2003.

48. Robert Pear, "States Can Limit Emergency Access in Medicaid Cases," *New York Times,* 17 January 2003; "U.S. Nears Clash with Governors on Medicaid Cost," *New York Times,* 16 February 2004.

49. Total Medicaid spending increased from $119.3 billion in 1992 to $257.5 billion in 2002. See Kaiser Family Foundation, "Health Care Spending and Costs," *Trends and Indicators in the Changing Health Care Marketplace, 2004 Update,* exhibit 1.12: Total Medicaid Spending 1992–2002, http://www.kff.org/insurance/7031/ti2004-1-12.cfm (accessed 20 May 2004).

50. Syl Bolder, "Issues Facing Rural Health Care Finances," in *Financing Rural Health Care,* ed. LaVonne A. Straub and Norman Walzer (New York: Praeger, 1988), 25–41; Ira Moscovice, "The Future of Rural Hospitals," in Straub and Walzer, *Financing Rural Health Care,* 65–81.

51. Spencer Rich, "Health Care: An Era of Consolidation," *National Journal,* 15 July 2000, pp. 2296–97.

52. Patricia Simms, "Non-Urgent Patients Are Flocking to the ER," *Wisconsin State Journal,* 23 April 2002.

53. Tim Size, executive director, Rural Wisconsin Health Cooperative, interview by author, 20 June 2000; "Rural Wisconsin Health Cooperative: Overview, Innovation and Action Since 1979," http://www.rwhc.com/papers/overview.html (accessed 5 May 2004).

54. Greg Nycz, interview by author, 8 February 1995.

55. Ibid.

56. Bradford H. Gray and Catherine Rowe, "Safety-Net Health Plans: A Status Report," *Health Affairs* 19 (January–February 2000): 185–202.

57. Michael K. Gusmano, Gerry Fairbrother, and Heidi Park, "Exploring the Limits of the Safety Net: Community Health Centers and Care for the Uninsured," *Health Affairs* 22 (November–December 2002): 188–194.

58. Nycz interview, 19 May 1999.

59. Ibid.

60. *Marshfield Clinic Pulse,* 4 January 2001.

61. Dave Bushee, director of FHC Pharmacy Services at Marshfield Clinic, interview by author, 18 May 2004.

62. For example, see Nycz testimony before House Committee on Ways and Means, Subcommittee on Health, *Hearings on Health Care Service Delivery Infrastructure in Inner City and Rural Communities,* 93d Cong., 1st sess., 24 June 1993.

63. *Marshfield Clinic Pulse,* 5 October 1995.

64. Ibid., 18 May 2000.

65. Ibid., 1 March 1999.

66. Ibid., 15 August 2002.

67. Ibid., 6 May 2003.

68. Ibid., 3 June 2004.

69. Nycz interview, 20 July 2003.

70. Ibid.; Association of State and Territorial Health Officials, "Health Disparities Collaboratives and Medicaid Disease Management: Tracking Trends Affecting Public Health," February 2002, http://www.neclinicians.org/pdf/asthocoll.pdf (accessed 1 May 2004).

71. Social Security Administration, "Hospital Insurance and/or Supplemental Medical Insurance: Number of Enrollees Aged 65 or Older . . . July 1, 1980-202," table 8B3a, and "Hospital Insurance and/or Supplemental Medical Insurance: Number of Disabled Enrollees . . . July 1, 1980-202," table 8B3b, *Annual Statistical Supplement—Medicare Enrollment, 2003*, http://www.ssa.gov/policy/docs/statcomps/supplement/2003/8b.pdf (accessed 2 May 2004).

72. National Academy of Social Insurance, "National Academy of Social Insurance Sourcebook/Medicare," no date, p. 8, http://www.nasi.org/publications 3901/publications_show.htm?slide_id=8&cat_id=76 (accessed 1 May 2004).

73. Marilyn Moon, " Health Policy 2001: Medicare," *New England Journal of Medicine* 344 (22 March 2001): 928–31.

74. Commonwealth Fund, "Medicare+Choice Enrollees Faced Rising Premiums, Benefits Cuts and Increased Costs in 2002," 1 November 2002, http://www.cmwf.org/media/releases/achmangold575580_release11012002.asp (accessed 3 May 2004).

75. Dana P. Goldman and Julie M. Zissimopoulos, "High Out-of-Pocket Spending by the Elderly," *Health Affairs* 22 (May–June 2003): 194–202.

76. Gerald F. Riley, Melvin J. Ingber, and Cynthia G. Tudor, "Disenrollment of Medicare Beneficiaries from HMOs," *Health Affairs* 16 (September–October 1997): 117–24.

77. Lyle Nelson et al., "Access to Care in Medicare HMOs," *Health Affairs* 16 (March–April 1997): 148–56.

78. Robert H. Miller and Harold S. Luft, "Does Managed Care Lead to Better or Worse Quality of Care?" *Health Affairs* 16 (September–October 1997): 7–25.

79. Marilyn Werber Serafini, "Managed Medicare," *National Journal*, 15 April 1995, pp. 920–23.

80. David R. Graber and Anne Osborne Kilpatrick, "Health Care Organization and Incentives Under Emerging Models of Elderly Health Care," *Journal of Public Administration and Management*, 1996, http://www.pamij.com/elderly.html (accessed 20 April 2004).

81. Timothy D. McBride, "Disparities in Access to Medicare Managed Care Plans and Their Benefits," *Health Affairs* 17 (November–December 1998): 170–80.

82. House Ways and Means Committee, "Medicare Beneficiaries in Urban and Rural Locations Who Are Enrolled in Risk HMOs, June 1996," *Medicare and Health Care Chartbook, May 17, 1999,* p. 168, fig. 4.4.

83. Alice Ann Love, "HMOs Cut Benefits to People on Medicare: Higher Costs, Lower Rate Increases Lead to Changes," *Wisconsin State Journal,* 26 December 1997; Peter T. Kilborn, *New York Times* News Service, "Big HMOs Backing away from Medicare Patients," *Wisconsin State Journal,* 6 July 1998; Robert Pear, "As HMOs Drop Medicare, Many Are Left in Quandary," *New York Times,* 19 October 1998.

84. John K. Iglehart, "The American Health Care System," *New England Journal of Medicine* 340 (28 January 1999): 327–32.

85. Marilyn Werber Serafini, "The HMO Exodus: Round Two," *National Journal,* 15 May 1999, p. 1337.

86. "HMOs Pull Out of Medicaid and Medicare in Some States," *New York Times,* 12 July 1998.

87. Dan Morgan, "More Health Plans Quit Medicare," *Washington Post,* 30 June 2000.

88. Paul Johnson, "State May Attract Medicare HMOs," *Wisconsin State Journal,* 7 November 1998; Donna E. Shalala and Uwe E. Reinhardt, "Viewing the U.S. Health Care System from Within; Candid Talk from HHS," *Health Affairs* 18 (May–June 1999): 47–55.

89. Jim Malone and Dan Stier, "Disparity in Medicare Rates Hurts Wisconsin," 17 February 2000 press release, Wisconsin Department of Health and Family Services (HFS); Jim Malone, HFS administrative manager of public affairs, interview by author, 24 February 2000.

90. Robert Kuttner, "The Risk-Adjustment Debate," *New England Journal of Medicine* 339 (24 December 1998): 1952–56; Jerome P. Kassirer and Marcia Angell, "Risk Adjustment or Risk Avoidance?" *New England Journal of Medicine* 339 (24 December 1998): 1925–26; Health Care Financing Administration, "Medicare+Choice Rates 45-Day Notice," 15 January 1999, http://www.cms.hhs .gov/healthplans/rates/2000/45day-00.asp (accessed 5 May 2004).

91. Penny H. Feldman, "Issues in Equalizing Medicare Expenditures: The Devil Is in the Details," *American Journal of Public Health* 87 (October 1997): 1595–96.

92. Shalala and Reinhardt, "Viewing the U.S. Health Care System," 50; Stuart M. Butler et al., "Crisis Facing CMS & Millions of Americans," *Health Affairs* 18 (January–February 1999): 8–10. The fourteen signatories were Stuart M. Butler of the Heritage Foundation; Patricia M. Danzon and Mark V. Pauly of the University of Pennsylvania; Bill Gradison of the Health Insurance Association of America; Robert Helms of the American Enterprise Institute; Marilyn Moon of

the Urban Institute; Joseph P. Newhouse of Harvard University; Martha Phillips of the Concord Coalition; Uwe E. Reinhardt of Princeton University; Robert D. Reischauer of the Brookings Institution; William L. Roper of the University of North Carolina at Chapel Hill; John Rother of AARP; Leonard D. Scheffer of WellPoint Health Networks, Inc.; and Gail R. Wilensky of Project Hope.

93. Marilyn Werber Serafini, "A Windfall for Medicare Providers," *National Journal*, 24 June 2000, pp. 1998–99.

94. *Milwaukee Journal/Sentinel*, 27 March 2000; Tania Anderson, "Medicare Parity Is a Tough Sell," *Wisconsin State Journal*, 3 April 2000.

95. Gloria Lau, "Golden Oldies," *Forbes*, 10 February 1997, pp. 60, 62.

96. Wisconsin Department of Justice, "Attorney General Files Suit Against Medicare Program: Doyle Says Federal Formula Hurts Senior Citizens in Wisconsin," http://www.doj.state.wi.us/news/nr031500.htm (accessed 2 July 2000); Tim Size, executive director, Rural Wisconsin Health Cooperative, "Medicare: A $2 Billion State Biennial Shortfall," testimony prepared for a public hearing before the Special Committee on Capture of Federal Resources, Madison, Wisconsin, 18 November 1998.

97. Conrad de Fiebre, "Judge Rejects Hatch, Senior Suit over Medicare Payments," *(St. Paul, Minn.) Star Tribune*, 8 July 2000; Minnesota Senior Federation, "Medicare Lawsuit Dismissed," http://www.mnseniors.org/mjchearing.html (accessed 12 July 2000).

98. Richard B. West, policy analyst, Wisconsin Department of Justice, personal communication, 27 October 2000; "Metro Region to Appeal Medicare Inequity Ruling," *Minnesota Senior News*, September 2000.

99. *Minnesota Senior Federation v. United States*, 273 F.3d 805 (8th Cir. 2002).

100. House Ways and Means Committee, "Beneficiaries Enrolled in Medicare Risk HMOs, 1990–2000."

101. Linda Boone Hunt, "Hurting in the Heartland," *Modern Physician*, September 2000, pp. 67–70, 80.

102. Jim Coleman et al., "Medicare Risk Contracting—A Partial Solution for Increasingly Restrictive Medicare Payment Policies," Marshfield Clinic Medicare Risk Contracting Workgroup, 10 December 1997; Jim Coleman et al., "Medicare Risk Contracting Workgroup Report on Reevaluation of Marshfield Clinic/SHP Risk Contracting Option," April 28, 1999; Nycz interview, 18 April 2000.

103. Nycz interview, 20 July 2003.

104. Scott Polenz, SHP director of government services, interview by author, 12 April 2002.

105. Linda Schuetz, "Profits at State HMOs Rose in 2001," *Wisconsin State Journal*, 6 April 2002; Marsha Gold, "Can Managed Care and Competition Control

Medicare Costs?" *Health Affairs* Web Exclusive 22 (May–June 2003): 11. Web Exclusive, http:www.content.healthaffairs.org/contents-by-date.0.shtml (accessed 10 June 2004).

106. Robert J. Blendon et al., "Common Concerns amid Diverse Systems: Health Care Experiences in Five Countries," *Health Affairs* 22 (May–June 2003): 106–21.

107. Robert A. Berenson and Jane Horvath, "Confronting the Barriers to Chronic Care Management in Medicare," *Health Affairs* 22 (March–April 2003): 11.

108. Steven M. Lieberman, Julie Lee, Todd Anderson, and Dan L. Crippen, "Reducing the Growth of Medicare Spending: Geographic Versus Patient-based Strategies," *Health Affairs* Web Exclusive (10 December 2003): 603–13. Web exclusive, see endnote 105 for URL.

109. J. F Jencks, E. D. Huff, T. Cuerdos, "Change in the Quality of Care Delivered to Medicare Beneficiaries, 1998–1999 to 2000–2001," *Journal of the American Medical Association* 289 (12 January 2003): 305–12.

110. Genny Becker Jacks, "How Do Your Physician's Earnings Compare to MGMA Survey Results?" *Medical Group Management Journal* 37 (July–August 1990) : 73–79; William C. Hsaio et al., *Managing Reimbursement in the '90s* (New York: McGraw-Hill, 1990), 5–13.

111. David W. Lee and Kurt D. Gillis, "Physician Responses to Medicare Physician Payment Reform: Preliminary Results on Access to Care," *Inquiry* 30 (Winter 1993): 417–28.

112. Henry G. Dove, "Use of Resource-Based Relative Value Scale for Private Insurers," *Health Affairs* 13 (Winter 1994): 193–210; M. R. Nuwer and B. Sigsbee, "Medicare's Resource-Based Relative Value Scale, a De Facto National Fee Schedule," *Neurology* 50 (June 1998): 1930; M. F. Berlin, B. P. Faber, L. M. Berlin, and M. F. Budzynski, "RVU Costing Applications," *Health Care Financing Management* 51 (November 1997): 73–74, 76.

113. Kickham and Clark, "Cost Containment and Access," 69–91; Norbert Goldfield, "Understanding Your Managed Care Practice," in *The Physician's Guide to Managed Care,* ed. David B. Nash (Gaithersburg, Md.: Aspen, 1994), 190–213; J. P. Weiner et al., "Risk-Adjusted Medicare Capitation Rates Using Ambulatory and Inpatient Diagnoses," *Health Care Financing Review* 17 (Spring 1996): 77–99.

114. Robert B. Doherty, "Washington Perspective," *ACP Observer,* July–August 1998, http://www.acponline.org/journals/news/jul98/pepfair.htm (accessed 2 May 2004); and Volume-and-Intensity Response Team, Office of the Actuary, "Physician Volume and Intensity Response Memorandum," 13 August 1998, Center for Medicare and Medicaid Services, http://www.cms.hhs.gov/statistics/actuary/physicianresponse/ (accessed 2 May 2004).

115. Douglas Holtz-Eakin, testimony before House Subcommittee on Health,

Committee on Energy and Commerce hearings on *Medicare's Physician Fee Schedule,* 108th Cong., 2d sess., May 5, 2004, http://www.cbo.gov/showdoc .cfm?index=5416&sequence=0 (accessed 17 October 2004).

116. Dana Gelb Safran et al., "Primary Care Quality in Medicare Program: Comparing the Performance of Medicare Health Maintenance Organizations and Traditional Fee-for-Service Medicare," *Archives of Internal Medicine* 162 (8 April 2002): 757–65.

117. *Arthur Andersen Washington Health Care Newsletter,* February 2000.

118. Gail R. Wilensky, "The Implications of Regional Variations in Medicare—What Does It Mean for Medicare? *Annals of Internal Medicine* 138 (18 February 2003): 350–51; Elliott S. Fisher et al., "The Implications of Regional Variations in Medicare Spending, Part 2: Health Outcomes and Satisfaction with Care," *Annals of Internal Medicine* 138 (18 February 2003): 288–98.

119. Centers for Medicare and Medicaid Services, "2003 Data Compendium," November 2003, http://www.cms.hhs.gov/researchers/pubs/datacompendium/ current/, then click link to Medicare and Prepaid Enrollment Distribution (accessed 14 May 2004).

120. Medical News Service, "December Medicare+Choice Special Enrollment Period Means More Options for People with Medicare," *FIRSTGOV for Seniors,* 4 December 2001, http://www.medicalnewsservice.com/ARCHIVE/ MNS598.cfm (accessed 5 May 2004).

121. Bob Herbert, "Stalking the Giant Chicken Coop," *New York Times,* 8 December 2003.

122. Edmund Walsh and Bill Brubaker, "Help for Everybody—at a Price," *Washington Post Weekly Edition,* 1–7 December 2003; "The Facts About Upcoming New Benefits in Medicare," Center for Medicare and Medicaid Services Publication No. CMS 11054, 17 February 2004.

123. Robert Pear, "Medicare to Monitor Prices in New Drug Plan," *New York Times,* 10 December 2003.

124. Edmund Walsh and Bill Brubaker, "Help for Everybody—at a Price."

125. Ibid., Lauran Neergaard, Associated Press, "U.S. Generic Drugs Often Still Best Buy," *Wisconsin State Journal,* 18 January 2004; Ramin Mojtabai and Mark Olfson, "Medication Costs, Adherence, and Health Outcomes Among Medicare Beneficiaries," *Health Affairs* 22 (July–August 2003): 220–29; Gardiner Harris, "Medicare Law Might Limit Drug Discounts for Insurers," *New York Times* (24 December 2003).

126. Albert B. Crenshaw, "Investing for Health: Tax-free Saving Covers Expenses," *Washington Post Weekly Edition,* 8–14 December 2003; Marsha Gold, "Can Managed Care and Competition Control Medicare Costs?" *Health Affairs,* 22 (May–June 2003): 11, Web Exclusive, http://content.healthaffairs.org/ contents-by-date.0.shtml (accessed 10 June 2004).

127. "CMS Announces 2005 Medicare Advantage Payment Rates and New Results on Beneficiary Savings from Medicare Advantage," Centers for Medicare and Medicaid Services, 10 May 2004, http://www.cms.hhs.gov/media/press/release.asp?Counter=1040 (accessed 18 May 2004); Associated Press, "Medicare Law Shortchanges State's Elderly, *Wisconsin State Journal,* 11 March 2004; Jeff Zriny, director of government services, Security Health Plan, interview, 28 May 2004.

12. HMO Enrollment Growth in the Private Sector in the 1990s

1. Private-sector spending on health care, nearly all of which is funded by employers, increased from $45.5 billion in 1970 to $416.2 billion in 1990 (Centers for Medicare and Medicaid Services, "National Health Expenditures by Type of Service and Source of Funds, Calendar Years 1960–2002," file nhe02.zip, *Health Accounts,* http://www.cms.hhs.gov/statistics/nhe/default.asp? (accessed 6 May 2004); David A. Kindig, *Purchasing Population Health: Paying for the Results* (Ann Arbor: University of Michigan Press, 1997), 1.

2. Robert Kuttner, "Must Good HMOs Go Bad? Part I: The Commercialization of Prepaid Group Health Care," *New England Journal of Medicine* 338 (21 May 1998): 1558–63; *Market Facts, February 1998* (Menlo Park, Calif.: Henry J. Kaiser Foundation, 1998).

3. Greeta Sharma-Jensen, "Health Networks Virtually Cut Out Insurers," *Wisconsin State Journal,* 4 December 1994; David R. Olmos, *Los Angeles Times* News Service, "Eyes on Minnesota Health Care Experiment," *Denver Post,* 27 October 1996; Thomas Bodenheimer and Kip Sullivan, "How Large Employers Are Shaping the Health Care Marketplace," *New England Journal of Medicine* 338 (9 August 1998): 1084–87; James Maxwell et al., "Managed Competition in Practice: 'Value Purchasing' by Fourteen Employers," *Health Affairs* 17 (May–June 1998): 216–26.

4. Jon R. Gabel, Paul B. Ginsburg, Heidi H. Whitmore, and Jeremy D. Pickreign, "Withering on the Vine: the Decline of Indemnity Health Insurance," *Health Affairs* 19 (September–October 2000): 152–57.

5. *New York Times,* 16 February 1995.

6. *Source Book of Health Insurance Data, 1996* (Washington, D.C.: Health Insurance Association of America, 1996).

7. Spencer Rich, "Health Care: An Era of Consolidation," *National Journal,* 15 July 2000, pp. 2296–97.

8. J. D. Kleinke, "Why Merger Mania Is Unhealthy for HMOs," *Wall Street Journal,* 17 August 1998.

9. Kennett Lynn Simmons, "Managed Health Care: Right Idea—Wrong

Rules" (Ph.D. diss., University of Texas at Austin, August 1992); Kuttner, "Must Good HMOs Go Bad? Part 1," 1558–63. Eli Ginzberg, "The Uncertain Future of Managed Care," *New England Journal of Medicine* 340 (14 January 1999): 144–46.

10. Daniel P. Gitterman et al., "The Rise and Fall of a Kaiser Permanente Expansion Region," *Milbank Quarterly* 81 (2003): 567–601.

11. Julie Appleby, "Aetna Cut Jobs, Customers in Effort to Boost Profit," *USA Today,* 19 December 2000.

12. James C. Robinson, "From Managed Care to Consumer Health Insurance: The Fall and Rise of Aetna," *Health Affairs* 23 (March–April 2004): 43–55.

13. Simmons, "Managed Health Care," 444; Irwin Miller, *American Health Care Blues: Blue Cross, HMOs and Pragmatic Reform Since 1960* (New Brunswick, N.J.: Transaction, 1996), 121.

14. Miller, *American Health Care Blues,* 113–19; Donald Light, letter to the editor, *New York Times,* 29 June 1993.

15. Miller, *American Health Care Blues,* 120; General Accounting Office, *Blue Cross and Blue Shield: Experience of Weak Plans Underscores the Role of Effective State Oversight* (Washington, D.C.: General Accounting Office, April 1994).

16. Jeff Cole, "Blue Cross Changes Its Approach," *Milwaukee Sentinel,* 1 March 1995.

17. William R. Wineke, "Falling HMO Stock," *Wisconsin State Journal,* 1 June 1995.

18. "Stock in the News: United Wisconsin Service," *Wisconsin State Journal,* 18 February 2000; "United Wisconsin Sees Loss," *Wisconsin State Journal,* 5 May 2000; Patricia Simms, "HMO Extends Its Losing Streak," *Wisconsin State Journal,* 3 November 2000.

19. "Blue Cross Unit Gets $40 Million Pact," *Wisconsin State Journal,* 2 December 2000.

20. Associated Press, "Health Merger Moves Forward: Move Is Last Step in Blue Cross Conversion," *Wisconsin State Journal,* 23 December 2000.

21. Philip R. Alper, "Flu Vaccine and What Happened to Social Responsibility," *Internal Medicine World Report* 15 (December 2000): 10; Rhonda L. Rundle, "Calling the Shots: California Health Plan Thrives, But Doctors Claim Care Suffers," *Wall Street Journal,* 31 May 2000.

22. Associated Press, "WellPoint Health Will Buy Cobalt," *Wisconsin State Journal,* 5 June 2003.

23. Milt Freudenheim, "A Big Merger in Health Care Arouses Suspicions That Insurers May Soon Cease to be Masters of Pricing," *New York Times* (30 October 2003); "Government Approves Merger of Big Health Insurers," *New York Times,* 28 February 2004.

24. Rich, "Health Care: An Era of Consolidation," 2296–97.

25. *Federal Trade Commission v. Mylan Laboratories,* Civ. 98-CV03114 (TFH) (29 November 2000), http://www.ftc.gov/os/2000/11/mylanordandstip .htm (accessed 15 May 2004).

26. Kaiser Family Foundation, "Health Insurance Enrollment," *Trends and Indicators in the Changing Health Care Marketplace,* exhibit 1.17: Relative Contributions of Utilization, Types of Prescription Drugs Used, and Price to Rising Prescription Drug Expenditure, 1993 vs. 1997–2002, http://www.kff.org/ insurance/7031/ti2004–1-17.cfm (accessed 5 May 2004).

27. Centers for Medicare and Medicaid Services, "Health Care Spending Reaches $1.6 Trillion in 2002," http://www.cms.hhs.gov/media/press/release.asp ?Counter=935 (accessed 5 May 2004).

28. "Drug Costs to Rise 20 Percent," *Internal Medicine World Report* 15 (December 2000): 4–5; Gary Plank, director of pharmacy services, Security Health Plan, interview in *Marshfield Clinic Pulse,* 11 October 2001.

29. Frank R. Lichtenberg, "Are the Benefits of Newer Drugs Worth Their Cost? Evidence from the 1996 MEPS," *Health Affairs* 20 (September–October 2001): 241–51; J. D. Kleinke, "The Price of Progress: Prescription Drugs in the Health Care Market," *Health Affairs* 20 (September–October 2001): 43–66; David M. Cutler and Mark McClellan, "Is Technological Change in Medicine Worth It?" *Health Affairs* 20 (September–October 2001): 11–29.

30. Frank Davidoff, "The Heartbreak of Drug Pricing," *Annals of Internal Medicine* 134 (5 June 2001): 1068–69.

31. Tony Pugh, "New Prescription Drugs May Not Be Better," Knight Ridder Newspapers Report, *Wisconsin State Journal,* 29 May 2002.

32. Frank Davidoff et al., "Sponsorship, Authorship, and Accountability," *New England Journal of Medicine* 345 (13 September 2001): 825–27.

33. Institute of Policy Innovation, "Consumer Advertising Doesn't Hike Drug Prices," IPI Policy Report Release no. 151, 6 January 2001, http://www.ipi.org/ ipi\IPIPressReleases.nsf/PublicationLookupPressRelease/E844061937516FBB 86256A630061DA2C? (accessed 5 May 2004); Plank interview.

34. Lauran Neergaard, AP medical writer, "TV's Role in Impacting Drug Sales Under Study," *Wisconsin State Journal,* 30 April 2002.

35. Kaiser Family Foundation, "Health Insurance Enrollment," *Trends and Indicators in the Changing Health Care Marketplace,* exhibit 1.20: Trends in Promotional Spending for Prescription Drugs, 1996–2002, http://www.kff.org/ insurance/7031/ti2004–1-20.cfm (accessed 5 May 2004).

36. Kaiser Family Foundation, "Health Care Spending and Costs," *Trends and Indicators in the Changing Health Care Marketplace, 2004 Update,* exhibit 1.5: Distribution of National Health Expenditures by Type of Service, 1992 and 2002, http://www.kff.org/insurance/703/ti2004/1-5.cfm (accessed 20 May 2004).

37. David Dranove and William D. White, *How Hospital Survived: Competition and the American Hospital* (Washington, D.C.: AEI Press, 1999), 19–20, 61. http://www.kff.org/insurance/7031/ti2004-1-5.cfm (accessed 20 May 2004).

38. Rich, "Health Care: An Era of Consolidation," 2296–97.

39. Glen Melnik, Emmett Keeler, and Jack Zwanziger, "Market Power and Hospital Pricing," *Health Affairs* 18 (May–June 1999): 167–73.

40. Steffie Woolhandler and David U. Himmelstein, "When Money Is the Mission: The High Costs of Investor Owned Care," *New England Journal of Medicine* 341 (5 August 1999): 444–46.

41. P. J. Devereaux et al., "A Systematic Review and Meta-analysis of Studies Comparing Mortality Rates of Private For-Profit and Private Not-for-Profit Hospitals," *Canadian Medical Association Journal* 166 (28 May 2002): 1399–1406.

42. Robert Pear, "Revolution in Health Care Industry Means Big Business for Specialist Lawyers," *New York Times,* 13 January 1995.

43. William M. Sage, David A. Hyman, and Warren Greenberg, "Why Competition Law Matters to Health Care Quality," *Health Affairs* 22 (March–April 2003): 31–44.

44. Robert J. Samuelson, *The Good Life and Its Discontents: The American Dream in the Age of Entitlement, 1945–1995* (New York: Times Books, 1995), 104–11.

45. Ibid., 113–18.

46. Marshfield Clinic report prepared for visit by Wisconsin governor Tommy Thompson, 14 August 2000, hereafter referred to as "Report for governor's visit"; "Marshfield Clinic 2000 System Review," October 2003, both in Marshfield Clinic corporate files; Reed Hall interview, 20 October 2004.

47. *Marshfield Clinic Pulse,* 9 January 1997.

48. Report for governor's visit.

49. *Marshfield Clinic Pulse,* 12 October 1995.

50. Ibid., 23 March 2000; "Marshfield Clinic 2000 System Review," October 2001.

51. *Marshfield Clinic Pulse,* 15 August 2002.

52. Jeff Zriny, director of government services, Security Health Plan, interview, 11 May 2001; John Smiley, director, Security Health Plan, interview, 4 June 2004.

53. Report for governor's visit; *Marshfield Clinic Pulse,* 11 May 2000; Kuttner, "Must Good HMOs Go Bad? Part 1," 1562–63.

54. Author's notes of remarks by Dr. Fredric Westbrook, Marshfield Clinic president, Marshfield Clinic meeting, 18 May 2000.

55. Kuttner, "Must Good HMOs Go Bad? Part 1," 1559–60.

56. Ibid., 1560.

57. Ibid., 1561.

58. David M. Lawrence, Patrick H. Mattingly, and John M. Ludden, "Trusting in the Future: The Distinct Advantage of Nonprofit HMOs," *Milbank Quarterly* 75 (March 1997): 5.

59. Mark Schlesinger and Bradford Gray, "A Broader Vision for Managed Care, Part 1: Measuring the Benefit to Communities," *Health Affairs* 17 (May–June 1998): 152–68; Mark Schlesinger et al., "A Broader Vision for Managed Care, Part 2: A Typology of Community Benefits," *Health Affairs* 17 (September–October 1998): 26–49.

60. The eight study sites were Allina Health System in Minneapolis, Minnesota; Baptist Health in Little Rock, Arkansas; BJC Health System in St. Louis, Missouri; Cambridge Hospital Community Health Network in Cambridge, Massachusetts; Harvard Pilgrim Health Care in Boston; Henry Ford Health System in Detroit; Mount Sinai Health System in Chicago; and Riverside Methodist Hospitals (later Grant–Riverside Methodist Hospitals) in Columbus, Ohio. See Thomas J. Chapel, Paul V. Stange, Randolph L. Gordon, and Adam Miller, "Private Sector Health Care Organizations and Essential Public Health Services: Potential Effects on the Practice of Local Public Health," *Journal of Public Health* 4 (4 January 1998): 36–44.

61. Glen P. Mays, Paul K. Halverson, and Rachel Stevens, "The Contributions of Managed Care Plans to Public Health Practice: Evidence from the Nation's Largest Local Health Departments," *Public Health Reports* 116 (2001 Supplement): 50–67.

13. Demands for Accountability

1. Associated Press, "Health Care Knowledge Lacking," *Wisconsin State Journal,* 12 November 1996.

2. Louise Kertesz, "HMO Makeover," *Modern Healthcare,* 12 May 1997, pp. 36–46.

3. Jerome P. Kassirer, "Managing Managed Care's Tarnished Image," *New England Journal of Medicine* 337 (31 July 1997): 338–39.

4. Alain C. Enthoven and Sara J. Singer, "The Managed Care Backlash and the Task Force in California," *Health Affairs* 17 (July–August 1998): 95–110.

5. "Bill on Maternity Coverage Ignites Managed-Care Debate," *Boston Globe,* 14 November 1995; David J. Casarett and John D. Lantos, "Have We Treated AIDS Too Well? Rationing and the Future of AIDS Exceptionalism," *Annals of Internal Medicine* 128 (1 May 1998): 756–59.

6. John Iglehart, "Markets and Regulation," *Health Affairs* 16 (November–December 1997): 6; David A. Rochefort, "The Role of Anecdotes in Regulating Managed Care," *Health Affairs* 17 (November–December 1998): 142–49.

7. Linda A. Johnson, Associated Press, "Couple Hopes to Strip HMOs of Suit Shield," *Wisconsin State Journal,* 4 December 2000.

8. Enthoven and Singer, "Managed Care Backlash," 95–110.

9. Ibid.

10. Several surveys are cited in "HMO Fact Sheet," published by the Group Health Association of America, Washington, D.C., January 1995. Other studies were reported by Paul Johnson, "State Workers Like Their HMOs," *Wisconsin State Journal,* 24 October 1996, and Will Lester, Associated Press, "Poll Finds Satisfaction on Health Insurance," *Wisconsin State Journal,* 6 February 1999.

11. Enthoven and Singer, "Managed Care Backlash," 95–110.

12. Board of Neuroscience and Behavior Health, Institute of Medicine, *Health Literacy: A Prescription to End Confusion* (Washington, D.C.: National Academies Press, 2004).

13. David B. Bernard and David J. Skulkin, "The Media vs. Managed Health Care: Are We Seeing a Full Court Press?" *Archives of Internal Medicine* 158 (26 October 1998): 2109–11.

14. Norman Daniels and James Sabin, "The Ethics of Accountability in Managed Care Reform," *Health Affairs* 17 (September–October 1998): 50–64.

15. Robert Kuttner, "Must Good HMOs Go Bad? Part II: The Search for Checks and Balances," *New England Journal of Medicine* 338 (21 May 1998): 1635–39; John La Puma and David Schiedermayer, "Ethical Issues in Managed Care and Managed Competition: Problems and Promises," in *The Physician's Guide to Managed Care,* ed. David B. Nash (Gaithersburg, Md.: Aspen, 1994), 31–53.

16. M. Susan Marquis and Stephen H. Long, "Trends in Managed Care and Managed Competition," *Health Affairs* 18 (November–December 1999): 75–88; Uwe E. Reinhardt, "Employer-Based Health Insurance: A Balance Sheet," *Health Affairs* 18 (November–December 1999): 124–32.

17. Amy B. Bernstein and Anne K. Gauthier, "Choice in Health Care: What Are They and What Are They Worth?" *Medical Care Research and Review* 56 (1999): 5–22, supplement 2; J. S. Lubalin, L. D. Harris-Kojetin, J. A. Meyer, and A. Lifson, "What Do Consumers Want and Need to Know in Making Health Care Choices?" *Medical Care Research and Review* 56 (1999): 67–107, supplement 2.

18. Daniels and Sabin, "The Ethics of Accountability," 50–64.

19. Michael M. Weinstein, "Managed Care's Other Problem: It's Not What You Think," *New York Times,* 28 February 1999.

20. *Pegram v. Herdich,* 120 S. Ct. 2143 (2000); Laurie Asseo, Associated Press, "Court Curbs Federal Suits against HMOs," *Wisconsin State Journal,* 12 June 2000.

21. M. Gregg Bloche and Peter D. Jacobson, "The Supreme Court and Bedside Rationing," *Journal of the American Medical Association* 284 (6 December 2000): 2776–79, especially 2776.

22. Katherine Swartz and Troyen A. Brennan, "Integrated Health Care, Capitated Payment and Quality: The Role of Regulation," *Annals of Internal Medicine* 124 (15 February 1996): 443–48.

23. David M. Studdert and Troyen A. Brennan, "The Problems with Punitive Damages in Lawsuits Against Managed Care Organizations," *New England Journal of Medicine* 342 (27 January 2000): 280–84.

24. Marilyn Werber Serafini, "Up Against ERISA," *National Journal,* 11 February 1995, pp. 349–52.

25. Eliza Newlin Carney, "Are HMOs off the Critical List?" *National Journal,* 15 August 1998, pp. 1920–21.

26. Robert J. Samuelson, "Myth of the Managed Care Monster," *Washington Post*, 29 July 1998, reprinted in Samuelson, *Untruth: Why the Conventional Wisdom Is (Almost Always) Wrong* (New York: Random House, 2001), 159–62.

27. David S. Broder, Washington Post Writers Group, "Health Policy Debate Getting More Absurd," *Wisconsin State Journal*, 29 July 1998.

28. Samuelson, "Myth of Managed Care Monster"; Richard Lamb, "Government Does, Indeed, Ration Health Care," *National Conference of State Legislators,* April 1999; Studdert and Brennan, "Problems with Punitive Damages," 283.

29. Phil Galewitz, Associated Press, "Survey: Health Plans at Risk," *Wisconsin State Journal,* 20 January 2000.

30. Clive Crook, "A Bill of Rights, Or a Bill of Goods?" *National Journal* (1 August 1998), p. 1797.

31. William Neikirk, "HMOs a Step Ahead of Patients' Right Bill," *Chicago Tribune,* 2 July 2001; "Patients Need Better Care from Senators," editorial, *Wisconsin State Journal,* 5 July 2001.

32. Kaiser Family Foundation, "Many Americans Dissatisfied with Managed Care, But Most Would Accept Limits on Patients' Rights Bill, Survey Finds, 31 August 2001, *Daily Health Policy Report,* www.kaisernetwork.org (accessed 22 April 2004).

33. Free information about filing a grievance concerning a health plan is available in the Consumer Advice area of the *Consumer Reports* website at www.ConsumerReports.org (accessed 22 April 2004).

34. Associated Press, "Reviews Help Health-Insurance Claims," *Wisconsin State Journal,* 13 June 2003.

35. Mark Schlesinger, Shannon Mitchell, and Brian Elbel, "Voices Unheard: Barriers to Expressing Dissatisfaction to Health Plans," *Milbank Quarterly* 80 (December 2002): 709–55; Amy Goldstein, "For Patients' Rights, a Quiet Fadeaway; Hill Partisanship and HMO Changes Cooled a Crusade," *Washington Post,* 12 September 2003.

36. Troyen A. Brennan and Donald M. Berwick, *New Rules: Regulations, Mar-*

kets, and the Quality of American Health Care (San Francisco: Jossey-Bass, 1996), 171–72.

37. *Kentucky Association of Health Plans Inc. v. Miller,* 123 S. Ct. 1471(2003); *Law Watch: A Legal Newsletter from Foley & Lardner,* 8 April 2003, pp. 1–3; Gina Holland, Associated Press, "States Are Given Power over HMOs," *Wisconsin State Journal,* 3 April 2003.

38. Charles Ornstein, Knight Ridder Newspapers, "Courts Rule Differently on HMO Issue," *Wisconsin State Journal,* 27 October 2000.

39. Gina Holland, Associated Press, "Second Opinions on HMOs Upheld," *Wisconsin State Journal,* 21 June 2002; Linda Greenhouse, *New York Times,* "Suits on HMO Coverage Rejected," *Wisconsin State Journal,* 22 June 2004; M. Gregg Bloche and David M. Studdert, "A Quiet Revolution: Law as an Agent of Health System Change," *Health Affairs* 23 (March–April 2004): 29–42.

40. James C. Robinson, "The End of Managed Care," *Journal of the American Medical Association* (23–30 May 2001): 2622–28.

41. Agency for Healthcare Research and Quality (AHRQ), "Health Insurance Premiums Rose More Than 30 Percent Between 1996 and 2000," *AHRQ Public Affairs,* 12 September 2002. According to Lauren A. McCormack et al., "Trends in Retiree Health Benefits," *Health Affairs* 21 (November–December 2002): 169–76, numerous indicators suggested a further and accelerating decline in retiree coverage.

42. "HMO Fact Sheet," 2–4.

43. Dana Gelb Safran, Alvin R. Tarlov, and William H. Rogers, "Primary Care Performance in Fee-for-Service and Prepaid Health Care Systems: Results from the Medical Outcome Study," *Journal of the American Medical Association* 271 (25 May 1994): 1579–86.

44. John E. Ware Jr. et al., "Differences in Four-Year Health Outcomes for Elderly and Poor, Chronically Ill Patients Treated in HMO and Fee-for-Service Systems," *Journal of the American Medical Association* 276 (2 October 1996): 1039–47; James P. Hadley and Kathryn Langwell, "Managed Care in the United States: Promises Evident to Date and Future Directions," *Health Policy* 19 (December 1991): 91–118; Fred J. Hellinger, "The Effect of Managed Care on Quality: A Review of Recent Evidence," *Archives of Internal Medicine* 158 (27 April 1998): 833–41; Benjamin G. Druss and Mark Schlesinger, "Chronic Illness and Plan Satisfaction Under Managed Care," *Health Affairs* 19 (January–February 2000): 203–9.

45. Kathryn A. Phillips et al., "Use of Preventive Services by Managed Care Enrollees: An Updated Perspective," *Health Affairs* 19 (January–February 2000): 102–16.

46. U.S. Preventive Services Task Force, *A Guide to Clinical Preventive*

Services: Report of U.S. Preventive Task Force, 2d ed. (Baltimore, Md.: Williams and Wilkins, 1996).

47. William R. Wineke, "Emphasis on Health Lifestyle," *Wisconsin State Journal,* 1 June 1995.

48. Michael L. Millenson, *Demanding Medical Excellence: Doctors and Accountability in the Information Age,* 2d ed. (Chicago: University of Chicago Press, 1999), 226–80.

49. Stephen H. Long and M. Susan Marquis, "Pooled Purchasing: Who Are the Players?" *Health Affairs* 18 (July–August 1999): 105–11.

50. Judy Cahill, senior vice president, Group Health Association of America, interview by author, 11 May 1995.

51. Millenson, *Demanding Medical Excellence,* 341–42.

52. Ibid.; Cahill interview.

53. Brennan and Berwick, *New Rules,* 159–62; Swartz and Brennan, "Integrated Health Care," 443–48; "Wide Variety of Standards Found in HMOs," *Boston Globe,* 24 February 1995.

54. Arnold Epstein, "Performance Reports on Quality—Prototypes, Problems and Prospects," *New England Journal of Medicine* 333 (6 July 1995): 57–61; Kuttner, "Must Good HMOs Go Bad? Part 2," 1635–36

55. Shoshanna Sofaer, "Aging and Primary Care: An Overview of Organizational and Behavioral Issues in the Delivery of Healthcare Services to Older Americans," *Health Services Research* 33 (June 1998): 298–321.

56. John Iglehart, "Health Policy Report: The American Health Care System," *New England Journal of Medicine* 326 (2 April 1992): 962–67. The web address for the Foundation for Accountability is http://www.facct.org/facct/site/facct/facct/home (accessed 7 May 2004).

57. "Paying for Performance: Medicare Should Lead," *Health Affairs* 22 (November–December 2003): 8–10. The signatories included Donald M. Berwick, Institute for Healthcare Improvement; Nancy Ann DeParle. J. P. Morgan Partners; David M. Eddy, a health policy advisor, Aspen, Colorado; Paul M. Ellwood, Jackson Hole Group; Alain C. Enthoven, Stanford University; Kenneth W. Kizer, National Quality Forum; Elizabeth A. McGlynn. Rand; Uwe E. Reinhardt, Princeton University; Robert D. Reischauer, Urban Institute; John W. Rowe, Aetna; Leonard D. Schaeffer, WellPoint Health Networks; John E. Wennberg, Dartmouth Medical School; and Gail R. Wilensky, Project HOPE.

58. David Dranove, Daniel Kessler, Mark McClellan, and Mark Satterhwaite, "Is More Information Better? The Effects of 'Report Cards' on Health Care Providers," National Bureau of Economic Research, Working Paper No. 8697, January 2002.

59. Kevin Fiscella, Peter Franks, Marsha R. Gold, and Carolyn M. Clancy, "Inequality in Quality: Addressing Socioeconomic, Racial and Ethnic Disparities

in Health Care," *Journal of the American Medical Association* 283 (17 May 2000): 2579–84.

60. Health Administration Responsibility Project, "HMO Executive Salaries, Reprinted from Families USA," http://www.harp.org/hmoexecs.htm (accessed 15 June 2004). Based on 1996 filings to the Securities and Exchange Commission, Stephen Wiggens, the former CEO of Oxford Health Plans topped his counterparts with an annual salary of $29.1 million in 1996. Trailing far behind were Wilson Taylor, chairman and CEO of CIGNA Corporation ($11.6 million) David Snow, executive vice president of Oxford Health plans ($10.4 million); Robert Smoler, executive vice president of Oxford Health Plans ($10.1 million); William Sullivan, president of Oxford Health Plans ($8.8 million); Joseph Sebastianelli, president of Aetna ($7.3 million); Michael Cardillo, executive vice president of Aetna ($7 million); and Leonard Schaffer, chairman and CEO of WellPoint Health Networks ($7 million). Not counting unexercised stock options, executives at the nine highest-paying companies received a total of $153.8 billion dollars in salaries.

61. Susan Brink and Nancy Shute, "America's Top HMOs: Are HMOs the Right Prescription?" *U.S. News and World Report,* 13 October 1997, pp. 60–78; Kuttner, "Must Good HMOs Go Bad? Part 2," 1637; Robert Kuttner, "Must Good HMOs Go Bad? Part I: The Commercialization of Prepaid Group Health Care," *New England Journal of Medicine* 338 (21 May 1998): 1562–63; David U. Himmelstein, Steffie Woolhandler, Ida Hellander, and Sidney M. Wolfe, "Quality of Care in Investor-Owned vs. Not-for-Profit HMOs," *Journal of the American Medical Association* 282 (14 July 1999): 159–63.

62. *Consumer Reports,* August 1996, pp. 40–41; *Comparing Medicare HMOs: Do They Keep Their Members?* (Washington, D.C.: Families USA, 1997), as reported in Kuttner, "Must Good HMOs Go Bad? Part I,"1562–63.

63. Ha T. Tu and James D. Reschovsky, "Assessments of Medical Care by Enrollees in For-Profit and Nonprofit Health Maintenance Organizations," *New England Journal of Medicine* 346 (25 April 2002): 1288–92.

64. *Marshfield Clinic Pulse,* 23 October 1997, 9 April 1998, and 19 August 1999.

65. Frederic J. Frommer, Associated Press, "Four State HMOs Rank Among Best in Country," *Wisconsin State Journal,* 19 September 2002.

66. Ibid.

67. NCQA's annual Health Plan Report Card rates plans in five key areas: access and service, qualified providers, staying healthy, getting better, and living with illness (NCQA, "NCQA Recognizes Nation's Best Health Plans with Introduction of New 'Excellent' Accreditation Status," *NCQA News,* 18 October 1999, http://www.ncqa.org/communications/news/excellentrel.htm (accessed 7 May 2004).

68. NCQA, "State of Managed Care Quality," 28 July 1999, http://www.ncqa .org/communications/news/somcqrel.html (accessed 7 May 2004).

69. Frederic J. Frommer, Associated Press, "Health and Science: Study Finds HMO Quality Still Improving," AP Online (18 September 2002).

70. Thomas Bodenheimer and Kip Sullivan, "How Large Employers Are Shaping the Health Care Marketplace," *New England Journal of Medicine* 338 (9 August 1998): 1086–87.

71. Reinhardt, "Employer-Based Health Insurance," 124; Donna E. Shalala and Uwe E. Reinhardt, "Viewing the U.S. Health Care System from Within: Candid Talk for HHS," *Health Affairs* 18 (May–June 1999): 47–55.

72. Thomas W. Still, "HMOs Can and Do Work When Consumers Insist on Quality," *Wisconsin State Journal,* 29 September 2000.

73. Cap Gemini Ernst & Young and National Business Coalition on Health, "New Patient Care Model Reduces Healthcare Costs and Improves Patient Care," National Business Coalition on Health, 21 May 2002, http://www.nbch .org/embargoed.pdf (accessed 7 May 2004).

74. Bruce Japsen, "Study: Poor Health Care Wasting Money," *Chicago Tribune,* 11 June 2002.

75. Millenson, *Demanding Medical Excellence,* 30–35, 131; C. David Naylor, "Grey Zones of Clinical Practice: Some Limits to Evidence-Based Medicine," *Lancet* 345 (1 April 1995): 840–42.

76. Institute of Medicine, Committee on Quality of Health Care in America, *To Err Is Human: Building a Safer Health System* (Washington, D.C.: National Academy Press, 2000).

77. Millenson, *Demanding Medical Excellence,* 350.

78. Steven H. Woolf, "Practice Guidelines: A New Reality in Medicine, Part I, Recent Developments," *Archives of Internal Medicine* 150 (September 1990): 1811–18; M. R. Chassin, "Practice Guidelines: Best Hope for Quality Improvement in the Future," *Journal of Occupational Medicine* 32 (December 1990): 1199–1206.

79. Kenneth M. Ludmerer, *Time to Heal: American Medical Education from the Turn of the Century to the Era of Managed Care* (New York: Oxford University Press, 1999), 363.

80. Agency for Health Care Policy and Research, "Notice of AHCPR Special Emphasis Area: Investigator-Initiated Grants: NIH Guide for Grants and Contracts," 23 December 1998, http://www.ahrq.gov/fund/99r036.htm (accessed 7 May 2004); National Library of Medicine, "Fact Sheet: National Information Center on Health Services Research and Health Care Technology," December 1998, updated 18 November 2002, http://www.nlm.nih.gov/pubs/factsheets/nichsr_ fs.html (accessed 26 May 2004); Bradford H. Gray, "The Legislative Battle over Health Services Research," *Health Affairs* 11 (Winter 1992) 33–66.

81. Agency for Healthcare Research and Quality, "AHRQ's Integrated Delivery System Research Network Starts First Studies," press release, 17 October

2000, http://www.ahrq.gov/news/press/pr2000/idsrn2pr.htm (accessed 7 May 2004); *Marshfield Clinic Pulse,* 30 November 2000.

82. For examples of professional resistance to practice guidelines, see Bureau of Health Maintenance Organization and Research Development, *Contracting Activities of HMOs and State Medicaid Agencies* (Rockville, Md.: U.S. Department of Health and Human Services, 30 August 1985); Steven H. Woolf, "Practice Guidelines: A New Reality in Medicine," *Archives of Internal Medicine* 153 (13 December 1993): 2646–55; David M. Mirvis and Cyril F. Chang, "Managed Care, Managing Uncertainty," *Archives of Internal Medicine* 157 (24 February 1997): 385–88.

83. Brennan and Berwick, *New Rules,* 185–97.

84. Odin W. Anderson, *Health Services in the United States: A Growth Enterprise Since 1875,* 2d ed. (Ann Arbor, Mich.: Health Administration Press, 1990), 261–62.

85. Health Insurance Association of America, "The Broad Reach of the Medical Malpractice Crisis," no date, http://www.publicforuminstitute.org/ext-content/hiaa-medmal.pdf (accessed 6 May 2004).

86. Michelle M. Mello, David M. Studdert, and Troyen A. Brennan, "The New Medical Malpractice Crisis," *New England Journal of Medicine* 348 (5 June 2003): 2282–84.

87. *Daubert v. Merrell-Dow Pharmaceuticals,* 509 U.S. 579 (1993); Charles Marwick, "Will Evidence-Based Practice Help Span Gulf Between Medicine and Law?" *Journal of the American Medical Association* 283 (7 June 2000): 2775–76.

88. Kate Johnson, "Medical Liability Reform Urged, *Ob. Gyn. News Online,* 1 June 2003, http://www2.eobgynnews.com/scripts/om.dll/serve?action=searchDB&searchDBfor=art&artType=fullfree&id=aqo030381101 (accessed 9 May 2004); "America Needs a New System of Medical Justice: Current Proposals Are Not Enough," *Common Good Law and Healthcare Page,* 25 February 2003, http://cgood.org/medicine/ (accessed 9 May 2004).

89. Jesse J. Holland, Associated Press, "GOP Loses Vote on Medical Malpractice," *Wisconsin State Journal,* 8 April 2004.

90. Sofaer, "Aging and Primary Care," 298–321.

91. Sharon E. Straus and Finlay A. McAlister, "Evidence-Based Medicine: A Commentary on Common Criticisms," *Canadian Medical Association Journal* 163 (3 October 2000): 837–41.

92. Chassin, "Practice Guidelines: Best Hope," 1204–5; D. W. Shapiro, R. D. Lasker, A. B. Bindman, and P. R. Lee, "Containing Costs While Improving Quality of Care: The Role of Profiling and Practice Guidelines," *Annual Review of Public Health* 14 (1993): 219–41; Christel Mottur-Pilson, "Internists' Evaluation of Guidelines: The IMCARE Practice Guidelines Network," *International Journal for Quality in Health Care* 7 (1995): 31–37; Donald W. Moran, "Health Infor-

mation Policy: On Preparing for the Next War," *Health Affairs* 17 (November–December 1998): 9–22; Ewan B. Ferlie and Stephen M. Shortell, "Improving the Quality of Health Care in the United Kingdom and the United State: A Framework for Change," *Milbank Quarterly* 79 (2001): 281–311.

93. Elizabeth A. McGlynn et al., "The Quality of Health Care Delivered to Adults in the United States," *New England Journal of Medicine* 348 (26 June 2003): 2635–45.

94. John E. Wennberg et al., "Use of Hospitals, Physician Visits, and Hospice Care During Last Six Month of Life Among Cohorts Loyal to Highly Respected Hospitals in the United States," *British Medical Journal* 328 (13 March 2004): 607–10; David J. Hunter, "Commentary: Getting a Grip on Clinical Variations in Hospital Services," *British Medical Journal* 328 (13 March 2004): 610.

95. Michael L. Millenson, "The Silence," *Health Affairs* 22 (March–April 2003): 103–12.

96. *Marshfield Clinic Pulse,* 26 September 1996.

97. R. Adams Dudley and Harold S. Luft, "Health Policy 2001: Managed Care in Transition," *New England Journal of Medicine* 344 (5 April 2001): 1087–92.

98. Jon B. Christianson, Douglas R. Wholey, Louis Warrick, and Paula Henning, "How are Health Plans Supporting Physician Practice? The Physician Perspective," *Health Affairs* 22 (January–February 2003): 181–89.

99. Brian S. Armour et al., "The Effect of Explicit Financial Incentives on Physician Behavior," *Archives of Internal Medicine* 161 (28 May 2001): 1261–66.

100. Julia E. McMurray et al., "Physician Job Satisfaction: Developing a Model Using Qualitative Data," *Journal of General Internal Medicine* 12 (November 1997): 711–14; Mark Linzer et al., "Managed Care, Time Pressure, and Physician Job Satisfaction: Results from the Physician Worklife Study," *Journal of General Internal Medicine* 15 (July 2000): 441–49.

101. David Mechanic, D. D. McAlpine, and M. Rosenthal, "Are Patients' Office Visits with Physicians Getting Shorter?" *New England Journal of Medicine* 344 (18 January 2001): 198–204.

102. Matthew K. Wynia, D. S. Cummins, J. B. VanGeest, and I. B. Wilson, "Should Physicians Manipulate Reimbursement Rules to Benefit Patients?" *Journal of the American Medical Association* 284 (20 September 2000): 1382–83.

103. Gina Holland, Associated Press, "Second Opinions on HMOs Upheld," *Wisconsin State Journal,* 21 June 2002; Bruce Japsen, "HMO Ruling Worries Corporations," *Chicago Tribune,* 21 June 2002.

104. Wynia, Cummins, VanGeest, and Wilson, "Should Physicians Manipulate Reimbursement Rules?" 1858–65.

105. Milt Freudenheim, "Some Doctors Letting Patients Skip Co-Payments," *New York Times,* 27 December 2003.

106. Steffie Woolhandler and David U. Himmelstein, "Extreme Risk: The New Corporate Proposition for Physicians," *New England Journal of Medicine* 333

(21 December 1995): 1706–7; J. P. Kassirer, "Managed Care and the Morality of the Marketplace," *New England Journal of Medicine* 333 (6 July 1995): 50–52.

107. Charles W. Wrightson Jr., *HMO Rate Setting and Financial Strategy* (Ann Arbor, Mich.: Health Administration Press, 1990), 64–65.

108. Robert Pear, *New York Times* News Service, "Feds Regulate HMO Bonuses to Doctors," *Wisconsin State Journal,* 26 December 1996.

109. Karen Ignagni, "Covering a Breaking Revolution: The Media and Managed Care," *Health Affairs* 17 (January–February1998): 26–34.

110. Kuttner, "Must Good HMOs Go Bad? Part II," 1637.

111. Sara Rosenbaum, K. Silver, and E. Wehr, *An Evaluation of Contracts Between Managed Care Organizations and Community Mental Health and Substance Abuse Treatment and Prevention Agencies,* Managed Care Technical Assistance Series (Washington, D.C.: U.S. Department of Health and Human Services, 1997); U.S. General Accounting Office, *Managed Care: Explicit Gag Clauses Not Found in HMO Contracts, but Physician Concerns Remain,* GAO/HEHS-97–175 (Washington, D.C.: Government Printing Office, 29 August 1997); David Mechanic, "The Managed Care Backlash: Perceptions and Rhetoric in Health Care Policy and the Potential for Health Care Reform," *Milbank Quarterly* 79 (2001): 35–54.

112. La Puma and Schiedermayer, "Ethical Issues in Managed Care," 50.

113. José Escarce, Kanika Kapur, Geoffrey Joyce, and Krista A. Van Vorst, "Expenditures for Physician Services under Alternative Models of Managed Care," *Medical Care Research and Review* 57.2 (June 2000): 161–81.

114. Steven Jonas, "Health Manpower: With an Emphasis on Physicians," in *Health Care Delivery in the United States,* ed. Anthony R. Kovner, 4th ed. (New York: Springer, 1990), 50–86. R. S. Miller, M. R. Dunn, T. H. Richter, and M. E. Whitcomb, "Employment-seeking Experience of Resident Physicians Completing Training During 1996," *Journal of the American Medical Association* 280 (2 September 1998): 777–83.

115. Kuttner, "Must Good HMOs Go Bad? Part II," 1638; Lindsey Tanner, Associated Press, "Worried AMA Wants to Beef Up Membership," *Wisconsin State Journal,* 11 June 2000; Marilyn Weber Serafini, "Physicians, Unite!" *National Journal,* 5 June 1999, pp. 1524–28.

116. Tanya Albert, "NLRB Ruling Gives Physician Unions Impetus," *American Medical News,* 25 February 2002 http://www.ama-assn.org/amednews/2002/02/25/prsc0225.htm (accessed 12 June 2004).

117. Serafini, "Physicians, Unite!" 1528.

118. Tanner, "Worried AMA Wants to Beef Up Membership."

119. Dean Land, "Medical School Prepares Students for Managed Care," *Wisconsin Week,* 2 March 1999, p. 7; "Changes in Medical Education," *Wall Street Journal,* 27 February 1995.

120. James C. Robinson and Lawrence P. Casalino, "The Growth of Medical

Groups Paid Through Capitation in California," *New England Journal of Medicine* 33 (21 December 1995): 1684–87.

121. Dudley and Luft, "Health Policy 2001," 1089.

122. Thomas Bodenheimer, "The American Health Care System," *New England Journal of Medicine* 340 (19 February 1999): 584–88; Hasan, "Let's End the Nonprofit Charade," *New England Journal of Medicine* 334 (18 April 1996), 1055–57; Iglehart, "Health Policy Report: The American Health Care System," 962–67; Hadley and Mitchell, "Effects of HMO Market Penetration," 99–111; Anita Clark, "Doctors' Incomes Decline: Locally and Across the Nation, HMOs Push for Lower Costs," *Wisconsin State Journal*, 20 October 1996.

123. Mark A. Hall, Elizabeth Dugan, Beiyao Zheng, and Aneil K. Mishra, "Trust in Physicians and Medical Institutions: What Is It, Can It Be Measured, and Does It Matter?" *Milbank Quarterly* 79 (4 November 2001): 613–39.

124. National Center for Health Statistics, V. M. Freid, K. Praeger, A. P. MacKay and H. Xia, *Health, United States, 2003* (Hyattsville, Maryland: National Center for Health Statistics, 2003), Table 132. Health maintenance organizations (HMO) and enrollment, according to the model type, geographic region and Federal program, United States, selected years, 1976–2002, p. 339, http://www.cdc.gov/nchs/products/pubs/pubd/hus/trendtables.htm (accessed 12 June 2004).

14. Critics and Would-be Reformers

1. Frank Davidoff and Robert D. Reinecke, "The Twenty-eighth Amendment," *Annals of Internal Medicine* 139 (20 April 1999): 692.

2. Mark A. Goldberg, Theodore R. Marmor, and Joseph White, "The Relation Between Universal Health Insurance and Cost Control," *New England Journal of Medicine* 332 (16 March 1995): 744.

3. David Mechanic, "The Managed Care Backlash: Perceptions and Rhetoric in Health Care Policy and the Potential for Health Care Reform," *Milbank Quarterly* 79 (January 2001): 50–51.

4. Robert Kuttner, "The Risk-Adjustment Debate," *New England Journal of Medicine* 339 (24 December 1998): 1956.

5. Donald W. Light, "Good Managed Care Needs Universal Health Insurance," *Annals of Internal Medicine* 139 (20 April 1999): 689.

6. Mark R. Chassin, Robert W. Galvin, and the National Roundtable on Health Care Quality, "The Urgent Need to Improve Health Care Quality," *Journal of the American Medical Association* 280 (16 September 1998): 1000–1005.

7. Institute of Medicine, Committee on Quality of Health Care in America, *Crossing the Quality Chasm: A New Health Care System for the Twenty-first Century* (Washington, D.C.: National Academy Press, 2001).

8. U.S. Census Bureau, "Income, Poverty and Health Insurance in the United

States: 2003," http://www.census.gov/prod/2004pubs/p60-226.pdf (accessed 20 October 2004); Associated Press, "Many Lack Health Insurance," *Wisconsin State Journal,* 16 June 2004; Robert Wood Johnson Foundation, 20 July 2003, http://www.rwjf.org/news/special/ctuWeek.jhtml (accessed 28 April 2004).

9. Robert Steinbrook, "Disparities in Health Care—From Politics to Policy," *New England Journal of Medicine* (8 April 2004) 350(15):1486–88; and M. Gregg Bloche, "Sounding Board: Health Disparities—Science, Politics, and Race," ibid., 1568–70.

10. Norman Daniels, "Justice, Health, and Healthcare," *American Journal of Bioethics* 1 (Spring 2001): 2–16, esp. 3.

11. Jack Hadley and John Holahan, "How Much Medical Care Do the Uninsured Use, and Who Pays for It?" *Health Affairs* 22 (March–April 2003): 13; Hadley and Holahan, "Covering the Uninsured: How Much Would It Cost?" *Health Affairs* 22 (July–August): 11.

12. Marilyn Werber Serafini, "One in Six, and Counting," *National Journal,* 17 July 1999), pp. 2066–72.

13. John Sheils and Paul Hogan, "Cost of Tax-Exempt Health Benefits in 1998," *Health Affairs* 18 (March–April 1999): 181.

14. John K. Iglehart, "Changing Health Insurance Trends," *New England Journal of Medicine* 347 (19 September 2002): 956–62.

15. In "Surprise: Workers, Not Their Bosses, Pay for Health Coverage," *Health Affairs* 17 (May–June 1998): 273–74, Jack A. Meyer reviews Mark V. Pauly's book, *Health Benefits at Work: An Economic and Political Analysis of Employment-Based Health Insurance* (Ann Arbor: University of Michigan Press, January 1999); Thomas Bodenheimer and Kip Sullivan, "How Large Employers Are Shaping the Health Care Marketplace," *New England Journal of Medicine* 338 (9 April 1998): 1084–87.

16. Victor R. Fuchs, "The Clinton Plan: A Researcher Examines Reform," *Health Affairs* 13 (Spring 1994): 110.

17. "Sick Days for Health Insurance Coverage," *U.S. News and World Report,* 25 June 2001, p. 10.

18. William S. Custer, Charles N. Kahn III, and Thomas F. Wildsmith IV, "Why We Should Keep the Employment-Based Health Insurance System," *Health Affairs* 18 (November–December 1999): 115–23.

19. Jon Gabel et al., "Job-Based Health Insurance in 2000: Premiums Rise Sharply While Coverage Grows," *Health Affairs* 19 (September–October 2000): 144–51.

20. William S. Custer and Pat Ketsche, "Health Insurance Coverage and the Uninsured, 1990–1998," 2004, membership.hiaa.org/pdfs/apps/custer.pdf (accessed 11 May 2004).

21. Randolph E. Schmid, Associated Press, "Uninsured Found to Be Dying Sooner," *Wisconsin State Journal,* 27 May 2002.

22. Diane Stafford, Knight Ridder Newspapers, "Scope of Employee Health Care Coverage Shrinking, Report Says," *Wisconsin State Journal*, 5 October 2003;Victor R. Fuchs, "What's Ahead for Health Insurance in the United States?" *New England Journal of Medicine* 346 (6 June 2002): 1822–24.

23. Iglehart, "Changing Health Insurance Trends."

24. Alain C. Enthoven and Sara J. Singer, "Markets and Collective Action in Regulating Managed Care," *Health Affairs* 16 (November–December 1997): 26–32.

25. Ibid.

26. William Sage, David A. Hyman, and Warren Greenberg, "Why Competition Law Matters to Health Care Quality," *Health Affairs* 22 (March–April 2003): 41–42.

27. M. L. Berk and A. C. Monheit, "The Concentration of Health Expenditure: An Update," *Health Affairs* 11 (Winter 1992): 145–49.

28. Deborah Chollet, "Expanding Individual Health Insurance Coverage: Are High-Risk Pools the Answer?" *Health Affairs* (23 October 2002) 349–52, Web Exclusive, http://content.healthaffairs.org/webexclusives/index.dtl?year=2002 (accessed 12 June 2004).

29. Mark Pauly, Allison Percy, and Bradley Herring, "Individual Versus Job-Based Health Insurance: Weighing the Pros and Cons," *Health Affairs* 18 (November–December 1999): 28–44; Stuart Butler and David B. Kendall, "Expanding Access and Choice for Health Care Consumers Through Tax Reform," *Health Affairs* 18 (November–December 1999): 45–57.

30. Elliott S. Fisher et al., "The Implications of Regional Variations in Medicare Spending, Part 2: Health Outcomes and Satisfaction with Care," *Annals of Internal Medicine* 138 (18 February 2003): 288–98.

31. Jeff Goldsmith, "The Road to Meaningful Reform: A Conversation with Oregon's John Kitzhaber," *Health Affairs* 22 (January–February 2003): 144–124.

32. Richard D. Lamb, "The Ethics of Excess," *Public Health Reports* 111 (May–June 1996): 218–23.

33. Willard Gaylin, "Faulty Diagnosis: Why Clinton's Health Care Plan Won't Cure What Ails Us," *Harper's Magazine*, October 1993, pp. 57–62.

34. Robert H. Blank, introduction to *Emerging Issues in Biomedical Policy: An Annual Review*, vol. 1, ed. Robert H. Blank and Andrea L. Bonnicksen (New York: Columbia University Press, 1992), 77.

35. Harvard Community Health Plan, "The LORAN Commission: A Report to the Community," in Blank and Bonnicksen, *Emerging Issues in Biomedical Policy*, 64–81.

36. J. E. Rossouw et al., "Risks and Benefits of Estrogen plus Progesterone in Healthy Post Menopausal Women: Principal Results from the Women's Health Initiative Randomized Control Trial," *Journal of the American Medical Association* 288 (17 July 2002): 321–33.

37. J. Bruce Moseley et al., "A Controlled Trail of Arthroscopic Surgery for Osteoarthritis of the Knee," *New England Journal of Medicine* 37 (11 July 2002): 81–88.

38. Some critics faulted Clinton for failing to talk about rationing while preparing his reform package in the early 1990s, but the leadership of his Domestic Policy Taskforce believed such talk would be political suicide. See Arthur L. Caplan, "Straight Talk About Rationing," *Annals of Internal Medicine* 122 (15 May 1995): 795–96.

39. Uwe E. Reinhardt, "Economics: Markets Ration by Price and Ability to Pay," *Journal of the American Medical Association* 275 (19 July 1996): 1802–4; Uwe E. Reinhardt, "Rationing Health Care," in *Strategic Choices for Changing the Health Care System,* ed. Stuart H. Altman and U. W. Reinhardt (Chicago: Health Administration Press, 1996), 95.

40. David Eddy, "Rationing Resources While Improving Quality: How to Get More for Less," *Journal of the American Medical Association* 272 (May 1994): 817–24, especially 823.

41. C. Caleb Alexander, Rachel M. Werner, and Peter A. Ubel, "The Cost of Denying Scarcity," *Archives of Internal Medicine* 164 (22 March 2004): 593–96.

42. Phillip J. Longman and Shannon Brownlee, "The Genetic Surprise," *Wilson Quarterly* 24 (Autumn 2000): 40–50.

43. Stephie Woolhandler, D. U. Himmelstein, Marcia Angel, and Q. D. Young, "Proposal of Physicians' Working Group for Single-Payer National Health Care System," *Journal of the American Medical Association* 290 (13 August 2003): 798–805.

44. Michael McCarthy, "U.S. Doctors Group Calls for National Health-Care System: Plan Would Save Enough Money to Pay for Health Insurance for the 41 Million Uninsured Americans," *Lancet* 362 (23 August 2003): 621.

45. Danny McCormick, David U. Himmilstein, Steffie Woolhandler, and David H. Bor, "Single-Payer National Health Insurance: Physicians' Views," *Archives of Internal Medicine* 164 (9 February 2004): 300–304.

46. Chris Ham, "Retracing the Oregon Trail: The Experience of Rationing and the Oregon Health Plan," *British Medical Journal* 316 (27 June 1998): 1965–69.

47. Thomas Bodenheimer, "The Oregon Health Plan—Lessons for the Nation, Part I," *New England Journal of Medicine* 337 (28 August 1997): 651–55.

48. Jonathan Oberlander, Theodore Marmor, and Lawrence Jacobs, "Rationing Medical Care: Rhetoric and Reality in the Oregon Health Plan," *Canadian Medical Association Journal* 164 (29 May 2001): 1583–87.

49. Goldsmith, "Road to Meaningful Reform."

50. Oberlander, Marmor, and Jacobs, "Rationing Medical Care."

51. Trish Riley and Elizabeth Kilbreth, "Health Coverage in the States—Maine's Plan for Universal Access," *New England Journal of Medicine* 350 (22 January 2004): 330–32.

52. Robert Imrie, Associated Press, "Doyle Signs Bill That Creates Regional Health Insurance Pools," *Wisconsin State Journal,* 12 December 2003.

53. Huw T. O. Davies and Martin N. Marshall, "UK and US Health-Care Systems: Divided by More Than a Common Language," *Lancet* 355 (29 January 2000): 336.

54. Swedish Ministry of Health and Social Affairs, Health Care and Medical Priorities Commission, *No Easy Choices: The Difficult Priorities of Health Care* (Stockholm: Swedish Government Official Reports, 1993); Caplan, "Straight Talk About Rationing," 795–96.

55. John K. Iglehart, "Revisiting the Canadian Health Care System," *New England Journal of Medicine* 342 (29 June 2000): 2007–12.

56. Ibid.

57. Colleen Fuller, *Caring for Profit: How Corporations Are Taking Over Canada's Health Care System* (Vancouver, B.C.: New Star Books, 1998).

58. Richard Smith, "The Failings of NICE: Time to Start Work on Version 2," *British Medical Journal* 321 (2 December 2000): 1363–64; Roger Dobson Abergavenny, "Report More Honest Approach to Rationing," *British Medical Journal* 322 (10 February 2001): 316; Alan Maynard and Trevor Sheldon, letter to the editor, "Limits to Demand for Health Care: Rationing Is Needed in a National Health Service," and several other letters to the editor, *British Medical Journal* 322 (24 March 2001): 734–35.

59. Stephen Frankel, Shah Ebrahim, and George Davey Smith, "The Limits to Demand for Health Care," *British Medical Journal* 321 (1 July 2000): 40–44.

60. Richard G.A. Feachem, Neelam K. Sekhri, and Karen L. White, "Getting More for Their Dollar: A Comparison of the NHS with California's Kaiser Permanente," *British Medical Journal* 324 (19 January 2002): 135–141; commentaries by Jennifer Dixon, Donald M. Berwick, and Alain C. Enthoven, *British Medical Journal* 324 (19 January 2002): 142–43; numerous letters to the editor, *British Medical Journal* 324 (June 2002): 1332–35.

61. Jennifer Dixson, "Another Health Care Funding Review: More of the Same," *British Medical Journal* 322 (10 February 2001): 312–13.

62. Ross Kessel, "The BMA Addresses Britain's Rationing Problem at Last," *Hastings Center Report,* March–April 2001, p. 6.

63. Rudolf Klein, "Health Policy Report: Britain's National Health Service Revisited," *New England Journal of Medicine* 350 (26 February 2004): 937–42.

64. Robert J. Samuelson, *The Good Life and Its Discontents: The American Dream in the Age of Entitlement, 1945–1995* (New York: Times Books, 1995), 175–76.

65. David A. Kindig, *Purchasing Population Health: Paying for the Results* (Ann Arbor: University of Michigan Press, 1997), 99.

66. Fitzhugh Mullen, "A Founder of Quality Assessment Encounters a Troubled System Firsthand," *Health Affairs* 20 (January–February 2001): 137–41.

67. David Blumenthal, "Health Care Reform—Past and Future," *New England Journal of Medicine* 332 (16 February 1995): 465–68.

68. "Health Insurers Gain a Huge New Lobby," *New York Times*, 23 September 2003.

Bibliographic Resources
for American Health Care
History and Policy

Books

Anderson, Odin W. *The Uneasy Equilibrium: Private and Public Financing of Health Service in the United States, 1975–1965.* New Haven, Conn.: College and University Press, 1968.

———. *Blue Cross Since 1929: Accountability and the Public Trust.* Cambridge, Mass.: Ballinger, 1975.

———. *Health Services in the United States: A Growth Enterprise Since 1875.* Ann Arbor, Mich.: Health Administration Press, 1985.

Anderson, Odin W. et al., *HMO Development: Patterns and Prospects: A Comparative Analysis of HMOs.* Chicago: Pluribus, 1985.

Berkowitz, Edward D. *America's Welfare State from Roosevelt to Reagan.* Baltimore, Md.: Johns Hopkins University Press, 1991.

Blendon, Robert J., and Mollyann Brodie, eds. *Transforming the System: Building a New Structure for the New Century: The Future of Health Care.* Vol. 4. New York: Faulkner & Gray; Washington, D.C.: Healthcare Information Center, 1994.

Brennan, Troyen. *Just Doctoring: Medical Ethics in the Liberal State.* Berkeley: University of California Press, 1991.

Brennan, Troyen, and Donald M. Berwick. *New Rules: Regulations, Markets, and the Quality of American Health Care.* San Francisco: Jossey-Bass, 1996.

Brown, Lawrence D. *Politics and Health Care Organizations: HMOs as Federal Policy.* Washington, D.C.: Brookings Institution, 1983.

Cambridge Health Economics Group. *Managing Reimbursement in the '90s.* New York: McGraw-Hill, 1990.

Davic, Karen, G. F. Anderson, D. Rowland, and E. P. Steinberg. *Health Care Cost and Containment.* Baltimore, Md.: Johns Hopkins University Press, 1990.

Falk, Isidore S. *Security against Sickness.* New York: Doubleday, Doran, 1936. Reprint, New York: Da Capo, 1972. Citations are to the 1936 edition.

Fox, Daniel M. *The Failure and Future of American Health Policy.* Berkeley: University of California Press, 1993.

———. *Health Policies, Health Politics: The British and American Experience, 1911–1965.* Princeton, N.J.: Princeton University Press, 1986.

Fox, Daniel M., LuAnn Heinen, and Richard J. Steele. *Determinants of HMOs' Success.* Ann Arbor, Mich.: Health Administration Press Perspectives, 1987.

Greenberg, Warren. *Competition, Regulation and Rationing in Health Care.* Ann Arbor, Mich.: Health Administration Press, 1991.

Havighurst, Clark. *Deregulating the Health Care Industry: Planning for Competition.* Cambridge, Mass.: Ballinger, 1982.

———. *Health Care Choices: Private Contracts as Instruments of Health Reform.* Washington, D.C.: AEI Press, 1995.

Hendricks, Rickey. *A Model for National Health Care: The History of Kaiser Permanente.* New Brunswick, N.J.: Rutgers University Press, 1993.

Kindig, David A. *Purchasing Population Health: Paying for the Results.* Ann Arbor: University of Michigan Press, 1997.

Kovner, Anthony R., ed. *Health Care Delivery in the United States.* 4th ed. New York: Springer, 1990.

Law, Sylvia A. *Blue Cross: What Went Wrong?* New Haven, Conn.: Yale University Press, 1974.

Leavitt, Judith Walzer, and Ronald A. Numbers, eds. *Sickness and Health in America: Readings in the History of Medicine and Public Health.* Madison: University of Wisconsin Press, 1978.

Ludmerer, Kenneth M. *Time to Heal: American Medical Education from the Turn of the Century to the Era of Managed Care.* New York: Oxford University Press, 1999.

Luft, Harold S. *Health Maintenance Organizations: Dimensions of Performance.* New York: John Wiley and Sons, 1981.

Mackie, Dustin L., and Douglas I. Decker. *Group and IPA HMOs.* Rockville, Md.: Aspen Systems, 1981.

Millenson, Michael. *Demanding Medical Excellence: Doctors and Accountability in the Information Age.* Chicago: University of Chicago Press, 1999.

Miller, Irwin. *American Health Care Blues: Blue Cross, HMOs and Pragmatic Reform Since 1960.* New Brunswick, N.J.: Transaction, 1996.

Numbers, Ronald L. *Almost Persuaded: American Physicians and Compulsory Health Insurance, 1912–1920.* Baltimore, Md.: Johns Hopkins University Press, 1978

Rivlin, Alice M., and Joshua M. Weener. *Caring for the Disabled Elderly: Who Will Pay?* Washington, D.C.: Brookings Institution, 1988.

Roemer, Milton I. *Ambulatory Health Services in America: Past, Present, and Future.* Rockville, Md.: Aspen Systems, 1981.

———. *Rural Health Care.* St. Louis: C. V. Mosley Co., 1976.

Rosen, George, and Charles E. Rosenberg, eds. *The Structure of American Medical Practice, 1875–1941.* Philadelphia: University of Pennsylvania Press, 1983.

Rosenblatt, Rand E., Sylvia A. Law, and Sara Rosenbaum. *Law and the American Health Care System.* Westbury, N.Y.: Foundation Press, 1997.

Salmon, J. Warren, ed. *The Corporate Transformation of Health Care: Perspectives and Implications.* Amityville, N.Y.: Baywood, 1994.

Somers, Herman, and Anne Somers. *Medicare and the Hospitals.* Washington, D.C.: Brookings Institution, 1967.

Starr, Paul. *The Social Transformation of American Medicine.* New York: Basic Books, 1982.

Straub, LaVonne, and Norman Walzer, eds. *Financing Rural Health Care.* New York: Praeger, 1988.

——. *Rural Health Care: Innovation in a Changing Environment.* Westport, Conn.: Praeger, 1992.

Stevens, Rosemary. *In Sickness and in Wealth: American Hospitals in the Twentieth Century.* New York: Basic Books, 1989.

Wrightson, Charles W. Jr. *HMO Rate Setting and Financial Strategy.* Ann Arbor, Mich.: Health Administration Press, 1990.

Reports

American Medical Association Council on Medical Services. *Health Maintenance Organizations: Background Information Supplement to the Council on Medical Services Report A.* Chicago: American Medical Association, June 1980.

Committee on the Cost of Medical Care. *Medical Care for the American People: The Final Report of the Committee on the Cost of Medical Care.* Chicago: University of Chicago Press, 1932.

Larson, Leonard. "Report on the Commission of Medical Care Plans: Findings, Conclusions, and Recommendations." *Journal of American Medical Association,* 17 (1959). Special edition.

Mechanic, David. *The Organization of Medical Practice and Practice Orientations Among Physicians in Prepaid and Non-Prepaid Primary Care Settings.* Research and Analytic Report Series. Madison: Center for Medical Sociology and Health Services Research, University of Wisconsin, 1974.

Nixon, Richard M. *Message from the President of the United States Relative to Building a National Health Strategy.* 92d Congress, 1st sess., Document No. 92-49.

U.S. Bureau of HMOs and Resource Development. *Considerations in Developing a Rural HMO.* Washington, D.C.: U.S. Department of Health and Human Services, 1985.

U.S. Congress. Office of Technology Assessment. *Health Care in Rural America.* Washington, D.C.: Government Printing Office, September 1990.

U.S. Institute of Medicine. National Academy of Sciences. *Health Maintenance*

Organizations: Toward a Fair Market Test. Washington, D.C.: National Academy of Sciences, May 1974.

———. *Informing the Future: Critical Issues in Health Care.* Washington, D.C.: Institute of Medicine, 2001.

U.S. Institute of Medicine. Committee on Implications of For-Profit Enterprise in Health Care, *For-Profit Enterprise in Health Care.* Edited by Bradford H. Gray. Washington, D.C.: National Academy Press, 1986.

———. Committee on Quality of National Health Care in America. *To Err Is Human: Building a Safer Health System.* Washington, D.C.: National Academy Press, 2000.

———. Committee on Quality of Health Care in America. *Crossing the Quality Chasm: A New Health System for the Twenty-first Century.* Washington, D.C.: National Academy Press, 2001.

———. Division of Health Care Services. Committee on Utilization Management by Third Parties. *Controlling Costs and Changing Patient Care? The Role of Utilization Management.* Edited by Bradford H. Gray and Marilyn J. Field. Washington, D.C.: National Academy Press, 1989.

Periodicals

American Journal of Law and Medicine
American Journal of Public Health
Archives of Internal Medicine
British Medical Journal
Bulletin of the History of Medicine
Canadian Medical Association Journal
Group Practice (Journal)
Health Affairs
Healthcare Financial Management
Health Care Management Review
Health Services Research
Journal of Health Politics, Policy and Law
Journal of Medicine and Philosophy
Journal of the American Medical Association
Lancet
Medical Care Research and Review
Medical Economics
Medical Group Management
Milbank Quarterly
Modern Healthcare
National Journal
New England Journal of Medicine

Index